CONCEPTS OF
PHYSICAL FITNESS
WITH LABORATORIES

SIXTH EDITION

CONCEPTS OF
PHYSICAL FITNESS
WITH LABORATORIES

CHARLES B. CORBIN
Arizona State University

RUTH LINDSEY
California State University, Long Beach

wcb
WM. C. BROWN PUBLISHERS
DUBUQUE, IOWA

Book Team

Editor *Chris Rogers*
Developmental Editor *Raphael Kadushin*
Designer *Julie E. Anderson*
Production Editor *David A. Welsh*
Photo Research Editor *Michelle Oberhoffer*
Visuals Processor *Reneê Pins*
Product Manager *Kathy Law Laube*

wcb

Chairman of the Board *Wm. C. Brown*
President and Chief Executive Officer *Mark C. Falb*

wcb group

Wm. C. Brown Publishers, College Division

Executive Vice-President, General Manager *G. Franklin Lewis*
Editor in Chief *George Wm. Bergquist*
Executive Editor *John Woods*
Director of Production *Beverly Kolz*
National Sales Manager *Bob McLaughlin*
Marketing Research Manager *Craig S. Marty*
Manager of Design *Marilyn A. Phelps*
Production Editorial Manager *Colleen A. Yonda*
Photo Research Manager *Faye M. Schilling*

Cover photo by Cliff Hollenbeck

New illustrations rendered for this text by Ruth Krabach; Rolin
Graphics; and Sanchez Graphics. Figure 6.3a, page 45 (right):
© David Corona; Figures 6.3b and 6.4, page 45 (left): © Tom
Ballard/EKM-Nepenthe.

Library of Congress Catalog Card Number: 87–071178

ISBN 0–697–07281–9

Printed in the United States of America by Wm. C. Brown Publishers
2460 Kerper Boulevard, Dubuque, IA 52001

10 9 8 7 6

TABLE OF CONTENTS

THE LABS

APPENDICES

PREFACE

Concepts of Physical Fitness is designed primarily for an introductory course at the college level. In it we have attempted to provide the reader with the best scientific evidence in physical fitness—particularly in the area of health-related physical fitness. The text is appropriate for both men and women.

An outline format is used to give the reader a concise and factual presentation with regard to the *why, how,* and *what* of exercise and physical activity for fitness. Discussion is kept to a minimum; references and suggested readings are provided for the reader who wishes to pursue a specific topic.

This sixth edition has many new and updated features, but retains all of the important features that made previous editions of *Concepts of Physical Fitness* such a success. In addition to the update of the facts, based on the most recent research evidence, portions of the book have been reorganized and new materials have been added, based on user suggestions.

The first section of the book, entitled "Physical Fitness and Programs of Exercise," includes concepts that elaborate on the need for fitness, distinguish between health-related fitness and skill-related fitness, and present the various components of fitness. Information is included for such important concepts as warm-up, cool down, and fitness target zones. Section I has been expanded to include specific exercise programs immediately after the concepts to which they are most related. For example, aerobic and anaerobic exercises now follow cardiovascular fitness; strength and muscular endurance exercises now follow the concepts on muscle fitness; stretching exercises immediately follow the concept on flexibility; and nutrition now follows the concept on body composition. This organizational change was made to make the first section of the book easier to use and to make practical information on exercise more accessible to the reader.

Also included in this Preface (p. ix) is an illustration containing the major muscle groups of the body to help the reader better understand the muscle system, particularly when reading the concepts on strength, muscular endurance and power, and flexibility. New exercises are included in these concepts for isokinetic strength devices, an extensive discussion of muscle power has been added, and a new updated and more accurate terminology for flexibility accepted by clinicians worldwide, has been introduced. Finally, as noted in a special discussion in Concept 2, the rating scales for each component of fitness have been modified for this edition. The intent is to focus attention on the amount of fitness necessary for good health rather than for physical performance.

The expanded second section of the book, "Important Fitness Factors," contains six concepts involving factors that must be considered in any health-related fitness program. These include facts about dangerous exercises, the care of the back, good posture, the relief of stress and tension, the avoidance of risk factors (especially for cardiovascular disease), and the role of exercise in daily life—"from the cradle to the grave." The third section, "Planning for Fitness," contains strategies on exercise motivation and techniques for making exercise more enjoyable. This section also includes what is perhaps the most important concept in the text: how to plan an individualized program for yourself based on your needs and interests. The program you plan is based on the self-tests you perform in the laboratory experiences. Finally, the last concept in Section 2 tells the reader how to avoid the rip-offs and quackery so frequently found in the fitness industry.

There are a total of twenty-five concepts and thirty-seven accompanying laboratories. The labs are numbered with special color tabs to correspond with the concepts that they supplement. This was done to make lab sheets and lab resource materials easy to locate.

The laboratories are on tear-out pages so that they can be completed and handed into the instructor. Much of the Lab Resource Materials necessary to complete the tear-out lab sheets is included in the Concept section of the text. This was done so that important information would not be torn from the book and would be available for future reference. When possible, charts and rating scales are presented in both the Lab Resource Materials and in the tear-out lab sheets. An understanding and appreciation of the information presented in these pages should provide the foundation for an intelligent selection of activities and health practices to aid you in leading a useful and productive life.

A NOTE TO THE READER

Concepts of Physical Fitness is unlike other textbooks you may have used in the past. To make the book as easy to use as possible, we have organized it in a unique way.

First, the text has an outline format. For this reason, it does not read like most texts. However, the information is useful and precise. Secondly, references are listed to support the facts presented in the text. While we do not expect you to look up each reference, we do want you to know where to look for more information. Two or three references in each concept are designated as "suggested readings" by an asterisk (*). The text also contains a list of terms at the beginning of each Concept. Each term is explained at this point and is then later boldfaced where it is first mentioned in the concept.

Another important feature of *Concepts of Physical Fitness* is the tear-out lab sheets. These sheets have been perforated so that you can hand them in to your instructor if requested to do so. Important testing or exercise information is included in the concept to which each lab pertains. This section of the concept, Lab Resource Materials, has been positioned here because we

feel certain that you will want to keep this information for future use. And as an added convenience, rating charts and scales are presented in both the tear-out labs and the Lab Resource Materials. Finally, special tables are included in the appendixes at the end of the book.

Concepts of Physical Fitness is intended to help you make important decisions about your personal exercise program and your personal physical fitness both now and during the rest of your life. We trust that you will find the book interesting and useful.

A NOTE TO THE INSTRUCTOR

A comprehensive instructor's manual is available to teachers who adopt *Concepts of Physical Fitness*. This manual includes suggestions for organizing the classes, grading, lecture outlines, and laboratory instructions, as well as suggested supplementary activities. It explains how to use only the part of these concepts in the text that fit your particular course. A master set of illustrations suitable for transparencies is available to accompany the lectures.

Other important instructor support materials available with the *Concepts of Physical Fitness* book include two different and updated computer software packages and a video cassette. The first of the two computer software diskettes includes exam questions and a program for creating your own exams in a user-friendly way. The second diskette has been expanded to include four different programs: (1) a self-evaluation profile, which aids students in fitness self-testing and program planning; (2) an on-screen attitude test, which allows students to take and score their personal attitudes about fitness; (3) a risk profile, which allows students to determine cardiovascular risks; and (4) a program that determines the students' threshold and target heart rates.

The video cassette contains a discussion of fitness testing philosophy, descriptions of each self-test in the book, and a sample dance aerobics program. The video can be used by instructors when preparing for class, by instructors and students in class, or by students on an individual basis.

If you have used previous editions, particularly the widely adopted fifth edition, you will notice that we have retained many of the features of that edition, but have made some changes at the recommendations of users. Most of these are outlined earlier in the preface. Particularly useful to the instructor, we think, is the expansion of Section I to include exercise programs immediately after the concept most related to those exercises. This format is more logical and more useful for both the student and instructor. It is hoped that this new organization and the other changes as previously noted, as well as the addition of new teacher support materials, will make this already "easy-to-use" book, even more easy to use.

We wish to extend our thanks to the many reviewers who have helped to make the book a success over the years. We particularly would like to acknowledge the following people for their effort and insight that helped guide us through the years:

Jimmy Jones, Henderson State University; James B. Angel, Samford University; Stanely R. Brown, University of British Columbia; Jeanne A. Ashley, Greenfield Community College; James R. Marett, Northern Illinois University; Sister Janice Iverson, South Dakota State University; Al Leister, Mercer County Community College; David Laurie, Kansas State University; Bo Fernhall, University of Rhode Island; Dr. Larry Gay Reagan, Volunteer State Community College; Paul H. Todd, Polk Community College; Patricia J. McSwegin, Emporia State University; Sandra Morgan, San Jacinto College; and Richard Krejci, Columbia College.

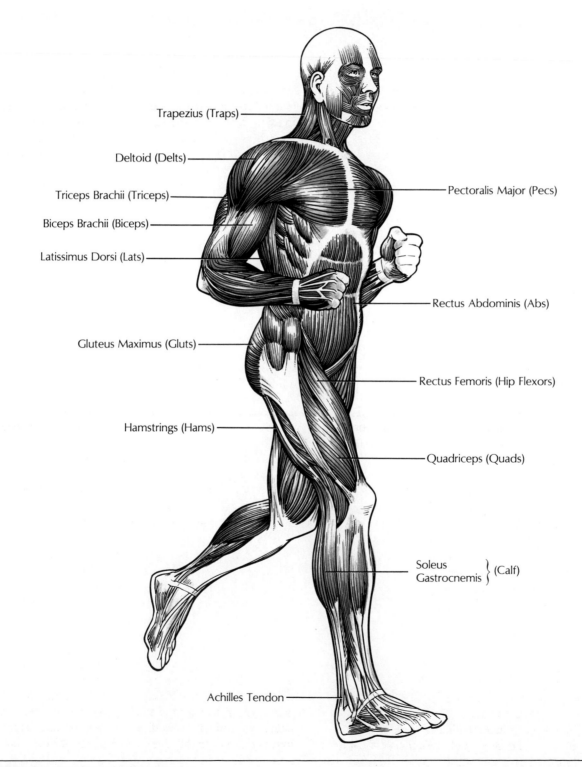

Trapezius (Traps)

Deltoid (Delts)

Triceps Brachii (Triceps)

Biceps Brachii (Biceps)

Latissimus Dorsi (Lats)

Gluteus Maximus (Gluts)

Hamstrings (Hams)

Achilles Tendon

Pectoralis Major (Pecs)

Rectus Abdominis (Abs)

Rectus Femoris (Hip Flexors)

Quadriceps (Quads)

Soleus
Gastrocnemis } (Calf)

FIGURE P.1 The Major Muscle Groups

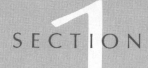

SECTION 1

PHYSICAL FITNESS AND PROGRAMS OF EXERCISE

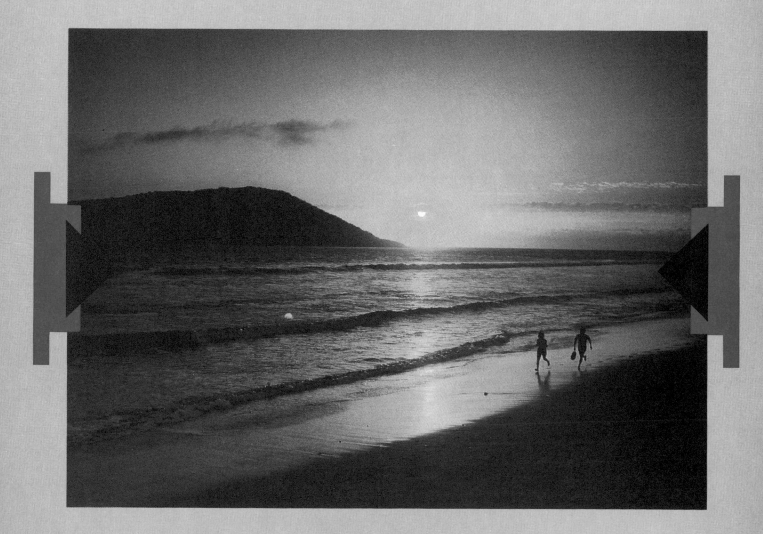

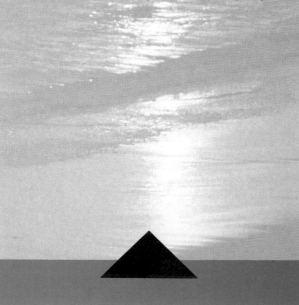

1

INTRODUCTION

CONCEPT 1

Regular exercise is important for all people.

INTRODUCTION

The human organism was designed to be active. Anthropologists indicate that the need to be active is associated with the "fight or flight" response. In search of food, primitive people sometimes had to fight with other predators or to flee for safety. In either case, the response was often vigorous activity. Even our more recent ancestors were required to do vigorous activity as a relatively major part of their normal daily routine. However, automation and technology have freed modern civilization from the exhausting physical labor required of earlier generations. The heavy physical work of the farmer and manual laborer is less and less likely to be a part of the normal daily routine of the average North American. Statistics indicate that in the past 100 years, the average workweek has been greatly reduced, thereby netting the average person many hours of free time annually.

Even though exercise has become less necessary as a part of the normal work of many adults, the need for regular exercise has not decreased. If anything, it has increased. Though we do not have to flee from saber-toothed tigers or fight wild animals for our food, our bodies still respond with the fight or flight response. The business person's stomach "churns" before the important meeting and the anxious sports fan's heartbeat increases during the close contest. The body is readied for activity, but the activity never comes. As a result, many Americans lack physical fitness and suffer from hypokinetic disease, or diseases associated with inactivity.

The need for good physical fitness and accompanying mental and physical health is vital for everyone. The human's need for regular exercise is critical in modern society. We have the necessary free time to be active, and given adequate information, all of us can learn to make intelligent decisions about lifetime health, physical fitness, and exercise.

TERMS

Exercise—Exercise, as used in *Concepts of Physical Fitness,* means human movement or physical activity. This term includes such formal activities as calisthenics, movements done in sports, dance, and games, as well as less formal activities, such as walking, jogging, and swimming. In this book, exercise, physical activity, and human movement are used interchangeably and, in general, describe large muscle activities rather than highly specific, relatively nontaxing movements of small muscle groups.

Hypokinetic Disease or Condition—"Hypo" means
under or too little, and "kinetic" means energy or
activity. Thus, hypokinetic means "too little activity." A hypokinetic disease or condition is associated with lack of physical activity or too little
regular exercise. Examples of such conditions include heart disease, low back pain, adult-onset
diabetes, and obesity.

Physical Fitness—Physical fitness is the entire human
organism's ability to function efficiently and effectively. It is made up of at least eleven different components, each of which contributes to a person's
ability to work effectively, to enjoy leisure time, to
be healthy, to resist hypokinetic diseases, and to meet
emergency situations. Though the development of
physical fitness is the result of many things, optimal
physical fitness is not possible without regular exercise.

SOME DISCOURAGING FACTS (THE BAD NEWS)

*Too many North American adults are not as ac-
tive as they should be.*

Recent statistics indicate that only about one-third of
all adults **exercise** regularly enough to build optimal
fitness. As adults grow older, they tend to become less
active.

*Many North American children are not as fit as
they should be.*

The results of recent studies, including the National
Children and Youth study, the Nabisco/AAU study,
and a study done by the President's Council on Physical Fitness and Sports, reveal that more than one-half
of school-age children are not as fit as they should be.
This affects their health and their functioning for work
and play.

*Teenagers are especially likely to lack good fit-
ness.*

Of all groups studied, teenagers are more apt than any
other to be unfit. Too many teens decrease, rather than
increase, in fitness following elementary school. During
this time, proper exercise and a healthy life-style can
result in exceptional fitness gains. Instead, lack of exercise and improper nutrition often result in a fitness
decline at this age.

Adult women are often less active than adult men.

Recent studies indicate that considerably more men are
involved in regular physical activity than are women
even though all evidence indicates that the benefits of
exercise for women are similar to those for men.

*Too many adults suffer from **hypokinetic diseases.***

In 1961, Kraus and Raab coined the term "hypokinetic
disease." They pointed out that recent advances in
modern medicine had been quite effective in eliminating infectious diseases, but that degenerative diseases, characterized by sedentary or "take-it-easy"
living, had increased in recent decades. In fact, heart
disease is the leading cause of death in the United
States. High blood pressure afflicts an estimated 57
million adults; nearly 2 million have had strokes; and
almost 5 million suffer from coronary heart disease, including heart attacks. The leading medical complaint
(except for the common cold) in the United States is
low back pain, and nearly one-half of all North Americans are considered obese. Studies now show that the
symptoms of hypokinetic disease begin in youth. This
fact, plus the relatively low fitness levels of children,
suggests that the incidence of hypokinetic disease in our
culture will not be reduced without considerable life-
style change in people of all ages.

*Many people are ignorant of the facts about ex-
ercise and physical fitness.*

Unfortunately, many American adults hold misconceptions about health, fitness, and exercise. For example,
57 percent of inactive adults feel that such sports as
baseball and bowling provide enough exercise to develop good health and physical fitness. Although the
facts indicate otherwise, those who do not exercise regularly believe that they get all the exercise they need.
Interestingly, those who report that they participate in
regular exercise are also the ones who are likely to feel
that they do not get enough exercise for their own good.

SOME ENCOURAGING FACTS (THE GOOD NEWS)

*North Americans are becoming more active in re-
cent years.*

Surveys taken in the 1960s indicated that only about
24 percent of all adults exercise in some form during
their free time. Recent statistics indicate that as many
as 50 to 60 percent of Americans are now active on a
regular basis, though as previously noted, too many are
not active enough to promote optimal fitness. In
Canada, 56 percent of the total population over the age
of ten is active for at least three hours per week on a
regular basis.

*More people with disabilities are becoming ac-
tive.*

Recent surveys indicate that 50 percent of the people
classified as having a "disability" consider themselves
to be "active." Only 20 percent considered themselves
to be sedentary.

Most adults realize the value of exercise and physical fitness.

Current findings show that the interest in fitness and exercise generated among large numbers of North Americans in the 1960s and 1970s is still prevalent today. Almost all adults believe that exercise is important for good health and fitness, and that regular activity and sports are valuable for their children.

Increasing numbers of women are getting involved in regular exercise.

It is true that women are less likely than men to be active, but it is also true that they are becoming active in sports and physical activities at a distinctly more rapid rate than men. Also, activities previously considered to be "for women only," such as aerobic dance, are gaining in popularity among men.

Adults who learn the facts about exercise tend to be more active and have better attitudes than those who hold misconceptions.

Though too many adults are inactive and uninformed of the facts about fitness and exercise, those adults who have learned the facts tend to persist in activity over the years. Those who are well informed are able to make intelligent decisions about exercise, including the ultimate decision to participate in adequate regular exercise for developing optimal fitness.

Industry has recognized the importance of exercise programs to employee fitness and productivity.

Realizing that many jobs are not as active as they were prior to automation, industry has taken steps to provide on-the-job exercise and fitness programs for their employees. Because medical costs are skyrocketing; because hypokinetic diseases, such as back pain, account for a billion dollar annual loss in production; and because absenteeism can be reduced considerably by offering employees an exercise and fitness program, company officials endorse the fitness-in-industry movement. Evidence indicates that such programs are cost-effective as well as popular among employees. One company official notes, "It's the best fringe benefit we've offered."

The United States Army has recently implemented a program to teach the fitness facts to supplement physical training programs.

For years, the military has had physical training programs designed to "get people fit." Unfortunately, these programs sometimes resulted in only short-term fitness gains because they taught participants to "hate exercise." The new program recognizes the importance of learning the facts about fitness and the need for each individual to develop a personalized fitness program that can be used for a lifetime.

FACTS ABOUT WHY PEOPLE DO NOT EXERCISE

The number one reason people give for not exercising is, "I don't have the time."

More than one-half of those who do not exercise regularly reason that, "I don't have the time." Often in the same breath the person says, "I am too busy." Young people state that they will soon be established and able to take the time to exercise. Older people state that they wish they had taken the time when they were younger.

Another major reason people do not exercise is, "It's too inconvenient."

Many people who avoid exercise do so because it is inconvenient. They are exercise procrastinators. Specific reasons for procrastinating include: "It makes me sweaty"; "It messes up my hair"; and "I just can't find the energy." (It is interesting, though, that people who do exercise regularly report improvements in their appearance and a feeling of increased energy.)

Large numbers of adults are not active because they "just don't enjoy exercise."

The reasons some people do not enjoy exercise include: "People might laugh at me"; "Sports make me nervous"; and "I am not good at physical activities." These people often lack confidence in their own abilities. In some cases, this is because of their past experiences in physical education or in athletics. With properly selected activities, even those who have never enjoyed exercise can get "hooked."

Poor health is a reason some people avoid exercise.

Some people avoid exercise because of health reasons. Though it is true that there are good medical reasons for not exercising, many people with such problems can benefit from exercise if it is properly designed for them.

Lack of facilities and bad weather are reasons some do not exercise regularly.

Regular exercise is much more convenient if facilities are easy to reach and the weather is good. Still, recreational opportunities have increased considerably in recent years. Furthermore, some of the most popular activities for building fitness require very little equipment, can be done in or near the home, and are inexpensive.

FACTS ABOUT WHY PEOPLE DO EXERCISE

The number one reason people exercise regularly is "for health and physical fitness."

Ninety percent of all adults recognize the importance of exercise for good health and fitness. More than one national survey has shown that health and fitness is the single most important reason why people engage in regular exercise. Unfortunately, many adults say that a "doctor's order to exercise" would be the most likely reason to get them to begin a regular program. For some, however, waiting for a doctor's order may be too late.

Enjoyment is a major reason people exercise regularly.

A majority of adults say that "enjoyment" would be of paramount importance in deciding to exercise. This is not surprising, given statements from joggers that they began exercising for fitness but continue for such reasons as the "peak experience," the "runner's high," and "spinning free." In fact, movement can be an end in itself. Satisfaction can be derived from the mere involvement in the movement activity. The sense of fun, the feeling of well-being, and the general enjoyment associated with physical activity is well documented.

Relaxation and release from tension are important reasons given for doing regular exercise.

Relaxation and release from tension rank high as important reasons why people do regular exercise. Exercise, such as walking, jogging, or cycling, is a way of getting some "quiet time" away from the stress of the job. For years, it has been recognized that exercise in the form of sports and games provides a "catharsis," or outlet, for the frustrations of normal daily activities. Evidence indicates that regular exercise can help reduce depression and anxiety, both common symptoms in Western culture.

Physical activity can provide a way of meeting a challenge and developing a sense of personal accomplishment.

A sense of personal accomplishment associated with performing various physical activities is frequently a reason people exercise. In some cases, it is merely learning a new skill, such as racquetball or tennis; in other cases, it is running a mile or doing a certain number of sit-ups that provides this feeling of accomplishment. The challenge of doing something never done before is apparently a very powerful experience. Physical activities provide opportunities not readily available in other aspects of life.

An important reason many people exercise is the social experience of involvement.

Physical activity often provides the opportunity to be with other people. It is this social experience that many appreciate most about exercise. Frequent answers to the question, "Why do you exercise?" include: "It is a good way to spend time with other members of the family"; "It is a good way to spend time with close

friends"; and "Being part of the team is a satisfying feeling." Physical activity settings can also provide an opportunity for making new friends.

The competitive experience is an important reason people participate in sports and physical activities.

"The thrill of victory" and "sports competition" are two reasons often given by people who participate in physical activities. For many, the competitive experiences can be very satisfying.

Physical appearance is a reason given by many for doing regular exercise.

People indicate that an important reason for exercising is to improve their physical appearance. In our society, "looking good" is highly valued, thus physical attractiveness is another major reason why people participate in regular exercise. Of major importance to many adults is weight or fat control.

OTHER IMPORTANT FACTS

The most popular forms of exercise among adults require very little skill or equipment and are easily accessible.

Surveys consistently show that the most popular activities among adults are walking, swimming, bicycling, aerobic dance, calisthenics, and jogging/running. All these can be done in or near the home for little or no cost. None requires a high degree of physical skill in order for a person to be successful or to enjoy the benefits associated with regular involvement. These activities are not often those that people value for their children, nor those in which they themselves were involved as children. And although football, baseball, basketball, gymnastics, and boxing are the activities adults most enjoy watching, they often are not the ones in which these adults participate.

Exercise can be important for many reasons but it is not a cure-all, and if done improperly, it can be dangerous.

The many benefits of exercise are well documented in this book. As we point out in later sections of *Concepts of Physical Fitness,* however, certain types of exercise are contraindicated for certain people. Doing too much too soon can be dangerous for those who have not been involved in exercise on a regular basis. Those who exercise irregularly, such as the "weekend athlete" who exercises vigorously only on weekends or other "special occasions," may be asking for trouble. There is some evidence that even avid exercisers can become overly involved with their commitment to physical activity and develop an "activity neurosis." This condition can develop if an individual becomes irrationally concerned about his or her need for involvement in exercise.

There is no single best form of exercise for all people.

Different people participate in different types of exercise for different reasons, as has been previously discussed. This is as it should be. Evidence indicates that each person has his or her own unique movement personality: no two people move in the same way. Because movement personalities differ, there is a wide variety of leisure activities from which different individuals can select. The choice of exercise and physical activities should be made only after carrying out the following steps:

1. Assess your current health and physical fitness status to determine your individual needs.

2. Examine your current interests. (Exercise should be enjoyable.)
3. Acquire a knowledge and an understanding of the values of different activities.
4. Determine which activities will best meet your needs and interests.
5. Acquire skill and knowledge in the selected activities.

Exercise is for virtually everyone.

Exercise, whether it be sports or some other form of physical activity, should not be limited to those with good athletic ability. Regardless of age, sex, or athletic ability (if there is no serious medical limitation), there is some form of activity that everyone will find enjoyable and in which everyone can succeed.

▶ LAB RESOURCE MATERIALS (FOR USE WITH LAB 1, PAGE 209)

CHART 1.1 The Physical Activity Questionnaire

The term "physical activity" in the following statements refers to all kinds of activities, including sports, formal exercises, and informal activities, such as jogging and cycling. Check your answers first, then read the directions for scoring at the end of the questionnaire.

	Strongly Agree	Agree	Undecided	Disagree	Strongly Disagree	Score
1. Doing regular physical activity can be as harmful to health as it is helpful.	☐	☐	☐	☐	☐	_____
2. One of the main reasons I do regular physical activity is because it is fun.	☐	☐	☐	☐	☐	_____
3. Participating in physical activities makes me tense and nervous.	☐	☐	☐	☐	☐	_____
4. The challenge of physical training is one reason why I participate in physical activity.	☐	☐	☐	☐	☐	_____
5. One of the things I like about physical activity is the participation with other people.	☐	☐	☐	☐	☐	_____
6. Doing regular physical activity does little to make me more physically attractive.	☐	☐	☐	☐	☐	_____
7. Competition is a good way to keep a game from being fun.	☐	☐	☐	☐	☐	_____
8. I should exercise regularly for my own good health and physical fitness.	☐	☐	☐	☐	☐	_____
9. Doing exercise and playing sports is boring.	☐	☐	☐	☐	☐	_____
10. I enjoy taking part in physical activity because it helps me to relax and get away from the pressures of daily living.	☐	☐	☐	☐	☐	_____
11. Most sports and physical activities are too difficult for me to enjoy.	☐	☐	☐	☐	☐	_____
12. I do not enjoy physical activities that require the participation of other people.	☐	☐	☐	☐	☐	_____
13. Regular exercise helps me look my best.	☐	☐	☐	☐	☐	_____
14. Competing against others in physical activities makes them enjoyable.	☐	☐	☐	☐	☐	_____

Score the physical activity questionnaire as follows:
1. For items 1, 3, 6, 7, 9, 11, and 12, give one point for strongly agree, two for agree, three for undecided, four for disagree, and five for strongly disagree. Put the correct number in the blank to the right of the statements.
2. For items 2, 4, 5, 8, 10, 13, and 14, give five points for strongly agree, four for agree, three for undecided, two for disagree, and one for strongly disagree. Put the correct number in the blank to the right of the statements.
3. Determine each of the following seven scores by adding the numbers to the right of the items as indicated (two numbers for each score).

Health and fitness score	Item 1 _____ + Item 8 ____ = _____
Fun and enjoyment score	Item 2 _____ + Item 9 ____ = _____
Relaxation and tension release score	Item 3 _____ + Item 10 ____ = _____
Challenge and achievement score	Item 4 _____ + Item 11 ____ = _____
Social score	Item 5 _____ + Item 12 ____ = _____
Appearance score	Item 6 _____ + Item 13 ____ = _____
Competition score	Item 7 _____ + Item 14 ____ = _____

Total score _____

4. Determine your total score by adding each of the seven scores. Write your total score in the bottom blank.
5. Use chart 1.2 to determine your rating on each score.

CHART 1.2 Physical Activity Questionnaire *Rating Scale*

Classification	Each of Seven Scores	Total Score
Excellent	9–10	63–70
Good	7–8	50–62
Fair	6	42–49
Poor	4–5	30–41
Very poor	3 or less	29 or less

REFERENCES

American Heart Association. *1986 Heart Facts.* Dallas: American Heart Association, 1986.

American Heart Association. *1986 Stroke Facts.* Dallas: American Heart Association, 1986.

Blair, S. N., et al. "Public Health Intervention Model for Worksite Health Promotion," *Journal of the American Medical Association* 255(1986):921.

Cinque, C. "Are Americans Fit? Survey Data Conflict." *Physician and Sportsmedicine* 14(1986):24.

Corbin, C. B. "Self-Confidence of Women in Sports." In *Clinics in Sports Medicine: Women in Sports,* edited by W. M. Walsh. Philadelphia: W. B. Saunders Co., 1984.

*Corbin, C. B., and R. Lindsey. *The Ultimate Fitness Book.* New York: Leisure Press, 1984.

Csikzentmihaly, M. *Beyond Boredom and Anxiety.* San Francisco: Jossey-Bass, 1977.

Department of the Army. *The Individual's Handbook on Physical Fitness.* Washington: Department of the Army, 1983.

Fitness Canada. *Canada Fitness Survey—Highlights.* Ottawa, Ontario: Government of Canada, 1986.

Gilliam, T. B., et al. "Exercise Programs for Children: A Way to Prevent Heart Disease?" *Physician and Sportsmedicine* 10(1982):96.

Greist, J. H., et al. "Running Through Your Mind." In *Psychology of Running,* edited by M. H. Sacks and M. L. Sachs. Champaign, IL: Human Kinetics, 1981.

Harris, L., and Associates. *The Perrier Study: Fitness in America.* New York: Great Waters of France, 1979.

Kenyon, G. S. "Six Scales for Assessing Attitudes Toward Physical Activity." *Research Quarterly* 39(1968):566.

*Kraus, H., and W. Raab. *Hypokinetic Disease.* Springfield, IL: C. C. Thomas, 1961.

Little, J. C. "The Athlete's Neurosis—A Deprivation Crisis." In Sacks, M. H. and M. L. Sachs, *Psychology of Running.* Champaign, IL: Human Kinetics, 1981.

President's Council on Physical Fitness and Sports, *1985 School Fitness Survey.* Washington, D.C. PCPFS 1986.

Gallup, G. and Associates. "Annual Survey on Fitness and Exercise," 1986.

Nabisco/AAU. *Toasted Wheat and Raisins/AAU Fitness Profile of American Youth.* Chicago: Golin-Harris, 1983.

*Pollock, M. L., et al. *Exercise in Health and Disease.* Philadelphia: W. B. Saunders Co., 1984.

Research and Forecasts, Inc. *The Miller Lite Report on American Attitudes toward Sports.* Milwaukee: Miller Brewing Co., 1983.

Rider, R. A., et al. "Effects of Florida's Personal Fitness Course on Cognitive, Attitudinal, and Physical Fitness Measures of Secondary Students: A Pilot Study." *Perceptual and Motor Skills* 62(1986):548.

Ross, J. G., et al. "The National Children and Youth Fitness
    Study." *Journal of Physical Education, Recreation and
    Dance* 56(1985):24.
Simon, D. G., and J. G. Travell. "Myofascial Origins of Low Back
    Pain." *Postgraduate Medicine* 73(1983):66.
Slava, S., D. R. Laurie, and C. B. Corbin. "The Long-Term
    Effects of a Conceptual Physical Education Program."
    Research Quarterly for Exercise and Sports 55
    (1984):161.
Snyder, E. E., and E. Spreitzer. "Adult Perceptions of Physical
    Education in the Schools and Community Sports Programs
    for Youth." *The Physical Educator* 40(1983):88.
Stone, W. J. "Exercise and Long-Term CV Risk Reduction in
    Corporate Executives." *Health Education* 14(1983):26.
Thorland, W. G., and T. B. Gilliam. "Comparison of Serum Lipids
    between Habitually High and Low Active Pre-Adolescent
    Males." *Medicine and Science in Sports and Exercise*
    13(1981):316.
Villeneuve, K., et al. "Employee Fitness: A Bottom Line Payoff."
    Journal of Physical Education, Recreation and Dance
    54(1983):35.
Wicks, B. "Physical Fitness Programs in Business and Industry."
    National Intramural and Recreational Sports Association
    7(1983):31.

2

PHYSICAL FITNESS

CONCEPT 2

Physical fitness is not only one
of the most important keys to a healthy
body;
it is also the basis for dynamic
and creative activity.
— President John F. Kennedy, 1960

INTRODUCTION

Some people associate "good physical fitness" with being good at sports and games. It does take a certain degree of fitness to excel in these activities, but being able to perform specific skills may not be a good indicator of total physical fitness because some sports require only specific aspects of fitness.

Historically, physical fitness has often been misrepresented, at times identified exclusively with skill in sports, at other times identified too closely with only one of the many aspects of physical fitness. For example, in previous decades, fitness for men was often associated with muscle strength. This is evidenced by the popularity of programs such as Charles Atlas' Dynamic Tension Program advertised widely in magazines and comic books. In the 1960s and 1970s, with the popularity of jogging and other forms of aerobic exercise, many people associated physical fitness almost exclusively with cardiovascular fitness. Recently, research and popular literature has brought considerable attention to flexibility as an important component of fitness. It is true that each of these is important, but it cannot be overemphasized that physical fitness is not a single entity, but it consists of a number of different characteristics of which strength, cardiovascular fitness, and flexibility are only three. Each of the specific components of fitness is critical to developing optimal physical fitness and to achieving the benefits associated with being optimally fit.

HEALTH-RELATED FITNESS TERMS

Body Composition—The relative percentage of muscle, fat, bone, and other tissue of which the body is composed. A fit person has a relatively low, but not too low, percentage of body fat (body fatness).

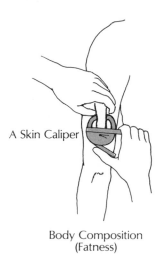

A Skin Caliper

Body Composition
(Fatness)

Cardiovascular Fitness—The ability of the heart, blood vessels, blood, and respiratory system to supply fuel, especially oxygen, to the muscles during sustained exercise. A fit person can persist in physical activity for relatively long periods of time without undue stress.

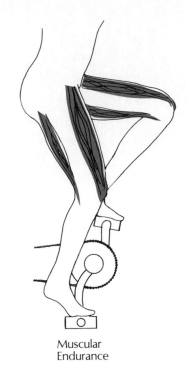

Cardiovascular
Fitness

Muscular Endurance—The ability of the muscles to repeatedly exert themselves. A fit person can repeat movements over a long period of time without undue fatigue.

Muscular
Endurance

Flexibility—The range of motion available in a joint. It is affected by muscle length, joint structure, and other factors. A fit person can move the body joints through a full range of motion in work and in play.

Flexibility

Strength—The ability to exert an external force or to lift a heavy weight. A fit person can do work or play that involves exerting force, such as lifting or controlling one's own body weight.

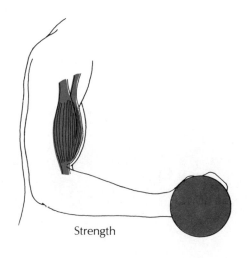

Strength

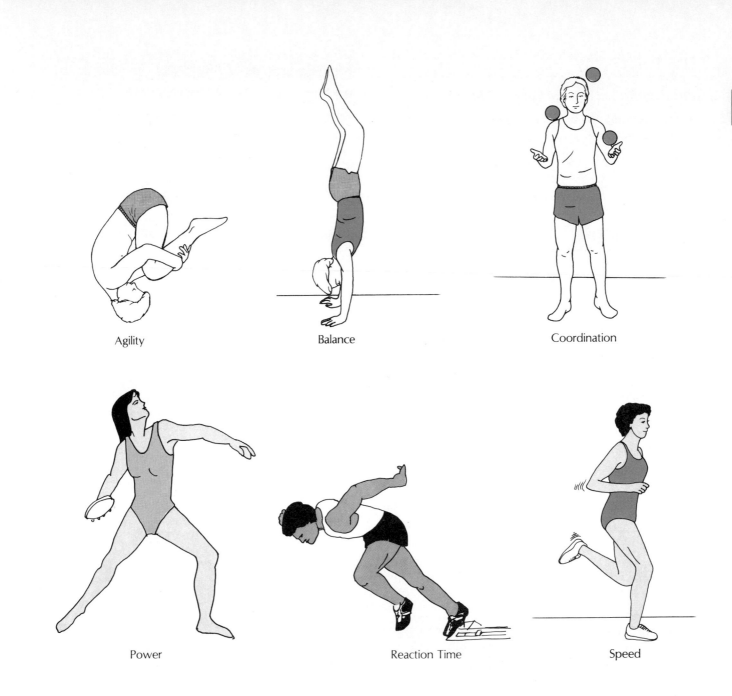

Agility

Balance

Coordination

Power

Reaction Time

Speed

SKILL-RELATED FITNESS TERMS

Agility—The ability to rapidly and accurately change the direction of the entire body in space. Soccer and wrestling are examples of activities that require exceptional agility.

Balance—The maintenance of equilibrium while stationary or while moving. Performing on the balance beam or working as a riveter on a high-rise building are activities that require exceptional balance.

Coordination—The ability to use the senses with the body parts to perform motor tasks smoothly and accurately. Juggling, batting a baseball, or kicking a ball are examples of activities requiring good coordination.

Power—The ability to transfer energy into force at a fast rate. Throwing the discus and putting the shot are activities that require considerable power.

Reaction Time—The time elapsed between stimulation and the beginning of reaction to that stimulation. Driving a racing car and starting a sprint race require good reaction time.

Speed—The ability to perform a movement in a short period of time. A runner on a track team or a wide receiver on a football team needs good foot and leg speed.

THE FACTS

Physical fitness is a part of total fitness.

Aspects of total fitness include emotional, social, spiritual, and mental fitness as well as physical fitness.

Physical fitness consists of many components, each of which is specific in nature.

Physical fitness is a combination of several aspects rather than a single characteristic. A fit person possesses at least adequate levels of each of the five health-related fitness components, and each of the six skill-related fitness components. People who possess one aspect of physical fitness do not necessarily possess all of the other aspects.

Each of the eleven components of physical fitness is separate and different from each of the others. Some relationship exists between different fitness characteristics, but people who possess exceptional strength do not necessarily have good cardiovascular fitness, and those who have good coordination do not necessarily possess good flexibility.

Body composition, cardiovascular fitness, flexibility, muscular endurance, and strength are the health-related components of physical fitness.

Because each fitness characteristic has a direct relationship to good health and lessens risk of hypokinetic disease, each is considered a part of health-related physical fitness.

Agility, balance, coordination, power, reaction time, and speed comprise the skill-related components of physical fitness.

Because each fitness characteristic is related to certain motor skills, such as those required in sports and in specific types of jobs, each is considered a part of skill-related physical fitness. Skill-related fitness is sometimes called "sports fitness" or "motor fitness."

Good physical fitness, particularly health-related fitness, is important to optimal health.

Optimal health is more than freedom from disease. According to the World Health Organization, health is "a state of complete physical, mental, and social well-being and not merely the absence of disease and infirmity." Good fitness can contribute to buoyant health, including feeling good, looking good, and enjoying life, as well as reduce the risk of certain diseases.

Good health-related physical fitness contributes to positive physical health, including a reduced risk of hypokinetic diseases.

Many of the contributions of health-related physical fitness are described in more detail later in this book. However, the physical health benefits associated with

TABLE 2.1 The Physical Health Benefits of Activity

Major Benefit	Related Benefits
Improved cardiovascular fitness	• Stronger heart muscle • Lower heart rate • Possible reduction in blood pressure • Reduced blood fat, including low density lipids (LDL) • Possible resistance to atherosclerosis • Possible improved peripheral circulation • Improved coronary circulation • Resistance to "emotional storm" • Less chance of heart attack • Greater chance of surviving a heart attack • Increased protective high density lipids (HDL) • Increased oxygen carrying capacity of the blood
Greater lean body mass and less body fat	• Greater work efficiency • Less susceptibility to disease • Improved appearance • Less incidence of self-concept problems related to obesity
Improved strength and muscular endurance	• Greater work efficiency • Less chance of muscle injury • Decreased chance of low back problems • Improved performance in sports • Improved ability to meet emergencies
Improved flexibility	• Greater work efficiency • Less chance of muscle injury • Less chance of joint injury • Decreased chance of low back problems • Improved sports performance
Other health benefits of exercise and physical activity	• Increased ability to use oxygen • Quicker recovery after hard work • Decreased chance of adult-onset diabetes

involvement in regular, properly planned exercises are summarized in table 2.1. Physical fitness also contributes to positive mental health. Mental illness is now recognized as a health problem, not as a personal weakness or a reason for social disgrace. The serious nature of mental health problems is illustrated by the following facts: approximately 25,000 suicides occur in the United States each year; doctors estimate that as many as 70 percent of all illnesses are psychosomatic, or emotionally related. Some mental health benefits that are derived from regular physical activity and good physical fitness are summarized in table 2.2.

TABLE 2.2 The Mental Health Benefits of Activity

Major Benefit	Related Benefits
Reduction in mental tension	• Relief of depression • Improved sleep habits • Fewer stress symptoms • Ability to enjoy leisure • Possible work improvement
Opportunity for social interactions	• Improved quality of life
Resistance to fatigue	• Ability to enjoy leisure • Improved quality of life • Improved ability to meet some stressors
Opportunity for successful experience	• Improved self-concept • Opportunity to recognize and accept personal limitations
Improved physical fitness	• Improved sense of well-being • Improved self-concept • Improved appearance

Good physical fitness can help an individual enjoy his or her free time.

A person who is not too fat, has no back problems, does not have to worry about high blood pressure, and has reasonable skills in different lifetime sports is more likely to get involved and stay regularly involved in leisure time activities than one who does not have these characteristics. It is said that enjoying your leisure time may not add years to your life, but can add life to your years.

Good physical fitness can help an individual work effectively and efficiently.

A person who can resist fatigue, muscle soreness, back problems, and other symptoms associated with poor health-related fitness is capable of working productively and having energy left over at the end of the day. Surveys of employees who have the opportunity to improve fitness through involvement in employee fitness programs indicate that 75 percent have an improved sense of well-being. Employers indicate that absenteeism decreased by up to 50 percent among program participants. People, with good skill-related fitness, may be more effective and efficient in performing specific motor skills required for certain jobs.

Good physical fitness is essential to effective living.

Although the need for each component of physical fitness is specific to each individual, every person requires enough fitness to perform normal daily activities without undue fatigue. Whether it be walking, performing household chores, or merely feeling good and enjoying the "simple things in life" without pain or fear of injury, good fitness is important to all people.

Good physical fitness may help you function safely and assist you in meeting unexpected emergencies.

Emergencies are never expected, but when they do arise, they often demand performance that requires good fitness. For example, flood victims may need to fill sandbags for hours without rest, and accident victims may be required to walk or run long distances for help. Also, good fitness is required for such simple tasks as safely changing a spare tire or loading a moving van without injury.

Physical fitness is the basis for dynamic and creative activity.

Though the following quotation by former President John F. Kennedy is now over twenty years old, it clearly points out the importance of physical fitness. "The relationship between the soundness of the body and the activity of the mind is subtle and complex. Much is not yet understood, but we know what the Greeks knew: that intelligence and skill can only function at the peak of their capacity when the body is healthy and strong, and that hardy spirits and tough minds usually inhabit sound bodies. Physical fitness is the basis of all activities in our society; if our bodies grow soft and inactive, if we fail to encourage physical development and prowess, we will undermine our capacity for thought, for work, and for the use of those skills vital to an expanding and complex America."

There is no substitute for regular exercise if achieving physical fitness is your goal.

There is no doubt that nutrition, sleep habits, job stress, and other environmental factors affect physical fitness, both positively and negatively. Of course, regular exercise is the single most critical factor associated with good fitness.

Heredity also plays an important role in the amount of physical fitness a person can attain. More than a few people have become discouraged after completing an exercise program only to find that they have scored lower on fitness tests than friends who are less active. Though it is clear that regular exercise is critical to optimal physical fitness, each person also has a hereditary predisposition to fitness. While achieving high scores on fitness tests is a desirable goal, it is important to understand that hereditary predispositions to fitness limit one's potential for achieving exceptionally high scores. Meeting standards for good health and improving personal fitness are more important than comparisons to other people. Many experts believe that people who exercise regularly but who do not have exceptionally high fitness scores are likely to resist hypokinetic diseases as well as, or better than, people who have high fitness scores but do no regular exercise. In other words, regular exercise, which leads to improved fitness, is at least as important, if not more important than high levels of fitness if the goal is to improve health and resist hypokinetic diseases.

There are some important guidelines that should be followed when doing personal fitness testing.

1. At some point, it is wise to have an expert test your fitness. This helps you get an accurate assessment of your current fitness level. *It is important, however, to learn to evaluate your own level of fitness.* Learning to evaluate your own fitness allows you to have a personal record of your fitness on a regular basis, keeps you from being dependent on others, and aids you in staying fit for a lifetime.

2. *Comparisons to health standards and improvement of your own fitness are more important than comparisons to other people.* In Western culture, we have a tendency to compare ourselves to others in almost all things we do. Rather than comparing your fitness scores to those of other people, you would be wise to concentrate on meeting "good fitness standards" and improving your personal fitness. Exceptionally high scores on fitness tests may improve performances in sports but probably are not necessary for good health. For example, a male having 10 to 15 percent body fat is considered to be more healthy than one having 25 to 30 percent body fat. However, having less than 10 percent of the body as fat is not necessarily more healthy than having 10 to 15 percent fat (though some people believe that low levels of fatness may enhance performance in some sports). As you will learn later in this book, having too little body fat can be harmful to good health.

3. *An assessment of all components of health-related fitness is important.* Because fitness has many different components, you will need to do many different self-tests if you are going to get an accurate picture of your total fitness. It is recommended that each person do *several* tests of fitness for each component of health-related fitness. Several tests will give you a more complete and accurate picture of your total physical fitness.

AN IMPORTANT NOTE ON PHYSICAL FITNESS TESTING

In this book, we present many different fitness self-tests. At the end of this chapter, we offer a series of stunts. These stunts are not intended as tests of fitness. They are presented to give you an idea of the nature of each component of fitness. In later chapters, many different tests are described. When possible, you should learn to give each test to yourself so that you can continue to reassess your fitness for lifetime. Tests such as skinfold measures are hard to administer to yourself, but you can learn to teach a friend or relative to measure you. You are encouraged to do as many tests as possible. For example, you may want to assess your cardiovascular fitness using all three tests described. You can use a summary of all tests to make accurate fitness assessments. Finally, you should know how to use the "Rating Scales" in each chapter to interpret your fitness results. If you score "low" in fitness, you are probably less fit than you should be for your own good health. "Marginal" scores indicate that some improvement is in order, but you are nearing minimal health standards set by experts. If you reach the "good fitness zone" you probably have enough of a specific fitness component to help reduce the risk of a specific hypokinetic condition, assuming that you maintain an active lifestyle. Even achievement in the good fitness zone may not result in optimal health benefits for inactive people. The "high performance zone" is also a good indicator of adequate fitness, but it is probably not necessary to reach this level to experience good health benefits. Achievement of high performance scores probably has more to do with performance on various physical tasks than it does with good health. For example, people who score in the high performance zone on a strength test may do well in a sport, such as weight lifting or putting the shot, but may not have less risk of hypokinetic conditions, such as back pain or poor posture, than people who score in the good fitness zone.

CHART 2.1 Physical Fitness Stunts

Item	Fitness Aspect	Pass
1. *One-foot balance.* Stand on one foot; press up so that the weight is on the ball of the foot with the heel off the floor. Hold the hands out in front and the other leg straight for ten seconds.	Balance	Yes ☐
2. *Long jump.* Stand with the toes behind a line; using no run or hop step, jump as far as possible. To pass, men must jump their height plus six inches. Women must jump their height only.	Power	Yes ☐
3. *Jack spring.* From a standing position, jump into the air, kick the legs up and out and touch the feet with the hands. Repeat two times, touching the floor once between jumps.	Agility	Yes ☐
4. *Paper drop.* Have a partner hold a sheet of notebook paper so that the side edge is between your thumb and index finger about the width of your hand from the top of the page. When your partner drops the paper, catch it before it slips through the thumb and finger. Do not move your hand lower to catch the paper.	Reaction time	Yes ☐

PHYSICAL FITNESS   15

CHART 2.1 *Continued*

Item	Fitness Aspect	Pass	
5. *Double heel click.* With the feet apart, jump into the air and tap the heels together twice before you hit the ground. You must land with your feet at least three inches apart.	Speed	Yes ☐	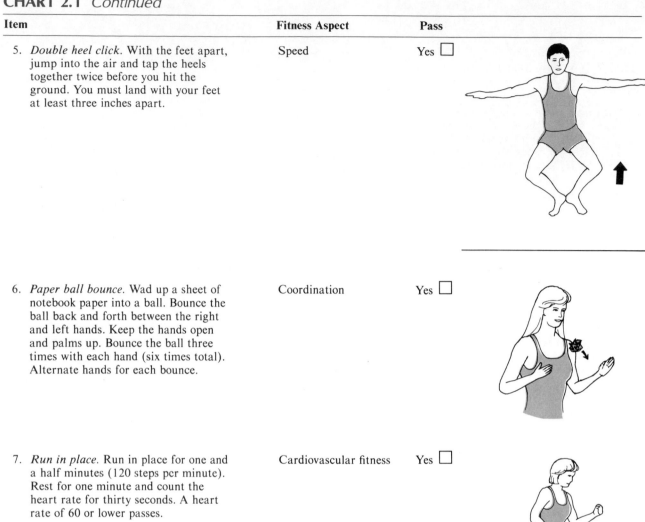
6. *Paper ball bounce.* Wad up a sheet of notebook paper into a ball. Bounce the ball back and forth between the right and left hands. Keep the hands open and palms up. Bounce the ball three times with each hand (six times total). Alternate hands for each bounce.	Coordination	Yes ☐	
7. *Run in place.* Run in place for one and a half minutes (120 steps per minute). Rest for one minute and count the heart rate for thirty seconds. A heart rate of 60 or lower passes.	Cardiovascular fitness	Yes ☐	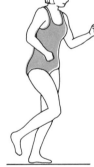
8. *Toe touch.* Sit on the floor with your feet against a wall. Keep the feet together and the knees straight. Bend forward at the hips. Reach forward and touch your closed fists to the wall. Bend forward slowly, do not bounce.	Flexibility	Yes ☐	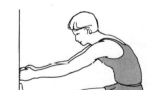

CHART 2.1 *Continued*

Item	Fitness Aspect	Pass
9. *The pinch.* Have a partner pinch a fold of skin on the back of your upper arm halfway between the tip of the elbow and the tip of the shoulder. Use your textbook to measure the skinfold width. Men: No greater than thickness of the textbook. Women: No greater than one and one-half the thickness of the textbook.	Body composition (body fatness)	Yes ☐
10. *High leg press up.* Start in the push-up position with a partner holding the legs off the ground. Keep the body straight, press off the floor until the arms are fully extended. Women repeat once, men three times.	Strength	Yes ☐
11. *Four-minute hop.* With the hands behind the head, pogo hop over a line as many times as possible in four minutes. Five hundred jumps over the line passes.	Muscular endurance and cardiovascular fitness	Yes ☐

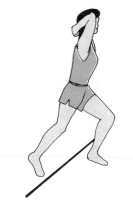

REFERENCES

*Blair, S. N. "Physical Activity Leads to Fitness and Pays Off." *Physician and Sportsmedicine* 13(1985):153.

Blair, S. N., et al. "A New Physical Fitness Test." *Physician and Sportsmedicine* 11(1983):87.

Blair, S. N., et al. "Public Health Intervention Model for Worksite Health Promotion." *Journal of the American Medical Association* 255(1986):921.

*Corbin, C. B., and R. Lindsey. *The Ultimate Fitness Book.* New York: Leisure Press, 1984.

Kennedy, J. F. "The Soft American." *Sports Illustrated* 13(December 1960):15.

Krahenbuhl, G. S., et al. "Developmental Aspects of Maximal Aerobic Power in Children." *Exercise and Sports Science Reviews* 13(1985):503.

*Paffenbarger, R. S., and R. T. Hyde. "Exercise as Protection Against Heart Attack." *New England Journal of Medicine* 302 (1980):1026.

Paffenbarger, R. S. "Exercise in the Primary Prevention of Coronary Heart Disease." In Pollock, M. L., et al., *Heart Disease and Rehabilitation.* New York: John Wiley, 1986.

Pate, R. R. "A New Definition of Youth Fitness." *Physician and Sportsmedicine* 11(1983):77.

Physician and Sportsmedicine. Published monthly, contains articles of all kinds on exercise, sports, and fitness.

*Pollock, M. L., et al. *Exercise in Health and Disease.* Philadelphia: W. B. Saunders Co., 1984.

Sherin, K. "Aerobic Exercise: Can You Answer the Questions Patients Ask?" *Postgraduate Medicine* 73(1983):157.

Wicks, B. "Physical Fitness Programs in Business and Industry." *National Intramural and Recreational Sports Association Journal* 7(1983):31.

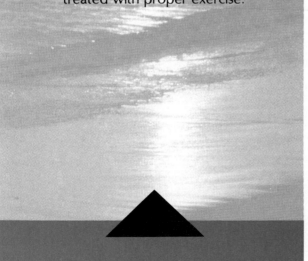

3

HYPOKINETIC DISEASE

CONCEPT 3

In many cases,
hypokinetic disease can be prevented or
treated with proper exercise.

INTRODUCTION

One of the ways that exercise, and the resulting health-related physical fitness, contributes to optimal health is by helping to reduce the risk of hypokinetic disease and related conditions. Given the epidemic proportions of heart disease, the prevalence of back pain as a major adult complaint, the high incidence of fatness and obesity among children as well as adults, and the dangers associated with the widespread existence of high blood pressure, ulcers, and mental disorders, the reduction of hypokinetic disease is a priority health concern for Western culture.

TERMS

Angina Pectoris—Chest or arm pain resulting from reduced oxygen supply to the heart muscle.

Arteriosclerosis—Conditions that cause the arterial walls to become thick, hard, and nonelastic; hardening of the arteries.

Atherosclerosis—The deposition of materials along the arterial walls; a type of arteriosclerosis.

Collateral Circulation—Development of auxiliary blood vessels that may take over coronary blood circulation to the heart muscle in the event that one or more of the coronary arteries becomes obstructed or has diminished blood flow.

Congestive Heart Failure—The inability of the heart muscle to pump the blood at a life-sustaining rate.

Coronary Occlusion—The blocking of the coronary blood vessels.

Emotional Storm—A traumatic emotional experience that is likely to affect the human organism physiologically.

Fibrin—The substance that, in combination with blood cells, forms a blood clot.

Hypertension—Another word for high blood pressure.

Lipid—All fats and fatty substances.

Lipoprotein—Fat-carrying proteins in the blood.

Lordosis—Excessive low back curve; swayback.

Parasympathetic Nervous System—Branch of the autonomic nervous system that slows the heart rate.

Referred Pain—Pain resulting from a problem in one part of the body, but felt at a different location.

Risk Factor—Any of the factors that increase the risk of hypokinetic diseases or conditions.

Sympathetic Nervous System—Branch of the autonomic nervous system that prepares the body for activity by speeding up the heart rate.

THE FACTS

The link between regular physical activity and good health is now well documented.

Based on the results of long-term research on large numbers of people, medical researchers have reached the following conclusion: "Evidence mounts that the relationship between exercise and good health is more than circumstantial. If some questions are not yet answered, they are far less important than those that have been" (Paffenbarger and Hyde, 1981). These researchers add that the true role of exercise has been known for centuries. In fact, several hundred years ago, John Dryden noted: "Better to hunt in fields, for health unbought, than fee the doctor for nauseous draught; the wise, for cure, on exercise depend; God never made his work for man to mend."

FACTS ABOUT EXERCISE, CARDIOVASCULAR FITNESS, AND HEART DISEASE

There are many different types of heart disease.

Hypertension (high blood pressure), **atherosclerosis, arteriosclerosis, coronary occlusion, angina pectoris,** and **congestive heart failure** are among the more prevalent forms of heart disease. Evidence indicates that inactivity may relate in some way to each of these types of heart disease.

A wealth of statistical evidence indicates that active people are less likely to have coronary heart disease than inactive people.

Much of the research relating inactivity to heart disease has come from occupational studies that show a high incidence of heart disease in people involved only in sedentary work. Even with the limitations inherent in these types of studies, the findings of more and more occupational studies present convincing evidence that the inactive individual has an increased risk of coronary heart disease.

Studies also indicate that people who are physically active in their leisure time have a reduced risk of coronary heart disease if the exercise they choose is done above the cardiovascular threshold of training and in the cardiovascular fitness target zones.

Recent evidence suggests that regular exercise can reduce risk of early death from heart disease.

A recent study of over 15,000 college alumni shows that those who do regular exercise have lower death rates from heart disease than those who are inactive.

Regular exercise is one effective means of rehabilitation for a person who has coronary heart disease or who has had a heart attack.

Not only does regular exercise seem to reduce the risk of developing coronary heart disease, there is also evidence that those who already have the condition may reduce the symptoms of the disease through regular exercise. For those who have had heart attacks, regular and progressive exercise can be an effective prescription when carried out under the supervision of a physician. Remember, however, that exercise is not the treatment of preference for all heart attack victims. In some cases, it may be contraindicated.

Recent decreases in the incidence of heart disease in the United States may be, in part, due to recent increases in activity levels of American adults.

In 1961, only 24 percent of Americans participated in regular physical activity. By 1980, more than twice as many American adults reported involvement in regular physical activity. During this same period of time, the incidence of heart disease decreased by 14 percent. Though heart disease is still present in epidemic proportions (one in three males will have a heart attack by age sixty), many experts feel that the increase in regular exercise by previously sedentary Americans is one reason for the modest decreases in heart disease in the last two decades.

Contrary to popular belief, exercise does not cause "athlete's heart" nor does it injure the hearts of children.

The term *athlete's heart* is a misnomer. Though some investigators have found increases in heart size as a result of training, this is not the pathological increase in size associated with heart disease. There is no evidence that heavy exercise injures a normal heart.

Many parents suggest that strenuous exercise is harmful to their children. To be sure, overstrenuous activity for long periods of time may have deleterious effects, but regular activity has no harmful effect on children's hearts.

There are many theories that attempt to explain the causes of coronary heart disease and the reasons regular exercise reduces the risk of this disease.

The six most plausible theories of heart disease are the Oxygen Pump Theory, the Lipid Deposit Theory, the Protective Protein Theory, the Fibrin Deposit Theory, the Coronary Collateral Circulation Theory, and the Loafer's Heart Theory. There is evidence that regular exercise relates in some way to each of these theories.

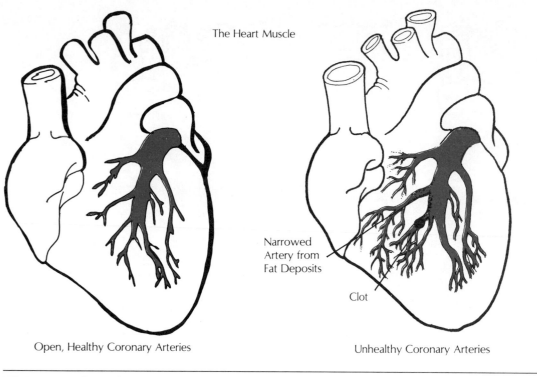

The Heart Muscle

Narrowed
Artery from
Fat Deposits

Clot

Open, Healthy Coronary Arteries

Unhealthy Coronary Arteries

FIGURE 3.1 Atherosclerosis

THE OXYGEN PUMP THEORY

There is evidence that regular exercise will increase the ability of the heart muscle to pump blood as well as oxygen.

The Oxygen Pump Theory suggests that a fit heart muscle is one able to handle any *extra* demands placed on it. Through regular exercise, the heart muscle gets stronger and therefore pumps more blood with each beat, resulting in a slower heart rate and a greater heart efficiency. Of importance is the fact that the heart is just like any other muscle—it must be exercised regularly if it is to stay fit. The fit heart pumps more blood, thus supplying more oxygen during physical exertion and times of emotional stress.

THE LIPID DEPOSIT THEORY

*There is evidence that exercise can reduce atherosclerosis from **lipid** deposits and thus help reduce the risk of heart disease.*

The heart has its own arteries that supply blood to the heart muscle. If these vessels become clogged, there is danger of a heart attack. The Lipid Deposit Theory of heart disease suggests that one of the causes of heart disease may be the narrowing of the arteries within the heart, resulting from fat or lipid deposits on the walls of these arteries (atherosclerosis). If the deposits on the inner walls of the arteries become excessive, there is a

diminished blood flow to the heart. Also, there is increased danger of a heart attack as a result of a clot lodging in the already narrowed coronary artery (coronary thrombosis). (Refer to figure 3.1.)

There are several kinds of fats in the bloodstream, including lipoproteins, phospholipids, triglycerides, and cholesterol. Whereas cholesterol is the most well-known fat, it may be no more a culprit than the other fats. Many blood fats are manufactured by the body itself, while others are ingested in high fat foods, particularly saturated fats (fats that are solid at room temperature). Whatever the source of the fat and the type of fat involved, the following two conclusions are justified by recent research.

1. Exercise can reduce blood fat levels, particularly for individuals who have above normal blood fat levels.
2. There is an increased risk of coronary heart disease with increased blood fat levels.

THE PROTECTIVE PROTEIN THEORY

There is evidence that exercise can increase levels of protective proteins in the blood and thus help reduce the risk of heart disease.

The Lipid Deposit Theory suggests that excess fats in the blood may result in atherosclerosis and may contribute to coronary heart disease. The Protective Protein Theory suggests that the levels of fat-carrying

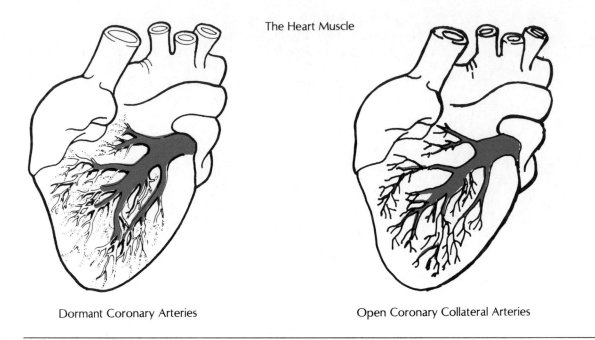

The Heart Muscle

Dormant Coronary Arteries

Open Coronary Collateral Arteries

FIGURE 3.2 Coronary Collateral Circulation

proteins (called **lipoproteins**) in the blood may be related to the incidence of coronary heart disease. Lipoproteins are of several sizes including large or very low density (VLDL), medium or low density (LDL), and small or high density (HDL). It appears that the medium-sized lipoproteins (LDL) are undesirable because they may be deposited on the wall of the artery just as other fats described in the Lipid Deposit Theory. It also appears that the small lipoproteins (HDL) are protective proteins. People who have high levels of small lipoproteins (HDL) in the blood have a lessened risk of coronary heart disease.

At this time, the best evidence suggests that high density lipoproteins (HDL), or protective blood proteins, pick up excess fats in the bloodstream and carry them to the liver where they are eliminated from the body. There is evidence that those who exercise regularly have higher levels of these proteins in the blood.

THE FIBRIN DEPOSIT THEORY

There is evidence that regular exercise can reduce atherosclerosis from fibrin deposits and thus help reduce the risk of heart disease.

Fibrin is a sticky, threadlike substance in the bloodstream that is important to the blood-clotting process. The Fibrin Deposit Theory of heart disease suggests that the narrowing of the wall of an artery (atherosclerosis) may result from fibrin deposits. A heart attack may result from the diminished flow of blood to the heart caused by the fibrin deposits or by a clot lodged in the *now* narrowed artery.

The fibrin and lipid deposit theories are compatible, because the deposits of both sticky fibrin and fat may be responsible for atherosclerosis. If this is correct, exercise may help prevent a heart attack. The following research findings form the basis for this statement:

1. Exercise causes the breakdown of fibrin in the blood, thus reducing its level in the blood.
2. Reduced blood fibrin may diminish the chances of development of fibrin atherosclerosis.
3. Reduced blood fibrin as a result of exercise may reduce the chance of a clot forming in the blood vessel.

THE CORONARY COLLATERAL CIRCULATION THEORY

*There is evidence that regular exercise can improve coronary **collateral circulation** and thus reduce the risk of heart disease.*

Within the heart, there are many tiny branches extending from the coronary arteries that supply blood to the heart muscle, as can be seen in figure 3.2. These interconnecting arteries can supply blood to any region of the heart as it is needed. If a person is relatively inactive, these interconnecting arteries are functionally closed. During regular exercise, these extra blood vessels are opened up to provide the heart muscle with the necessary blood and oxygen. For a person with atherosclerosis (evidence suggests most of us have some atherosclerosis beginning early in life) or a person who has suffered a heart attack, coronary collateral circulation may be very important. There is also evidence that the size of the coronary arteries increase as a result of exercise.

Improved coronary circulation may provide protection against a heart attack because a larger artery would require more atherosclerosis to occlude it. In addition, the development of collateral blood vessels supplying the heart may diminish the effects of an attack if one does occur. These "extra" (or collateral) blood vessels may take over the function of regular blood vessels during a heart attack.

THE LOAFER'S HEART THEORY

The heart of the inactive person is less able to resist stress and is more susceptible to "an emotional storm" that may precipitate a heart attack.

The heart is rendered inefficient by the following circumstances: high heart rate, high blood pressure, and excessive stimulation. Any of these conditions requires the heart to use more oxygen than is normally necessary and decreases its ability to adapt to stressful situations.

The "loafer's heart" is one that beats rapidly because it is dominated by the **sympathetic nervous system,** which speeds up the heart rate. Thus, the heart continuously beats rapidly, even in resting situations, and never has a true rest period. Further, high blood pressure makes the heart work harder and contributes to its inefficiency.

Research indicates the following concerning exercise and the loafer's heart.

1. Regular exercise leads to **parasympathetic** dominance rather than to sympathetic dominance; thus the heart rate is reduced and the heart works efficiently.
2. Regular exercise helps the heart rate return to normal faster after emotional stress.
3. Regular exercise strengthens the loafer's heart, making the heart better able to weather emotional storms.
4. Regular exercise may be one effective method of reducing high blood pressure.
5. Regular exercise decreases sympathetic dominance and its associated hormonal effects on the heart, thus lessening the chances of altered heart contractibility and the likelihood of the circulatory problems that accompany this state.

The theories of heart disease are compatible, and it is likely that most cases of coronary heart disease are related in some way to more than one theory.

It is likely that all the listed theories are correct and that exercise may help reduce the incidence of coronary heart disease in several ways. Because recent evidence indicates a decreased age for the onset of coronary heart disease, it seems especially important to consider any factor that might reduce heart attacks.

There is no single cause or prevention of coronary heart disease. However, exercise is one of several factors that relates significantly to the incidence of coronary heart disease. Also, benefits to the circulatory system, other than those already described, may result from regular exercise.

1. Regular exercise may be *one* effective method of reducing high blood pressure (hypertension).
2. Regular exercise is necessary for the efficient return of venous blood to the heart after it is pumped to the body parts. People in standing occupations, such as barbers and dentists, can improve venous return by regular exercise, especially by exercise of the leg muscles. Excessive pooling of blood in the legs resulting from inactivity may cause varicose veins.
3. There is some evidence that regular exercise may improve peripheral circulation (circulation to the arms, legs, and body parts other than the heart).
4. There is evidence that regular exercise may result in greater blood volume and in a greater number of red blood cells, thus making the delivery of oxygen to the body more efficient.

THE FACTS ABOUT EXERCISE, MUSCLE FITNESS, AND BACK PAIN

Active people, who possess good flexibility, strength, and muscular endurance, are less likely to have back problems than inactive and unfit people.

Because few people die from it, back pain does not receive the attention heaped on such medical problems as heart disease and cancer. But back pain is considered the number one medical complaint in the United States, resulting in millions of hours of lost work annually, not to mention the hours of discomfort for those who are afflicted.

Over twenty-five years ago, medical doctors began to associate back problems with the lack of physical fitness. At least 85 percent of the common complaints are a result of poor muscle fitness, including poor flexibility, strength, and muscular endurance according to researchers. Early tests done on patients complaining of back problems showed that they were exceptionally low in fitness. Results of similar fitness tests given to schoolchildren showed that nearly 60 percent of American children failed compared to less than 10 percent of children in four other countries. Current evidence indicates that as many as 50 percent of American children are still lacking in muscle fitness.

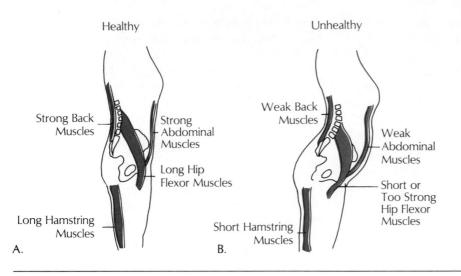

Healthy   Unhealthy

Strong Back Muscles

Strong Abdominal Muscles

Long Hip Flexor Muscles

Long Hamstring Muscles

A.

Weak Back Muscles

Weak Abdominal Muscles

Short or Too Strong Hip Flexor Muscles

Short Hamstring Muscles

B.

FIGURE 3.3 *(a)* Healthy and *(b)* Unhealthy Back

Inactivity statistics among adults in North America suggest that back problems will continue to be a problem until good muscle fitness becomes the rule rather than the exception. People who exercise in the target zones for building flexibility, strength, and muscular endurance can reduce the risk of musculoskeletal problems.

Regular exercise and good muscle fitness are not the only factors associated with risk of back pain.

Though lack of fitness is probably the leading reason for back pain in Western society, there are many other factors that increase the risk of back ailment including poor posture, improper lifting and work habits, heredity, and other disease states, such as scoliosis and arthritis. Some of these are discussed in greater detail in Concepts 17 and 18.

There are many reasons why exercise can be effective in reducing the risk of back pain.

Proper exercise helps to prevent lordosis (excessive low back curve), muscle fatigue, referred pain, and muscle injury, all major factors in back pain.

Lordosis usually results from weak abdominals and short hip flexor muscles.

As can be seen in figure 3.3, the lower part of the back normally has a slight inward curvature. If the lower back curve is too great, the muscles of the low back are more easily fatigued, more likely to suffer muscle spasms, and more prone to injury.

The best way to prevent lordosis is to have strong abdominal muscles and long, but not too strong, hip flexor muscles. The strong abdominal muscles pull the bottom of the pelvis upward and help keep the top of the pelvis tipped backward, eliminating excessive back curve.

If the hip flexor muscles are too strong, or not long enough, they have the opposite effect of strong ab-

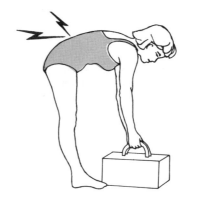

FIGURE 3.4 Muscle Spasms Result in Back Pain

dominal muscles; that is, they tip the top of the pelvis forward causing excessive low back curve (lordosis). This is why it is important to have long, but not too strong, hip flexor muscles. As a general rule, flexibility exercises to lengthen the hip flexor muscles, as well as strength and endurance exercises for the abdominal muscles, are recommended. For obvious reasons, exercises to increase the strength of the hip flexor muscles are not recommended for those with back pain.

People who sit most of the day are especially likely to have short, weak back muscles, especially if they do no special exercises to lengthen and strengthen them. Through disuse, the muscles become short and weak so that even the slightest strain, as from improper lifting or sudden vigorous exercise, could result in muscle injury.

Hours of standing, on the other hand, as is done by a dentist or a store clerk, can result in muscle fatigue. Muscle fatigue and muscle injury can each result in muscle spasms evidenced in back pain. Regular, well-planned exercise to strengthen and lengthen the back muscles is important in the prevention of such pain. (See figure 3.4.)

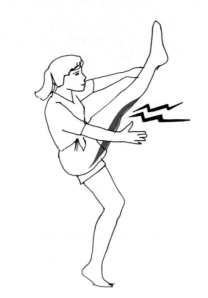

FIGURE 3.5 Referred Pain

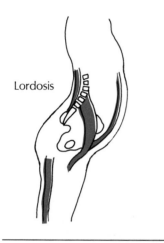

Lordosis

FIGURE 3.6 Back Pain Caused by Protruding Abdomen

***Referred pain** from short leg muscles can result in back pain.*

Inactive people, especially those who sit a lot, are likely to have short muscles in the back of the upper leg (hamstring muscles). When short hamstring muscles are overstretched, spasms or injury may occur (see figure 3.5). Often the pain from hamstring muscle soreness can be referred to the low back and result in low back pain. Referred pain, or pain felt in an area other than where the pain originates, can be reduced by doing regular exercise to lengthen the short muscles.

Protruding abdomen can increase the risk of back pain.

If the abdomen or "gut" sticks out too far over the belt line, problems with the back muscles can result. The extra weight of the protruding gut can cause lordosis by pulling the top of the pelvis forward. This can result

in extra strain on the low back muscles and can precipitate muscle fatigue, soreness, or injury. Strengthening of the abdominal muscles and a loss of body fat are advised for those with this problem (fig. 3.6).

Back pain caused by muscle spasms can usually be reduced or relieved with static stretching of back and leg muscles.

A stretch held for twenty to sixty seconds can break what is known as the "spasm cycle," helping to relieve the muscle pain. (See Concept 18, exercises 9–14.)

THE FACTS ABOUT EXERCISE, HEALTH-RELATED FITNESS, AND OTHER HYPOKINETIC CONDITIONS

Many musculoskeletal problems, including poor posture, neck, leg, and foot pain are associated with inactivity and poor health-related physical fitness.

Regular exercise, particularly exercise designed to increase strength, muscular endurance, and flexibility, can help alleviate neck, leg, and foot pain and can help improve posture. Slow stretching and tension reduction exercises, such as those described in Concept 20, can help relieve the symptoms of muscle tension.

Obesity, as well as lesser degrees of fatness, is not a disease state in itself, but is a hypokinetic condition associated with a multitude of far-reaching complications.

Obesity is associated with serious organic impairments, shortened life, psychological maladjustments, poor relationships with peers (especially among children), awkward physical movement, and lack of achievement in athletic activities. Obesity can be both a cause and an effect of physical unfitness. Those who are overfat have a higher risk of respiratory infections; are prone to developing high blood pressure, atherosclerosis, and disorders of the circulatory, respiratory, and kidney systems; and have greater than normal risk of some forms of cancer. The symptoms of adult-onset diabetes are associated with excessive fatness. (Fortunately, fat loss to normal levels is usually followed by remission of diabetic symptoms.) Because exercise, together with sound nutritional management, is an effective means of lowering body fat, it can be helpful in reducing the risks of those conditions associated with fatness and obesity.

Diabetes is often considered a hypokinetic condition because of the important role exercise plays in managing the disease.

As already noted, exercise can be effective in managing adult-onset diabetes by helping to keep body fatness at reasonable levels. Together with sound nutritional habits and proper medication, exercise can also be useful in the management of other types of diabetes.

Bone degeneration due to atrophy (osteoporosis) can be considered a hypokinetic condition.

Studies indicate that excessive bed rest can result in deterioration of the bones. When the long bones do not bear weight, they lose calcium and become porous and fragile. Even excessive sitting can result in bone deterioration, regardless of age. Bones are strengthened, not only by bearing weight, but by the pull of active muscles. Regular exercise is as necessary for healthy bone development as it is for healthy muscle development. The osteoporosis commonly seen in older adults (especially in women) is caused by a loss of hormone, as well as by lack of activity.

Common stress-related disorders can be considered hypokinetic conditions.

Some stress-related conditions prevalent in modern society are discussed in Concept 20. However, a few that are associated with inactive lifestyles are noted here.

Insomnia is a condition that afflicts many people in our culture and one that is often stress related. Results from a survey of American adults indicates that 52 percent feel regular exercise helps them to sleep better.

Depression is another stress-related condition experienced by many adults. In fact, one study showed that 33 percent of inactive adults often felt depressed. For some, depression is a serious psychosis and exercise alone will not cure it; however, recent research does indicate that exercise, combined with other forms of therapy, can be effective in its treatment. For those with minor depression, exercise may also be helpful. Thirty-four percent of those considered very active in one study feel that regular exercise helps them to better cope with life's pressures.

Even more common than depression and insomnia is the condition called *Type A behavior.* "Type A personalities" are stress-prone individuals with a greater than normal incidence of diseases. A Type A person is tense, overly competitive, and worried about meeting time schedules. Regular exercise can be of special benefit to the Type A person, though noncompetitive exercise would probably be best.

In many cases, gastric ulcers may be a hypokinetic condition.

In their classic work, *Hypokinetic Disease,* Kraus and Raab (1961) theorized that gastric ulcers could be considered a hypokinetic condition because inactive individuals have a higher mortality rate from the condition than active people. Their conclusion must be considered tentative at best; however, the lower incidence of ulcer disease among active people, plus the fact that exercise can be effective in helping to manage stress and tension levels often associated with ulcer disease, suggest that regular exercise may be useful for some people in the prevention or management of gastric ulcer symptoms.

Regular exercise can have positive effects on some nonhypokinetic conditions.

Infectious diseases and cancer are not generally considered hypokinetic conditions. However, regular exercise that fosters good health may help you resist diseases resulting from lowered general resistance. On the other hand, when the body is fighting an infection, too much exercise can result in a lowered state of resistance.

There is now some evidence to indicate that inactivity is associated with a higher risk of cancer. Physically active men show lower colon cancer rates and athletic women show lower rates of breast and reproductive system cancer. Further there is evidence that exercise can help those with cancer lead more fulfilling and productive lives.

Hypokinetic diseases and conditions have many different causes.

Regular exercise is only one factor associated with reduced risk of hypokinetic diseases and conditions. Whereas exercise is the focus of this concept, nutrition (see Concept 14), smoking, lifestyles, heredity, stress (see Concept 20), age (see Concept 22), and environment cannot be overlooked as important **risk factors.** Many of these important hypokinetic disease risk factors are discussed in Concept 21.

CHART 3.1 Incidence of Hypokinetic Diseases and Conditions

Listed here are various hypokinetic diseases and conditions. In the column beside each condition or disease, place a check (✔) if you possess it, if one of your close relatives possesses it, or if one of your close friends possesses it. Close relatives are the four or five people you consider to be closest to you, whether parents, brothers, sisters, grandparents, spouse, or children. Close friends are the four or five nonrelatives you care about most. You need not live close to the individual to classify him or her as a close friend or relative.

The Hypokinetic Disease or Condition	Self	Close Relative	Close Friend
1. Heart disease	☐	☐	☐
2. High blood pressure	☐	☐	☐
3. Back pain or problems	☐	☐	☐
4. Overfat or obese	☐	☐	☐
5. Ulcer	☐	☐	☐
6. Diabetes	☐	☐	☐
7. Insomnia	☐	☐	☐
8. Depression	☐	☐	☐
9. Type A personality	☐	☐	☐
Column Totals	_____	_____	_____

REFERENCES

Anderson, K. M., et al. "Cholesterol and Mortality: Thirty Years of Follow-up from the Framingham Study." *Journal of the American Medical Association* 257(1987):2,176.

Blair, S. N., et al. "Changes in Coronary Heart Disease Risk Factors Associated with Increased Treadmill Time in 753 Men." *American Journal of Epidemiology* 118(1983):352.

Blair, S. N., et al. "Physical Fitness and Incidence of Hypertension in Healthy Normotensive Men and Women." *Journal of the American Medical Association* 252(1984):487.

Blair, S. N. and R. S. Paffenburger. "Physical Activity and Risk of Cancer." (Ab.) *Medicine and Science in Sports and Exercise* 19(1987):418.

Brewer, V., et al. "Role of Exercise in Prevention of Involutional Bone Loss." *Medicine and Science in Sports and Exercise* 15(1983):445.

Brownell, K. D., et al. "Changes in Plasma Lipid and Lipoprotein Levels in Men and Women after a Moderate Exercise Program." *Circulation* 65(1982):477.

Connor, J. F., et al. "Effects of Exercise on Coronary Collateralization: Angiographic Analysis of Six Patients in a Supervised Exercise Program." *Medicine and Science in Exercise and Sports* 8(1976):145.

Corbin, C. B., ed. *A Textbook of Motor Development.* Dubuque, IA: Wm. C. Brown Publishers, 1980.

Corbin, C. B. "Flexibility." In *Clinics in Sportsmedicine: Profiling,* edited by J. Nicholas and E. Hershman. Philadelphia: W. B. Saunders Co., 1984.

Duda, M. "The Role of Exercise in Managing Diabetes." *Physician and Sportsmedicine* 13(1985):164.

Dufaux, B., et al. "Plasma Lipoproteins and Physical Activity: A Review." *International Journal of Sports Medicine* 3(1982):123.

Duncan, J. J. "The Effects of Aerobic Exercise on Plasma Catacholamines and Blood Pressure in Patients with Mild Essential Hypertension." *Journal of the American Medical Association* 254(1985):2609.

Durrah, M. I., and R. L. Engen. "Beneficial Effects of Exercise on 1–Isoproterenol-Induced Myocardial Infarction in Male Rats." *Medicine and Science in Sports and Exercise* 14(1982):76.

Durstine, J. L., et al. "Increases in HDL-Cholesterol and the HDL/LDL Cholesterol Ratio During Prolonged Endurance Exercise." *Metabolism* 32(1983):993.

Felig, P., et al. "Hypoglycemia during Prolonged Exercise in Normal Men." *New England Journal of Medicine* 306(1982):895.

Frey, M. A., et al. "Exercise Training, Sex Hormones, and Lipoprotein Relationships in Men." *Journal of Applied Physiology* 55(1983):757.

*Friedman, M., and K. H. Rosenman. *Type A Behavior and Your Heart.* New York: A. A. Knopf, 1974.

Gibbons, L. W., et al. "Association Between Coronary Heart Disease Risk Factors and Physical Fitness in Healthy Adult Women." *Circulation* 67(1983):977.

Griest, J. H., et al. "Running Through Your Mind." In *Psychology of Running,* edited by M. H. Sacks and M. L. Sachs. Champaign, IL: Human Kinetics, 1981.

Hagan, R. D., and L. R. Gettman. "Maximal Aerobic Power, Body Fatness, and Serum Lipoproteins in Male Distance Runners." *Journal of Cardiac Rehabilitation* 3(1983):331.

Hall, J. A. "Effects of Diet and Exercise on Peripheral Vascular Disease." *Physician and Sportsmedicine* 10(1982):90.

Hartung, G. H., and W. G. Squires. "Exercise and HDL Cholesterol in Middle-Aged Men." *Physician and Sportsmedicine* 8(1980):74.

Hartung, G. H., et al. "Relation of Diet to High Density-Lipoprotein Cholesterol in Middle-Aged Marathon Runners, Joggers, and Inactive Men." *New England Journal of Medicine* 302(1980):357.

Haskell, W. L. "The Influence of Exercise on the Concentration of Triglycerides and Cholesterol in Human Plasma." *Exercise and Sports Science Reviews* 12(1984):205.

Heaton, W. H., et al. "Beneficial Effect of Physical Training on Blood Flow to the Myocardium Perfused by Chronic Collaterals in the Exercising Dog." *Circulation* 57(1978):575.

Jennings, G., et al. "The Effects of Changes in Physical Activity on Major Cardiovascular Risk Factors, Hemodynamics, Sympathetic Function, and Glucose Utilization in Man: A Controlled Study of Four Levels of Physical Activity." *Circulation* 73(1986):30–40.

Keim, H. A., and W. H. Kirkaldy-Willis. "Low Back Pain." *Clinical Symposia* 32(1980):6.

Knight, D. R., and H. L. Stone. "Alteration of Ischemic Cardiac Function in the Normal Heart by Daily Exercise." *Journal of Applied Physiology* 55(1983):52.

Kornitzer, M. "Belgian Heart Disease Prevention Project: Incidence and Mortality Results." *Lancet* 8333(1983):1066.

*Kraus, H., and W. Raab. *Hypokinetic Disease.* Springfield, IL: C. C. Thomas, 1961.

Lane, N. E., et al. "Long-Distance Running, Bone Density, and Osteoporosis." *Journal of the American Medical Association* 255(1986):1147.

LaRosa, J. C. "Effects of Long Term Moderate Physical Exercise on Plasma Lipoproteins: A National Exercise and Heart Disease Program." *Archives of Internal Medicine* 142(1982):2269.

Levy, R. "Declining Mortality in Cardiovascular Disease." *Atherosclerosis* 5(1981):312.

McCunney, R. J. "Fitness, Heart Disease, and High-Density Lipoproteins: A Look at Relationships," *Physician and Sportsmedicine* 15(1987):67.

Maciejko, J., et al. "Apolipoprotein A-I as a Marker of Angiographically Assessed Coronary-Artery Disease." *New England Journal of Medicine* 309(1983):385.

Mann, G. V. "The Influence of Obesity on Health." *New England Journal of Medicine* 291(1974):178.

Mayer, J. *Overweight Causes, Costs and Control.* Englewood Cliffs, NJ: Prentice-Hall, 1968.

Monahan, T. "Exercise and Depression: Swapping Sweat for Serenity." *Physician and Sportsmedicine* 14(1986):192.

Montoye, H. J., et al. "Bone Mineralization in Tennis Players." *Scandinavian Journal of Sport Science* 2(1980):26.

Multiple Risk Factor Intervention Trial Research Group. "Multiple Risk Factor Intervention Trial." *Journal of the American Medical Association* 248(1982):1465.

*Nash, H. J. "Can Exercise Make Us Immune to Disease?" *Physician and Sportsmedicine* 14(1986):250.

National Institutes of Health. "Health Implications of Obesity." *Contemporary Nutrition* 10(1985):9.

*Paffenbarger, R. S., and R. T. Hyde. "Exercise as Protection Against Heart Attack." *New England Journal of Medicine* 302(1980):1026.

Paffenbarger, R. S., et al. "Physical Activity, All-Cause Mortality, and Longevity of College Alumni." *New England Journal of Medicine* 314(1986):605.

*Pollock, M. L., et al. *Exercise in Health and Disease.* Philadelphia: W. B. Saunders Co., 1984.

Rose, G., et al. "The United Kingdom Heart Disease Prevention Project: Incidence and Mortality Results." *Lancet* 8333(1983):1062.

Ryan, A. "Heart Size and Sports." *Physician and Sportsmedicine* 8(1980):30.

Seals, D. R., et al. "Effects of Endurance Training on Glucose Tolerance and Plasma Lipid Levels in Older Men and Women." *Journal of the American Medical Association* 252(1984):645.

*Sherin, K. "Aerobic Exercise: Can You Answer Questions Patients Ask?" *Postgraduate Medicine* 73(1983):157.

Simons, D. G., and J. G. Travell. "Myofascial Origins of Low Back Pain." *Postgraduate Medicine* 73(1983):157.

Smith, E. L. "Exercise for Prevention of Osteoporosis: A Review." *Physician and Sportsmedicine* 10(1982):72.

Smith, M. P., et al. "Exercise Intensity, Dietary Intake and High-Density Lipoprotein Cholesterol in Young Female Competitive Swimmers." *American Journal of Clinical Nutrition* 36(1983):251.

Stillman, R. J. "Physical Activity and Bone Mineral Content in Women Aged 30 to 85 Years." *Medicine and Science in Sports and Exercise* 18(1986):576.

Storer, T. W., and R. O. Ruhling. "Essential Hypertension and Exercise." *Physician and Sportsmedicine* 9(1981):58.

Thompson, P. D., et al. "Incidence of Death during Jogging in Rhode Island from 1975 through 1980." *Journal of the American Medical Association* 247 (1982):2535.

Travell, J. G., and D. G. Simons. *Myofascial Pain and Dysfunction.* Baltimore: Williams and Williams, 1983.

West, R. R. "Changes in Life-Style After Early or Late Mobilization Following Acute Myocardial Infarction: A Ten-Year Follow-Up of a Randomized Controlled Trial." *Journal of Cardiopulmonary Rehabilitation* 6(1986):113.

Williams, P. T. "Lipoprotein Subfractions of Runners and Sedentary Men." *Metabolism* 35(1986):45.

Williams, R. S., et al. "Physical Conditioning Augments the Fibrinolytic Response to Venous Occlusion in Healthy Adults." *New England Journal of Medicine* 302(1980):987.

Winningham, M. L., and M. G. MacVicar. "Response of Cancer Patients on Chemotherapy to a Supervised Exercise Program." (abs.) *Medicine and Science in Sports and Exercise* 17(1985):292.

Winningham, M. L., et al. "Exercise for Cancer Patients: Guidelines and Precautions." *Physician and Sportsmedicine* 14(1986):125.

Zung, V. T., et al. "The Effects of Exercise on Blood Lipids and Lipoproteins: A Metaanalysis of Studies." *Medicine and Science in Sports and Exercise* 15(1983):393.

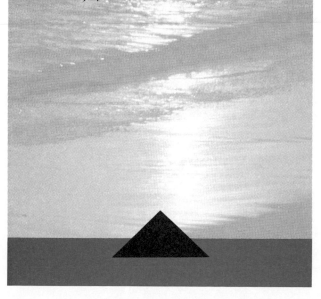

4

PREPARING
FOR EXERCISE

CONCEPT 4

Proper preparation can help make exercise
enjoyable, effective, and safe.

INTRODUCTION

More than at any other time in recent history, adults are engaging in some form of regular exercise during their free time. Unfortunately, all too often those who start an exercise program with good intentions "drop out" after a few days, weeks, or months. As noted in Concept 1, part of the problem is that people lack information concerning the correct way to exercise.

For those just beginning an exercise program, adequate preparation may be the key to persistence. It is hoped that a person armed with good information about preparing for exercise will become involved and stay involved with that exercise for a lifetime. To be effective, exercise must be something that is a part of a person's normal lifestyle. Some facts that will help you to prepare for exercise and make it part of your normal routine are presented in this concept.

TERMS

PAR-Q—The Physical Activity Readiness Questionnaire is designed to help you determine if you are medically suited to begin an exercise program.

PAR-X—The Physical Activity Readiness Examination is used by physicians to determine a person's readiness for a program of regular physical activity.

Achilles Tendon—The long tendon that attaches the calf muscles (the back of the lower leg) to the heel bone (on the back of the foot).

Warm-Up Exercise—Light to moderate activity, including stretching, done prior to serious exercise. Its purpose is to reduce the risk of injury and soreness and possibly to improve performance in a physical activity.

Cool-Down Exercise—Light to moderate tapering-off activity after vigorous exercise; often consisting of the same exercises used in the warm-up.

THE FACTS

Before beginning a regular exercise program, it is important to establish your medical readiness to participate.

There is no way to be absolutely sure that you are medically sound to begin an exercise program. Even a thorough exam by a physician cannot guarantee that a person does not have some limitations that may cause a problem during exercise. However, an exam is the surest way to make certain that you are ready to participate.

The American College of Sports Medicine, in its guidelines for evaluating health status for exercise participation, suggests that under certain circumstances people should have a preexercise exam, which includes an exercise test coupled with an EKG during exercise. Specifically, the college recommends a preexercise test for those forty-five and over; for those thirty-five years and over who have higher than normal risk of heart disease (see Lab 21 to check your risk); for those with symptoms of heart disease; and for those with known heart disease. Healthy people under forty-five need not have a preexercise exam but may wish to seek medical consultation when resuming exercise following injury or illness, when returning to an exercise program after an extended layoff, or when making significant modifications in exercise programs.

Recently the British Columbia (Canada) Ministry of Health conducted extensive research to devise a procedure that would help people know when it was advisable to seek medical consultation prior to beginning or altering an exercise program. The goal was to prevent unnecessary medical examinations, while at the same time to give a reasonable assurance that regular exercise was appropriate for an individual. The research resulted in the development of two questionnaires, both now used nationally in Canada. The first, the **PAR-Q,** consists of seven simple questions you can ask yourself to determine if medical consultation is necessary prior to exercise involvement. The second, the **PAR-X,** is a special form developed for use by physicians. It aids the physician in knowing what to include in a preexercise exam and in giving advice to prospective exercisers after an exam.

To help you decide whether to have a complete medical exam before you begin or modify your exercise program, or whether to adopt the American College of Sports Medicine guidelines, complete the PAR-Q provided in the Lab Resource Materials on page 34. Those who choose to seek medical consultation, including an examination, may wish to make the PAR-X form available to the examining physician (see Appendix A).

Young adults, such as college students, or older adults who plan to do intensive training (particularly for sports) may want to answer some additional questions concerning whether a medical exam is necessary before beginning (see chart 4.2).

It is important to dress properly for exercise.

The clothing you wear for exercise should be specifically for that exercise. It should be comfortable and not too tight or binding at the joints. Though appearance is important to everyone, comfort in exercise is more important than looks. Clothing should not restrict movement in any way. Preferably, the clothing that comes in direct contact with the body should be porous to allow for sweat evaporation. Some women, especially those who need extra support, should consider using an exercise bra, and men will need an athletic supporter. A warm-up suit over other exercise apparel is recommended because they can be removed during exercise if desired. Many exercise suits are nonporous so, by themselves, are not desirable for exercise.

Proper exercise footwear is important.

There are many types of exercise footwear. Jogging/ running shoes and multipurpose shoes are the most common, although some sports participants, such as basketball players, prefer a high top shoe. Jogging/ running shoes are specialty shoes designed specifically for jogging and running, although they are suitable for walking. These shoes should have a high back to support the **Achilles tendon;** a wide, cushioned, and elevated heel; good arch support; and adequate room for the toes. The exterior of the heel should be rounded and the exterior sole should be flexible with a rippled or dimpled tread.

A multipurpose shoe is not recommended for jogging and running, but is well suited for most court sports. It should have a cushioned heel, a good arch support, and adequate toe room. Unlike the running shoe, the multipurpose shoe should have a smooth or court sole tread and a narrower, nonelevated heel.

Regardless of the type of shoe worn, exercise shoes should generally be one-half size larger than your regular shoes. If you wear two pairs of socks while exercising, you should wear two pairs when trying on the shoes. It is important to try on the shoes and move around in them before making a purchase. Make sure they feel good to you. Quality should not be sacrificed for appearance or to save a few dollars. Good quality shoes can help prevent foot and leg problems that make exercise ineffective and unenjoyable.

Probably the biggest mistake is failure to replace shoes when they are worn out. The condition of the sole of the shoe is far less important than the breakdown of the heel (rundown to the inside or outside), or disproportionate wear that results in unusual movement patterns. It is better to replace shoes too soon than to risk injury from worn-out shoes.

It takes time for exercise to benefit health-related physical fitness.

Sometimes people just beginning an exercise program expect immediate results. They expect to see large losses in body fat in short periods of time, or great increases in muscle strength in just a few days. Evidence tells us, however, that improvements in health-related physical fitness and the associated health benefits take several weeks to become apparent. Though some people report psychological benefits, such as "feeling better" and a "sense of personal accomplishment" almost immediately after beginning regular exercise, the physiological changes will take considerably longer to be realized. Proper preparation for exercise includes learning not to expect too much too soon, nor to do too much too soon. Attempts to "overdo it" and to try to "get fit fast" will probably be counterproductive, resulting in soreness and even injury. The key is to start slowly, stay with it, and enjoy the exercise. Benefits will come to those who persist.

*A **warm-up** prior to exercise is important.*

There are two good reasons for warming up prior to exercise. The first is to stretch the skeletal muscles to help prevent muscle soreness and injury. The second is to prepare the heart muscle for exercise.

The skeletal muscle warm-up should include static stretching of the major muscle groups involved in the exercise that is to follow (see Concepts 11 and 12). It should be emphasized that even though warming up prior to an activity may help reduce the chance of muscle injury, it is not a substitute for a regular program of exercise designed to improve flexibility.

A warm-up designed to prepare the heart muscle for moderate to vigorous exercise should include approximately two minutes of walking, jogging, or mild exercise. Research shows that for some people, starting vigorous exercise abruptly is not wise. Apparently in some exercises, the increased blood flow to the heart and other muscles does not immediately increase when the exercise begins, at least not for all people. Adults who do this type of warm-up do not experience electrocardiogram abnormalities that are apparent in some people who do not warm up.

A warm-up that is suitable for walking, jogging, running, cycling, and even basketball is included here for your information and use. This warm-up can be used for other activities if stretching exercises for the major muscle groups involved in various activities are added. (Some good stretching exercises are described in Concept 12.) The cardiovascular warm-up is suitable for most activities, but other mild exercise such as a slow, two-minute swim for swimmers, or a slow, two-minute ride on a bicycle for cyclists, can be substituted.

Warm-up stretching can be done before or after the cardiovascular warm-up.

Some experts believe that the cardiovascular warm-up should precede the stretching warm-up because warm muscles stretch longer than those not previously exercised. However, it is acceptable to begin your warm-up with stretching as long as static stretches are used.

There is a minimal and an optimal amount of exercise for producing improvements in health-related physical fitness.

Each component of health-related physical fitness has a "threshold of training" (minimal amount of exercise) necessary for improvement. Each component also has a "target zone;" that is, an optimal frequency, intensity, and time (duration) of exercise necessary to produce fitness gains. A properly prepared program includes exercise *above* the threshold level and *in* the target zone for *each part of health-related fitness.* The general concepts of threshold of training and exercise target zones are covered in greater depth in Concept 5. Specific threshold and target zone recommendations for each of the five components of health-related fitness are included in Concepts 6–13.

*A **cool down** after exercise is important.*

Proper exercise planning is very important. One part of this planning is the organization of each exercise session. Each session should include a warm-up, a workout, and a cool down. The warm-up has already been discussed. The workout, or actual exercise, is discussed in greater detail in later concepts. The cool down is done immediately after the workout.

Like the warm-up, there are two principal components of a cool down: static muscle stretching and an activity for the cardiovascular system. Some experts believe that static muscle stretching *after* the workout is more important than stretching before because it can help reduce delayed localized soreness or muscle pain felt the day after exercise, as well as prevent shortening of the muscles in general. There is still some controversy about the best time to stretch and about the benefits of warming up and cooling down. However, given current evidence, both a warm-up and cool down seem wise.

A SAMPLE WARM-UP AND COOL DOWN FOR AN AEROBIC WORKOUT

The exercises shown here can be used before an aerobic workout as a warm-up, or after workout as a cool down. This sample program would be good before jogging, walking, or cycling. It includes slow cardiovascular exercise, as well as stretching for the lower and upper legs, the hip and back, and the trunk. If the activity you plan to do requires considerable use of different areas of the body, you should add stretching and circulatory exercises for those areas of the body (see Concept 12). Perform the exercises slowly. Do not bounce or jerk against the muscle. Hold each stretch for at least ten seconds. Perform each exercise at least once and up to three times. You may wish to have someone passively assist you in doing the exercise but, if so, you should read Concept 11 first.

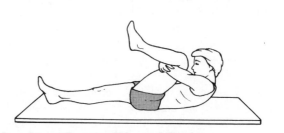

Leg Hug (For the Hip and Back)

Lie on your back. Bend one leg and grasp your thigh under the knee. Hug it to your chest. Keep the other leg straight and on the floor. Curl your head, then your shoulders, forward and upward. Hold. Repeat with the opposite leg.

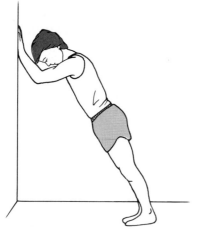

Calf Stretcher (For Back of Lower Leg)

Face a wall with your feet two to three feet away. Lean forward to allow both hands to touch the wall. Turn the toes inward slightly, keeping your heels on the ground, knees straight, and buttocks tucked in. Lean forward by bending your arms and allowing your head to move nearer the wall. Hold.

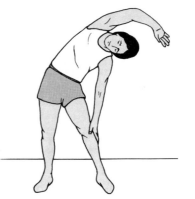

Side Stretch

With the feet apart approximately shoulder width, lean to one side. Reach down with the arm on that side and reach up over your head with the opposite arm. Let your body weight stretch the muscles as you lean downward. Do not twist. Hold. Repeat to the other side.

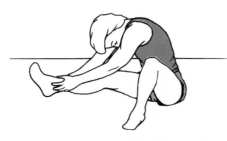

Back Saver Toe Touch (For Back of Upper Leg)

Sit on the floor. Spread your feet two to three feet apart. Bend at the hip and reach forward with both hands. Grasp one foot, ankle, or calf, depending upon how far you can reach. Pull forward with your arms trying to touch your head to your knee. Keep your knee relatively straight. Hold. Repeat with the opposite leg.

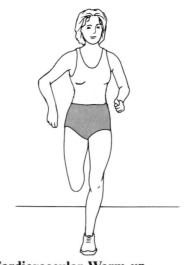

The Cardiovascular Warm-up

Before you perform a vigorous workout, walk or jog slowly for two minutes. After exercise, do the same.

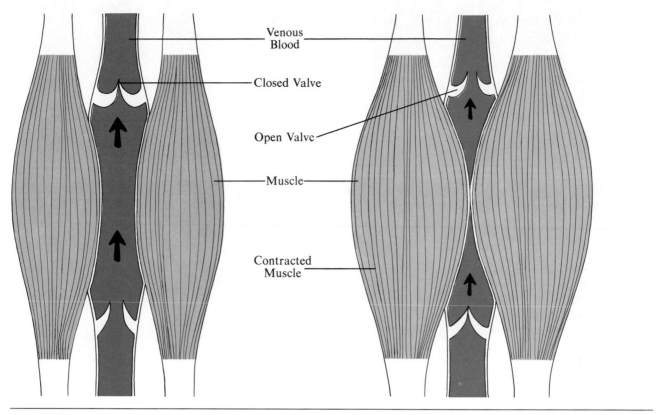

FIGURE 4.1 The Pumping Action of the Muscles

A cardiovascular cool down is also important. During exercise, the heart pumps a large amount of blood to the working muscles to supply the oxygen necessary to keep moving. The muscles squeeze the veins (fig. 4.1), which forces the blood back to the heart. Valves in the veins prevent the blood from flowing backward. As long as exercise continues, the blood is moved by the muscles back to the heart, where it is once again pumped to the body. If exercise is stopped abruptly, the blood is left in the area of the working muscles and has no way to get back to the heart. In the case of the runner, the blood pools in the legs. Because the heart has less blood to pump, blood pressure may drop. This can result in dizziness, and can even cause a person to pass out. The best way to prevent this problem is to taper off or slow down gradually after exercise. A cardiovascular cool down should include approximately two minutes of walking, slow jogging, or any nonvigorous activity that uses the muscles involved in the workout.

The same program used for the warm-up (see page 32) may be used to cool down after exercise. For variety, you can choose some of the stretching exercises included in Concept 12.

It may be necessary to alter exercise programs or adjust exercise schedules to accommodate the weather and environmental conditions.

Good preparation for exercise includes making adjustments in the content and the time of the exercise workout to account for cold, heat, humidity, and other environmental factors that might make exercise less enjoyable, less effective, or unsafe. For more information on appropriate dress and guidelines for working out in different climatic conditions, refer to Concept 19.

CHART 4.1 Physical Activity Readiness Questionnaire (PAR-Q)* A Self-Administered Questionnaire for Adults

PHYSICAL ACTIVITY READINESS QUESTIONNAIRE (PAR-Q)*
A Self-administered Questionnaire for Adults

PAR Q & YOU

PAR-Q is designed to help you help yourself. Many health benefits are associated with regular exercise, and the completion of PAR-Q is a sensible first step to take if you are planning to increase the amount of physical activity in your life.

For most people physical activity should not pose any problem or hazard. PAR-Q has been designed to identify the small number of adults for whom physical activity might be inappropriate or those who should have medical advice concerning the type of activity most suitable for them.

Common sense is your best guide in answering these few questions. Please read them carefully and check the ☑ YES or NO opposite the question if it applies to you.

YES NO

☐ ☐ 1. Has your doctor ever said you have heart trouble?

☐ ☐ 2. Do you frequently have pains in your heart and chest?

☐ ☐ 3. Do you often feel faint or have spells of severe dizziness?

☐ ☐ 4. Has a doctor ever said your blood pressure was too high?

☐ ☐ 5. Has your doctor ever told you that you have a bone or joint problem such as arthritis that has been aggravated by exercise, or might be made worse with exercise?

☐ ☐ 6. Is there a good physical reason not mentioned here why you should not follow an activity program even if you wanted to?

☐ ☐ 7. Are you over age 65 and not accustomed to vigorous exercise?

If You Answered

YES to one or more questions

If you have not recently done so, consult with your personal physician by telephone or in person BEFORE increasing your physical activity and/or taking a fitness test. Tell him what questions you answered YES on PAR-Q, or show him your copy.

programs

After medical evaluation, seek advice from your physician as to your suitability for:
- unrestricted physical activity, probably on a gradually increasing basis.
- restricted or supervised activity to meet your specific needs, at least on an initial basis. Check in your community for special programs or services.

NO to all questions

If you answered PAR-Q accurately, you have reasonable assurance of your present suitability for:
- A GRADUATED EXERCISE PROGRAM - A gradual increase in proper exercise promotes good fitness development while minimizing or eliminating discomfort.
- AN EXERCISE TEST - Simple tests of fitness (such as the Canadian Home Fitness Test) or more complex types may be undertaken if you so desire.

postpone

If you have a temporary minor illness, such as a common cold.

* Developed by the British Columbia Ministry of Health. Conceptualized and critiqued by the Multidisciplinary Advisory Board on Exercise (MABE).

Reference: PAR-Q Validation Report, British Columbia Ministry of Health, May, 1978.

* Produced by the British Columbia Ministry of Health and the Department of National Health & Welfare.

CHART 4.2 Physical Readiness for Sports or Vigorous Training

Answer the PAR-Q before using this chart. If you had one or more "yes" answers follow the directions for the PAR-Q concerning consultation with a physician. If you had all "no" answers on the PAR-Q, answer the additional questions below before beginning intensive training particularly for sports.

YES	NO	
☐	☐	1. Do you plan to participate on an organized team that will play intense competitive sports (i.e., varsity team, professional team)?
☐	☐	2. If you plan to participate in a collision sport (even on a less organized basis), such as football, boxing, rugby, or ice hockey, have you been knocked unconscious more than one time?
☐	☐	3. Do you currently have pain from a previous muscle injury?
☐	☐	4. Do you currently have symptoms from a previous back injury or do you experience back pain as a result of involvement in physical activity?
☐	☐	5. Do you have any other symptoms during physical activity that give you reason to be concerned about your health?

If your answer to any of these questions is "yes," then you should consult with your personal physician by telephone or in person to determine if you have a potential problem with vigorous involvement in physical activity.

REFERENCES

*American College of Sports Medicine. *Guidelines for Graded Exercise Testing and Exercise Prescription.* 3d ed. Philadelphia: Lea and Febiger, 1986.

*Barnard, R. J. "The Heart Needs a Warm-Up Time." *Physician and Sportsmedicine* 4(1976):40.

*Chisholm, D. M., et al. "Physical Activity Readiness." *British Columbia Medical Journal* 17(1975):375.

Chisholm, D. M., et al. *Par-Q Validation Report.* Victoria, British Columbia: British Columbia Ministry of Health, 1978.

Corbin, C. B. "Flexibility." *Clinics in Sports Medicine: Profiting,* edited by J. Nicholas and E. Hershman. Philadelphia: W. B. Saunders Co., 1984.

Howley, E. T., and B. D. Franks. *Health/Fitness Instructors Handbook.* Champaign, IL.: Human Kinetics, 1986.

Mead, W. F., and R. Hartwig. "Fitness Evaluation and Exercise Prescription." *Journal of Family Practice* 13(1981):1039.

*Shellock, F. G. "Physiological Benefits of Warm-Up." *Physician and Sportsmedicine* 11(1983):134.

Stone, W. J. *Adult Fitness Programs* (Glenview, Ill.: Scott, Foresman and Company, 1987).

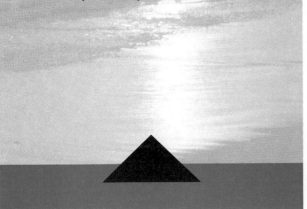

5

HOW MUCH EXERCISE IS ENOUGH?

CONCEPT 5

There is a minimal
and an optimal amount of exercise
necessary for developing
each of the health-related
aspects of physical fitness.

INTRODUCTION

Just as there is a correct dosage of medicine for treating an illness, there is a correct dosage of exercise for developing physical fitness. The minimum amount (dose) of exercise is called the threshold of training. The fitness target zone is the optimal amount of physical activity for developing physical fitness.

TERMS

Fitness Target Zone—A range of exercise from the minimum necessary to improve fitness to the maximum amount, beyond which exercise may be counterproductive. If you exercise above the minimum and below the maximum, you are exercising in the fitness target zone.

The Overload Principle—A basic principle that specifies that you must perform exercise in greater than normal amounts (overload) to get an improvement in physical fitness.

Threshold of Training—The minimum amount of exercise that will improve physical fitness.

THE FACTS

The overload principle is the basis for improving physical fitness.

In order for a muscle (including the heart muscle) to get stronger, it must be "overloaded," or worked against a load greater than normal. To increase flexibility, a muscle must be stretched longer than is normal. To increase muscular endurance, muscles must be exposed to sustained exercise for a longer than normal period. If overload is less than normal for a specific component of fitness, the result will be a decrease in that particular component of fitness. A normal amount of exercise will maintain the current fitness level.

There is no substitute for overload in developing physical fitness.

Many people do not overload enough to develop good fitness. Often the programs found in health clubs and in exercises described in popular books and magazines do not provide for adequate overload. Some people try exercise machines, special foods or medicines, or quack devices that violate the overload principle and are therefore ineffective.

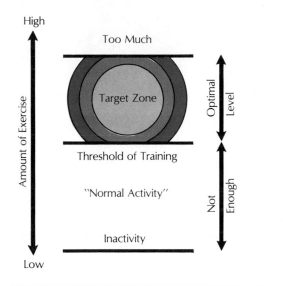

High

Too Much

Target Zone

Optimal Level

Threshold of Training

Amount of Exercise

"Normal Activity"

Not Enough

Inactivity

Low

FIGURE 5.1 Exercise Target Zones. *Adapted from Laurie, D. R., and Corbin, C. B.* How Much Exercise Is Enough? *Manhattan, KS: Master Teacher, 1980. An audiovisual program.*

To get fit, you must overload above the normal everyday level of activity.

The threshold of training is the minimum amount of exercise necessary to produce gains in fitness. What you normally do, or just a little more than your normal exercise, is not enough to cause improvements in fitness. Figure 5.1 shows the threshold of training and target zones for physical fitness improvement.

To get optimal benefits of regular exercise, you should exercise in the fitness target zone.

The fitness target zone begins at the threshold of training and stops at the point where the benefits of exercise become counterproductive, as shown in figure 5.1. This is the optimal level of exercise.

*The **principle of specificity** is an important law of exercise that should be observed if optimal fitness is to be obtained.*

The "principle of specificity" simply states that to develop a certain characteristic of fitness, you must overload specifically for that particular fitness component. For example, strength-building exercises may do little for developing cardiovascular fitness, and flexibility exercises may do little for altering body composition.

Just as overload is specific to each component of fitness, it is also specific to each body part. If you exercise the legs, you build fitness of the legs. If you exercise the arms, you build fitness of the arms. For this reason, it is not unusual to see some people with disproportionate fitness development. Some gymnasts, for example, have good upper body development but poor leg development, whereas some soccer players have well-developed legs but lack upper body development.

Specificity is important in designing your warm-up, cool down, and training program for specific activities. Training is most effective when it closely resembles the activity for which you are training. For example, if your goal is to improve your skill in putting the shot, it is not enough to overload the arm muscles. You should perform a training activity requiring overload while doing a putting motion that closely resembles what you use in the actual sport.

*There is a **threshold of training** and a **fitness target zone** for each component of fitness.*

Some people incorrectly associate the concepts of threshold of training and fitness target zones with only cardiovascular fitness. As the principle of specificity suggests, each component of fitness has its own threshold and target zone. Details for each of the health-related aspects of fitness are presented in Concepts 6–13.

*The **principle of progression** is an important corollary of the overload principle.*

The progression concept indicates that overload should not be increased too slowly nor too rapidly if fitness is to result. Obviously, the concepts of threshold of training and fitness target zones are based on the "progression principle." Beginners can exercise progressively by starting near threshold levels and gradually increasing in frequency, intensity, and time (duration) within the target zone. Exercise above the target zone is counterproductive and can be dangerous. For example, the "weekend" athlete who exercises vigorously only on weekends does not exercise often enough, and so violates the principle of progression. Approximately 30 percent of all Americans, or 50 percent of those who consider themselves to be regular exercisers, violate the principle of progression by failing to exercise above threshold levels and in the exercise target zone. Clearly, it is possible to do too little and too much exercise to develop optimal fitness.

The word FIT can help you remember the three important variables for determining threshold of training and fitness target zone levels.

For exercise to be effective, it must be done with enough Frequency, and Intensity, and for a long enough Time. The first letter of these three words spells FIT. The acronym FIT can help you remember these important factors.

1. Frequency (how often)—Exercise must be performed regularly to be effective. The number of days a person exercises per week is used to determine frequency. Exercise frequency depends on the specific component to be developed. However, most fitness components require at least three days and up to six days of activity per week.

2. Intensity (how hard)—Exercise must be hard enough to require more exertion than normal to produce gains in health-related fitness. The method for determining appropriate intensity varies with each aspect of fitness. For example, flexibility requires stretching muscles beyond normal length, cardiovascular fitness requires elevating the heart rate above normal, and strength requires increasing the resistance more than normal.

3. Time (how long)—Exercise must be done for a significant length of time to be effective. Generally, an exercise period must be at least fifteen minutes in length to be effective, while longer times are recommended for optimal fitness gains. As the length of time increases, intensities of exercise may be decreased. Time of exercise involvement is also referred to as exercise duration.

Threshold levels and target zones change as your fitness level changes.

As you become more fit by doing correct exercises, your threshold of training and fitness target zones may change. Likewise, if you stop exercising for a period of time, they will also change. Your threshold of training and fitness target zones are based on your current physical fitness levels and your current exercise patterns.

REFERENCES

American College of Sports Medicine. "Position Statement on the Recommended Quantity and Quality of Exercise for Developing and Maintaining Fitness in Healthy Adults." *Medicine and Science in Sports and Exercise* 10(1978):vii.

*American College of Sports Medicine. *Guidelines for Graded Exercise Testing and Exercise Prescription.* 3d. ed. Philadelphia: Lea and Febiger, 1986.

Gilliam, T. B., et al. "Physical Activity Patterns Determined by Heart Rate Monitoring in 6-7-Year-Old Children." *Medicine and Science in Sports and Exercise* 13(1981):65.

Hickson, R. C., and M. A. Rosenkoetter. "Reduced Training Frequencies and Maintenance of Increased Aerobic Power." *Medicine and Science in Sports and Exercise* 13(1981):13.

Laurie, D. R., and C. B. Corbin. "How Much Exercise Is Enough?" Manhattan, KS: Master Teacher, 1980.

*Pollock, M. L. "How Much Exercise Is Enough?" *Physician and Sportsmedicine* 6(1978):50.

*Pollock, M. L., and S. N. Blair. "Exercise Prescription." *Journal of Physical Education and Recreation* 52(1981):30.

Research and Forecasts, Inc. *The Miller Lite Report on American Attitudes toward Sports.* Milwaukee: Miller Brewing Co., 1983.

Van Camp, S. P. "The Fixx Tragedy: A Cardiologist's Perspective." *Physician and Sportsmedicine* 12(1984):153.

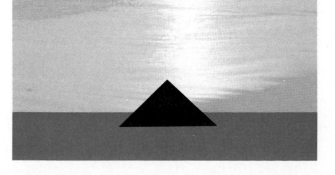

6

CARDIOVASCULAR FITNESS

CONCEPT 6

Cardiovascular fitness,
the ability of the blood, heart, lungs,
and other systems of the body
to effectively persist in effort,
is probably the most important aspect
of physical fitness and can be developed
and assessed in a number of ways.

INTRODUCTION

Cardiovascular fitness is frequently considered the most important aspect of physical fitness because those who possess it are likely to decrease their risk of coronary heart disease. Cardiovascular fitness is also referred to as cardiovascular endurance, cardiorespiratory capacity, and circulatory fitness. Regardless of the word used to describe it, cardiovascular fitness is complex because it requires fitness of several body systems.

TERMS

Aerobic Exercise—Exercise for which the body is able to supply adequate oxygen to sustain performance for long periods of time.

Anaerobic Exercise—Exercise that requires the use of the body's high-energy fuel. This type of exercise is of short duration and does not depend on the body's ability to supply oxygen.

Hemoglobin—Oxygen-carrying pigment of the red blood cells.

Liter—A metric measure of volume slightly larger than one quart.

Maximal Oxygen Uptake—A laboratory measure of fitness commonly held to be the best measure of cardiovascular fitness.

THE FACTS

Because of its importance to a healthy life, cardiovascular fitness is one of the most significant aspects of physical fitness.

A considerable amount of evidence indicates that people who exercise regularly have a lower incidence of heart disease, and that exercise is an effective prescription for those who have already suffered a heart attack.

Good cardiovascular fitness requires a fit heart muscle.

The heart is a muscle; to become stronger it must be exercised like any other muscle in the body. If the heart is exercised regularly, its strength increases; if not, it becomes weaker. Contrary to the belief that strenuous work harms the heart, research has found no evidence that regular, progressive exercise is bad for the normal heart. In fact, the heart muscle will increase in size and power when called upon to extend itself. The increase in size and power allows the heart to pump a greater volume of blood with fewer strokes per minute. For example, the average individual has a resting heart rate between seventy and eighty beats per minute, while it is not uncommon for a trained athlete's pulse to be in the low fifties or even in the forties.

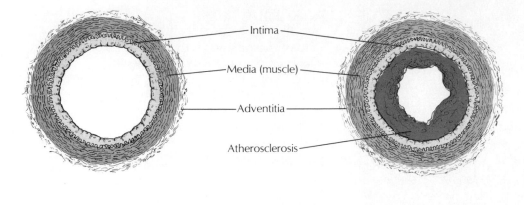

Intima

Media (muscle)

Adventitia

Atherosclerosis

FIGURE 6.1 *(a)* Healthy, Elastic Artery and *(b)* Unhealthy Artery

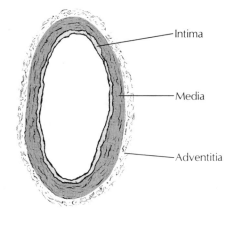

Intima

Media

Adventitia

FIGURE 6.2 Healthy, Nonelastic Vein

The healthy heart is efficient in the work that it does.

The fit heart can convert about half of its fuel into energy. An automobile engine in good running condition converts about one-fourth of its fuel into energy. By comparison, the heart is an efficient engine.

The heart of a normal individual beats reflexively about 40 million times a year. During this time, over 4,000 gallons or 10 tons of blood are circulated each day, and every night the heart's work load is equivalent to a person carrying a thirty-pound pack to the top of the 102-story Empire State Building.

Good cardiovascular fitness requires a fit vascular system.

Blood flows through a sequence of arteries to capillaries, to veins, and back to the heart. Arteries always carry blood away from the heart. Healthy arteries are elastic, free of obstruction, and expand to permit the flow of blood. Muscle layers line the arteries and control the size of the arterial opening on impulse from

nerve fibers. Unfit arteries may have a reduced internal diameter (atherosclerosis) because of deposits on the interior of their walls, or they may have hardened, nonelastic walls (arteriosclerosis).

Fit coronary arteries are especially important to good health. The blood in the four chambers of the heart does not directly nourish the heart. Rather, numerous small arteries within the heart muscle provide for coronary circulation. Poor coronary circulation precipitated by unhealthy arteries can be the cause of a heart attack (see figure 6.1).

Veins have thinner, less elastic walls than arteries as shown in figure 6.2. Also veins contain small valves to prevent the backward flow of blood. Skeletal muscles assist the return of blood to the heart. The veins are intertwined in the muscle; therefore, when the muscle is contracted, the vein is squeezed, pushing the blood on its way back to the heart. A malfunction of the valves results in a failure to remove used blood at the proper rate. As a result, venous blood pools especially in the legs causing a condition known as varicose veins.

Capillaries are the transfer stations where oxygen and fuel are released and waste products removed from the tissues. The veins receive the blood from the capillaries for the return trip to the heart.

Good cardiovascular fitness requires a fit respiratory system, fit blood, and fit muscles capable of using oxygen.

In order for a healthy heart to transmit oxygen through a healthy artery, the blood must also be healthy. It must contain adequate **hemoglobin** in the red blood cells (erythrocytes). Insufficient oxygen-carrying capacity of the blood is called anemia.

As fit blood travels through the lungs, adequate oxygen must be transmitted from the lungs to the blood. A limited respiratory system will limit cardiovascular fitness.

TABLE 6.1 Cardiovascular Fitness Threshold of Training and Target Zones for Aerobic Exercise*

	Threshold of Training	Target Zone
Frequency	• 3 days a week.	• At least 3 and no more than 6 days a week.
Intensity	• Elevate the heart rate to 60% of its working range.	• Elevate the heart rate to at least 60% and up to 80% of its working range. For most young adults, the average target zone is between 135 and 170 beats per minute. For older adults, the zone for most people is between 120 and 140 beats per minute.
Time	• Exercise at the proper intensity for *a minimum of 15-30 minutes.* Another way to determine the minimal length of time for exercise is counting the calories you expend. Exercise of the proper intensity and frequency that causes a calorie expenditure of 2,000 per week is enough to improve cardiovascular fitness. As the intensity of exercise increases, the length of exercise sessions can be decreased. Beginners may start with 500 or 600 calories expended per week and gradually increase to 2,000.	• Exercise at the proper intensity for *15-60 minutes or expend from 2,000-3,500 calories* per week at the correct intensity and frequency.

*The threshold of training and target zone values depicted in this table are for healthy young adults. Older people or those who have not been active recently should begin exercising below threshold values and increase exercise gradually. Those with known medical problems should consult a physician to determine appropriate exercise amounts.

If cardiovascular fitness is to be developed, you must regularly exercise above the cardiovascular threshold of training and in the cardiovascular fitness target zone.

Three factors must be considered in designing exercise programs for developing cardiovascular fitness: frequency, intensity, and time (see table 6.1).

*Cardiovascular fitness can be achieved by doing either **aerobic** or **anaerobic** exercise.*

Aerobic means "with oxygen." During aerobic exercise, the body can supply the oxygen it needs to function effectively; thus the name aerobic. Examples of aerobic exercise are walking, jogging, and swimming at moderate speeds. If exercise becomes more intense, it is likely to be at least partially anaerobic in nature. Anaerobic means "without oxygen." During anaerobic exercise, the body cannot supply adequate oxygen to meet the body's needs. For this reason, true anaerobic exercise can only be continued for less than a minute at a time. Examples of pure anaerobic exercises are all-out sprints in running or swimming.

Many activities, such as a mile run for time or a three-mile bicycle race, are part aerobic and part anaerobic. However, activities continuously performed for fifteen to sixty minutes without regular intervals of rest are primarily aerobic and are often referred to as aerobic exercise. Cooper (1982) and others advocate exercise that is principally aerobic, while Astrand (1986) and others recommend exercise that is principally anaerobic. Both can be effective in building cardiovascular fitness. Some advantages and disadvantages of each are presented in table 6.2.

TABLE 6.2 Advantages of Aerobic and Anaerobic Exercise

Aerobic	Anaerobic
• Is often done slowly and continuously, rather than in short vigorous bursts, therefore, many people consider aerobic exercise to be less demanding and more enjoyable.	• Is often done using short bursts of exercise alternated with rest periods. Some people find such varied schedules of exercise interesting.
• Is less intense and may be best for beginners, especially for those who are older and those who are just starting an exercise program after a long layoff.	• May be the best approach for those preparing for competition in events that require bursts of speed, such as track and swimming.
• Produces aerobic fitness, or the ability to do sustained exercise.	• Produces anaerobic fitness, or the ability to do short explosive bursts of exercise.
• Less risk to older people or to those with less than very good levels of fitness.	• Saves time—allows a person to do more work in a given period of time.

There is a threshold of training and a target zone for building cardiovascular fitness using aerobic exercise. Specific amounts of exercise necessary to achieve increases in cardiovascular fitness using aerobic exercise are outlined in table 6.1.

To determine the intensity of exercise for building cardiovascular fitness, it is important to know how to count your pulse. Each time the heart beats it pumps blood into the arteries. The surge of blood causes a pulse that can be felt by holding a finger against an artery.

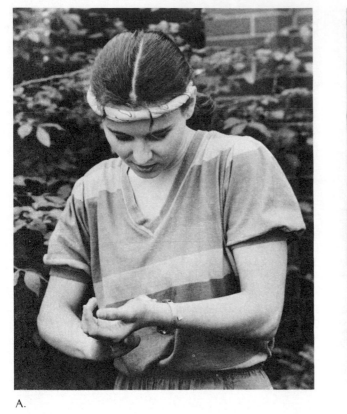
A.

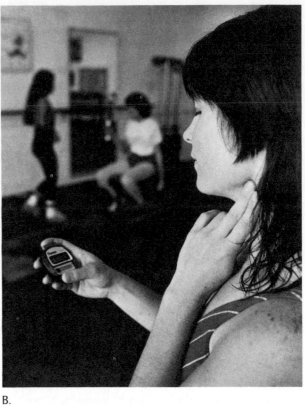
B.

FIGURE 6.3 Counting Your Own Pulse: *(a)* Wrist (Radial) and *(b)* Neck (Carotid)

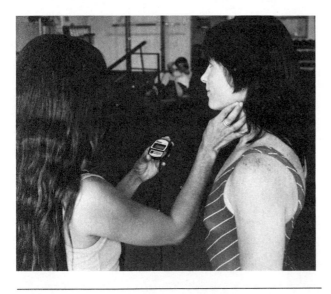

FIGURE 6.4 Counting Someone Else's Pulse: Neck (Carotid)

Major arteries that are easy to locate and are frequently used for pulse counts are the carotid (on either side of the Adam's apple), and the radial (just above the base of the thumb on the wrist). (See figures 6.3 and 6.4.) Heart rate (pulse) is important for determining the correct intensity of exercise for building cardiovascular fitness.

To count the pulse, simply place the finger tips (index and middle finger) over the artery at one of the previously mentioned locations. Move the fingers around until a strong pulse can be felt. Press gently so as not to cut off the blood flow through the artery. Counting the pulse with the thumb is not recommended because the thumb has a relatively strong pulse of its own. This could be especially confusing when counting another person's pulse.

Counting the pulse at the carotid artery is the most popular procedure probably because the carotid pulse is easy to locate. Some researchers suggest that caution should be used when taking carotid pulse counts because pressing on this artery can cause a reflex that slows the heart rate. This could result in incorrect heart rate counts. More recent research indicates that carotid palpations, when done properly, can be used safely to count heart rate for most people.

The radial pulse is a bit harder to find than the carotid pulse because of the many tendons near the wrist. Moving the fingers around to several locations just above the thumb on the wrist will help you locate this pulse. For older adults or those with known medical problems, this procedure is recommended.

Though less popular, the pulse can also be counted at the brachial artery. This is located on the inside of the upper arm just below the armpit.

Once the pulse is located, the heart rate can be determined in beats per minute. At rest, this is done simply by counting the number of beats in one minute. To determine exercise heart rate, it is best to count heart beats or pulses during exercise. However, to count the pulse during most activities is difficult. Machines do exist that can count heartbeats during exercise but they are not available to most people. The most practical method is to count the pulse immediately after exercise. During exercise, the heart rate increases; immediately after exercise, it begins to slow down or return to normal. In fact, the heart rate has already slowed considerably within one minute after exercise ceases. The key is to locate the pulse quickly and to count the rate for a short period of time. A full one-minute count after exercise does not give a good estimate of exercise heart rate, even if the pulse is quickly located, because the heart rate during the end of the count is much slower than it was during exercise. Keep moving while quickly locating the pulse, then stop and take a fifteen-second count. Multiply the number of pulses counted in a fifteen-second period by four to convert heart rate to beats per minute.

The pulse rate should be counted after regular exercise, not after a sudden burst of activity. Some runners sprint the last few yards of their daily run and then count their pulse. Such a burst of exercise will elevate the heart rate considerably. This gives a false picture of the actual exercise heart rate. It would be wise for every person to learn to determine resting heart rate accurately and to estimate exercise heart rate by quickly and accurately making pulse counts after exercise.

In order to plan aerobic exercise for building cardiovascular fitness, it is important to know how to calculate heart rate threshold levels and target zones.

In table 6.1, we noted that the threshold, or minimal heart rate intensity for building cardiovascular fitness, is based on a percentage of your working heart rate range. To calculate your working heart rate range, you must know your resting and your maximal heart rate.

The resting heart rate is easily determined by counting the pulse for one minute while sitting or lying. Ideally, this should be done early in the morning when you are rested, rather than late in the day when you have been involved in many activities.

Maximal heart rate is harder to determine. It could be measured by an electrocardiogram while exercising to exhaustion; however, for most people it is safer and better to estimate *maximal heart* rate by using a formula. This is done by subtracting your age from 220. Maximal heart rates are near 200 in young people but decrease with age. The formula for calculating your maximal heart rate and an example of the calculations for a twenty-two-year-old individual are shown in table 6.3.

TABLE 6.3 Formula and Example for Calculating Target Heart Rates (Example is for a twenty-two-year-old person with a resting heart rate of 68 bpm.)

Formula for Calculating Maximal Heart Rate	Example
220 − Age (in years) = Maximal Heart Rate	220 − 22 = 198 beats per minute

Formula For Calculating Working Heart Rate	Example
Maximal Heart Rate − Resting Heart Rate = Working Heart Rate	198 − 68 = 130

Formula for Calculating Threshold of Training Heart Rate	Example
Working Heart Rate	130
× .60	× .60
	= 78
+ Resting Heart Rate	+ 68
Threshold of Training Heart Rate	= 146

Formula for Calculating the Upper Limit of the Target Heart Rate Zone	Example
Working Heart Rate	130
× .80	× .80
	= 104
+ Resting Heart Rate	+ 68
= Upper Limit for Target Heart Rate Zone	= 172

The target zone for this twenty-two-year-old is 146–172 bpm.

The *working heart rate* range is determined by subtracting the resting heart rate from the maximal heart rate. The heart always works in this range because the resting is the lowest and the maximal is the highest rate of your pulse. The formula for calculating the working heart rate range and an example for the twenty-two-year-old with a resting heart rate of sixty-eight are also shown in table 6.3.

The *threshold of training, or minimum heart rate* for building cardiovascular fitness, is determined by calculating 60 percent of the working heart rate range then adding it to the resting heart rate. The upper limit of the target zone is 80 percent of the working heart rate range added to the resting heart rate. The formula for determining threshold and the upper limit of the target heart rate zone and examples for the hypothetical exerciser are shown in table 6.3.

TABLE 6.4 Cardiovascular Fitness Threshold of Training and Target Zones for Anaerobic Exercise*

	Threshold of Training	Target Zone
Frequency	• 3 days a week.	• 3-4 days a week.
Intensity	• Short Intervals — 100% of maximum speed running, swimming, or other exercise of short duration (10–30 seconds).	• Short Intervals — 100% of maximum speed running, swimming, or other exercise of short duration (10–30 seconds).
	• Long Intervals — 90% of maximum speed running, swimming, or other exercise (30 seconds–2 minutes).	• Long Intervals — 90%–100% of maximum speed running, swimming, or other exercise (30 seconds–2 minutes).
Time	• Short Intervals — Exercise 10 seconds, rest 10 seconds. Repeat 20 times.	• Short Intervals — Same as threshold but repeat up to 30 times.
	or	
	• Exercise 20 seconds, rest 15 seconds. Repeat 10 times.	• Same as threshold but repeat up to 20 times.
	or	
	• Exercise 30 seconds, rest 1–2 minutes. Repeat 8 times.	• Same as threshold but repeat up to 18 times.
	• Long Intervals — Exercise 1 minute, rest 3–5 minutes. Repeat 5 times.	• Long Intervals — Same as threshold but repeat up to 15 times.
	or	
	• Exercise 2 minutes, rest 5–15 minutes. Repeat 4 times.	• Same as threshold but repeat up to 10 times.

*The threshold of training and target zone values depicted in this table are for healthy, young adults. For older people, or those who have not been active recently, aerobic training is recommended. Those with known medical problems should consult a physician to determine appropriate exercise amounts.

You should learn to calculate your own threshold and target heart rate values. However, for convenient reference and so that you can check your calculations, chart 6B.1 in the Lab Resource Materials on page 45 includes threshold and target heart rates for people of all ages. Once you have determined your threshold and target heart rates, you should exercise vigorously enough to bring your heart rate above threshold and into the target zone. Count your fifteen-second heart rate immediately after exercise (and multiply by four) to see if your heart rate is in the proper range. You may have to adjust the intensity of your exercise if your heart rate is not in the target zone. The heart rate of the *hypothetical* twenty-two-year-old used in the previous example should be elevated to no less than 146 and up to 172 beats per minute for optimal cardiovascular fitness benefits.

There is a threshold of training and a target zone for developing cardiovascular fitness using anaerobic exercise.

Specific amounts of exercise necessary to increase cardiovascular fitness using anaerobic exercise are outlined in table 6.4.

Counting calories expended can be a useful way to determine if your regular exercise is enough to reduce risk of heart disease.

Scientific evidence suggests that people who expend 2,000 calories per week in exercise such as walking, stair climbing, and sports reduce death rates from heart disease by 25 to 33 percent compared to those who do not exercise. Death rates decreased with increased weekly calorie expenditure up to 3,500, after which there was no advantage to those who did more exercise. Keeping track of your weekly energy expenditure can be useful in determining if you do enough regular exercise to reduce your risk to various types of heart disease. (See Lab 6C.)

*Though cardiovascular fitness can be measured in many ways, **maximal oxygen uptake** is the best method of evaluation.*

A person's maximal oxygen uptake is determined in a laboratory by measuring how much oxygen can be used in one minute of maximal work. Great endurance athletes can extract five or six **liters** of oxygen per minute from the environment during an all-out treadmill run or bicycle ride, as opposed to the average person, who can extract only two or three liters. In order to extract a large amount of oxygen during maximal work, a person must have a fit heart muscle, capable of pumping large amounts of blood; fit blood, capable of carrying adequate amounts of oxygen; fit arteries, free from congestion and capable of carrying large amounts of blood; and fit muscles, capable of using the oxygen supplied to the muscle. Less sophisticated tests, such as the twelve-minute run, the step test, or the Astrand-Ryhming bicycle test, can also be used to measure cardiovascular endurance (see the Lab Resource Materials that follow).

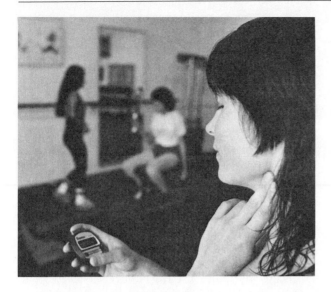

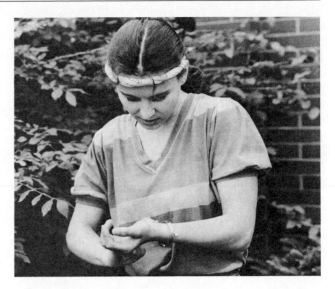

1. *Locating the Carotid Pulse*
   Place the index and middle fingers of one hand on one side of your throat about an inch to the side of your Adam's apple. Pressing lightly, you should feel the pulse with your fingers. If not, move the fingers to another spot in the area (but do not move the fingers above the level of the Adam's apple) until a strong pulse is felt. Do not press hard because this may restrict the movement of the blood through the carotid artery.

2. *Locating the Radial Pulse*
   Place the index and middle fingers of one hand on the palm side of the other wrist just above the base of the thumb. Pressing lightly, you should feel the pulse with your fingers. You may need to move the fingers to several spots in the area until a strong pulse is felt. Do not press hard because this may restrict the movement of the blood through the radial artery.

CHART 6B.1 Threshold of Training and Target Zone Heart Rates
(Heart rates necessary to produce improved cardiovascular fitness)*

Resting Heart Rate		Age									
		Less than 25	25–29	30–34	35–39	40–44	45–49	50–54	55–59	60–64	Over 65
below 50	Threshold	136	133	130	127	124	121	118	115	112	109
	Target zone	136–166	133–164	130–160	127–156	124–152	121–148	118–144	115–140	112–136	109–134
50–54	Threshold	138	135	132	129	126	123	120	117	114	111
	Target zone	138–167	135–165	132–161	129–157	126–153	123–149	120–145	117–141	114–137	111–135
55–59	Threshold	140	137	134	131	128	125	122	119	116	113
	Target zone	140–168	137–166	134–162	131–158	128–154	125–150	122–146	119–142	116–138	113–136
60–64	Threshold	142	139	136	133	130	127	124	121	118	115
	Target zone	142–169	139–167	136–163	133–159	130–155	127–151	124–147	121–143	118–139	115–137
65–69	Threshold	144	141	138	135	132	129	126	123	120	117
	Target zone	144–170	141–168	138–164	135–160	132–156	129–152	126–148	123–144	120–140	117–138
70–74	Threshold	146	143	140	137	134	131	128	125	122	119
	Target zone	146–171	143–169	140–165	137–161	134–157	131–153	128–149	125–145	122–141	119–139
75–79	Threshold	148	145	142	139	136	133	130	127	124	121
	Target zone	148–172	145–170	142–166	139–162	136–158	133–154	130–150	127–146	124–142	121–140
80–85	Threshold	150	147	144	141	138	135	132	129	126	123
	Target zone	150–173	147–171	144–167	141–163	138–159	135–155	132–151	129–147	126–143	123–141
85 and over	Threshold	152	149	146	143	140	137	134	131	128	125
	Target zone	152–174	149–172	146–168	143–164	140–160	137–156	134–152	131–148	128–144	125–142

Computed using 60%–80% of the working heart rate.

Evaluating Cardiovascular Fitness

For an exercise program to be most effective, it should be based on personal needs. Some sort of testing is necessary to determine your personal need for cardiovascular fitness. A treadmill test that includes continuous EKG monitoring or assessment of maximal oxygen uptake is the best test of cardiovascular fitness (see American College of Sports Medicine, 1986). However, there are some tests that do not require as much time and equipment and can be done to give you a good estimate of cardiovascular fitness. The twelve-minute run, the step test, and the Astrand-Ryhming bicycle test are such tests, all of which are described here. Prior to performing any of these, be sure that you are physically and medically ready (Concept 4). Prepare yourself by doing some regular exercise for three to six weeks before actually taking the tests. If possible, take more than one test and use the summary of your test results to make a final assessment of your cardiovascular fitness.

The Twelve-Minute Run Test

1. Locate an area where a specific distance is already marked, such as a school track or football field; or measure a specific distance using a bicycle or automobile odometer.

2. Use a stopwatch or wristwatch to accurately time a twelve-minute period.
3. For best results, warm up prior to the test, then run at a steady pace for the entire twelve minutes (cool down after the tests).
4. Determine the distance you can run in twelve minutes in fractions of a mile. Depending upon your age, locate your score and rating on Chart 6D.1.

The Step Test*

1. Prior to exercise, warm up, and after finishing, be sure to cool down.
2. Step up and down on a twelve-inch bench for three minutes at a rate of twenty-four steps per minute. One step consists of four beats, that is, "up with the left foot, up with the right foot, down with the left foot, down with the right foot."
3. Immediately after the exercise, sit down on the bench and relax. Don't talk.
4. Locate your pulse or have another person locate it for you.
5. Five seconds after the exercise ended, begin counting your pulse. Count the pulse for sixty seconds.
6. Your score is your sixty-second heart rate. Locate your score and your rating on the following chart.

CHART 6D.1* Twelve-Minute Run Test (Scores in Miles)

	Men (age)			
Classification	**17–26**	**27–39**	**40–49**	**50+**
High Performance Zone	1.80+	1.60+	1.50+	1.40+
Good Fitness Zone	1.55–1.79	1.45–1.59	1.40–1.49	1.25–1.39
Marginal Zone	1.35–1.54	1.30–1.44	1.25–1.39	1.10–1.24
Low Zone	<1.35	<1.30	<1.25	<1.10

	Women (age)			
Classification	**17–26**	**27–39**	**40–49**	**50+**
High Performance Zone	1.45+	1.35+	1.25+	1.15+
Good Fitness Zone	1.25–1.44	1.20–1.34	1.15–1.24	1.05–1.14
Marginal Zone	1.15–1.24	1.05–1.19	1.00–1.14	0.95–1.04
Low Zone	<1.15	<1.05	<1.00	<.94

Adapted from K. H. Cooper.

The Astrand-Ryhming Bicycle Test

1. Ride a stationary bicycle ergometer for six minutes at a rate of fifty pedal cycles per minute (one push with each foot per cycle). Prior to beginning, a stretching warm-up is recommended. The test itself will serve as a cardiovascular warm-up. Cool down after the test.
2. Set the bicycle at a work load between 300 and 1,200 kpm. For less fit or smaller people, a setting in the range of 300 to 600 is appropriate. Larger or fitter people will need to use a setting of 750 to 1,200. The work load should be enough to elevate the heart rate to at least 125 bpm but no more than 170 bpm during the ride.
3. During the sixth minute of the ride (if the heart rate is in the correct range—see step 2), count the heart rate for the entire sixth minute. The carotid or radial pulse may be used.
4. Use the nomogram to determine your predicted oxygen uptake score. Connect the point that represents your heart rate with the point on the right-hand scale that represents the work load you used in riding the bike (use the ♂ scale for men and the ♀ scale for women). Read your score at the point where a straight line connecting the two points crosses the Max VO_2 line. For example, the sample score for the woman represented by the dotted line is 2.55, or nearly 2.6. She had a heart rate of 150 and worked at a load of 600 kpm.
5. Determine your score in terms of VO_2 per kilogram of body weight by dividing your weight in kilograms into the score obtained from the nomogram. To compute your weight in kilograms, divide your weight in pounds by 2.2.
6. To determine your cardiovascular fitness rating on the bicycle test, look up your VO_2 per kilogram of body weight score on the following chart.

Nomogram

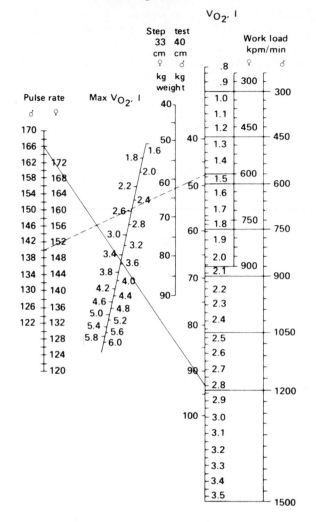

CHART 6D.2 Step Test Rating Chart

Classification	Sixty-Second Heart Rate
High Performance Zone	84 or less
Good Fitness Zone	85–95
Marginal Zone	96–119
Low Zone	120 and above

As you grow older you would want to continue to score well on this rating chart. Because your maximal heart rate decreases as you age, you should be able to score well if you exercise regularly.
*Adapted from Kasch, F. W., and Boyer, J. L. Adult Fitness: Principles and Practices. Palo Alto, Calif.: Mayfield Publishers, 1968.

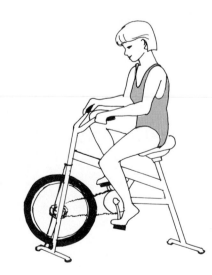

CHART 6D.3 Bicycle Test *Rating Scale* (ml/O₂ /kg)*

	Women				
Age	**17–26**	**27–39**	**40–49**	**50–59**	**60–69**
High Performance Zone	46+	40+	38+	35+	32+
Good Fitness Zone	36–45	33–39	30–37	28–34	24–31
Marginal Zone	30–35	28–32	24–29	21–27	18–23
Low Zone	<30	<28	<24	<21	<18

	Men				
Age	**17–26**	**27–39**	**40–49**	**50–59**	**60–69**
High Performance Zone	50+	46+	42+	39+	35+
Good Fitness Zone	43–49	35–45	32–41	29–38	26–34
Marginal Zone	35–42	30–34	27–31	25–28	22–25
Low Zone	<35	<30	<27	<25	<22

*Test adapted from P. O. Astrand, and K. Rodahl. Textbook of Work Physiology. *New York: McGraw-Hill, 1977.*

REFERENCES

American College of Sports Medicine. *Guidelines for Exercise Testing and Exercise Prescription.* 3d ed. Philadelphia: Lea and Febiger, 1986.

Astrand, P. O., and K. Rodahl. *Textbook of Work Physiology.* 3d ed. New York: McGraw-Hill, 1986.

Brooks, G. A., and T. D. Fahey. *Exercise Physiology.* New York: John Wiley, 1984.

*Cooper, K. H. *The Aerobics Program for Total Well-Being.* New York: M. Evans, 1982.

Cooper, K. H. *Running without Fear.*

*Couldry, W., C. B. Corbin, and A. Wilcox. "Carotid vs. Radial Pulse Counts." *Physician and Sportsmedicine* 10(1982):67.

deVries, H. A. *Physiology of Exercise.* 4th ed. Dubuque, IA: Wm. C. Brown Publishers, 1986.

*Mahurin, J., and T. P. Martin. "Anaerobic Threshold: A Trainable Component of Cardiovascular Fitness." *Motor Skills: Theory into Practice* 6(1982):41.

Olderidge, N. B., et al. "Carotid Palpation, Coronary Heart Disease, and Exercise Rehabilitation." *Medicine and Science in Sports and Exercise* 13(1981):6.

Paffenbarger, R. S., and R. T. Hyde. "Exercise as Protection Against Heart Disease." *New England Journal of Medicine* 302(1980):1026.

Paffenbarger, R. S., et al. "A Natural History of Athleticism and Cardiovascular Health." *Journal of the American Medical Association* 252 (1984):496.

Paffenbarger, R. S. "Exercise in the Primary Prevention of Coronary Heart Disease." In Pollock, M. L., et al., *Heart Disease and Rehabilitation.* 2d ed. New York: John Wiley, 1986.

*Pollock, M. L., and S. N. Blair. "Exercise Prescription." *Journal of Physical Education and Recreation* 52(1981):30.

Sedlock, D. A., et al. "Accuracy of Subject-Palpated Carotid Pulse after Exercise." *Physician and Sportsmedicine* 11 (1983):106.

Stone, W. J. *Adult Fitness Programs* (Glenview, Ill.: Scott, Foresman and Company, 1987).

Zohman, L. R. *Exercise Your Way to Fitness and Heart Health.* Englewood Cliffs, N.J.: CPC International, 1983.

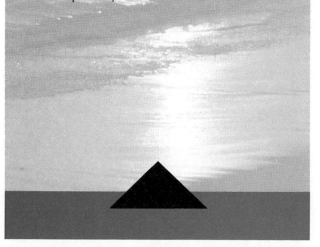

7

AEROBIC AND ANAEROBIC EXERCISE

CONCEPT 7

Both aerobic and anaerobic exercises are effective in developing health-related physical fitness, especially cardiovascular fitness.

INTRODUCTION

Both aerobic and anaerobic exercises are good methods of building cardiovascular fitness. Which you use depends on your personal needs and interests.

TERMS

Aerobic Exercise—Exercise for which the body is able to supply adequate oxygen to sustain performance for long periods of time.

Anaerobic Exercise—Exercise that requires the use of the body's high-energy fuel. This type of exercise can only be sustained for short periods of time without rest and does not depend on the body's ability to supply oxygen.

Continuous Exercise—Exercise that is done for relatively long periods of time without stopping.

Intermittent Exercise—Exercise that is done in short bursts followed by rest periods.

THE FACTS ABOUT AEROBIC EXERCISE

***Aerobic exercise** is a good way to develop several components of health-related physical fitness.*

When done in the cardiovascular fitness target zone, aerobic activities are excellent for building cardiovascular fitness. Because aerobic activities can be sustained for relatively long periods of time, they can result in considerable calorie expenditure and are very good for helping to control body fatness. Aerobic activities can also be of value in developing muscular endurance (usually in the leg muscles).

*Aerobic exercise can be **continuous** or **intermittent**.*

Anaerobic exercise cannot be done continuously. Because it is so intense, you must alternate vigorous anaerobic exercise with frequent rest periods. Aerobic exercise, on the other hand, can be done continuously or intermittently, but for best result, it should be done continuously. For information concerning the correct frequency, intensity, and time for aerobic exercise, refer to Concepts 6 and 13.

Not all aerobic exercise is effective in building health-related physical fitness.

Bowling is aerobic exercise. So is golf. Yet these activities may do very little to contribute to the development of health-related physical fitness. Those who popularized the term *aerobics* really meant *continuous* aerobic exercise that stressed the cardiovascular system when they spoke of the health benefits of aerobic activity. As the term is commonly used now, it means activities sustained for relatively long periods of time without rest intervals.

49

Some activities that are at least partially anaerobic, such as basketball and racquetball, can be considered aerobic if done continuously.

Because sports, such as basketball and racquetball, involve short, vigorous bursts of exercise followed by rest or recovery periods, they are at least in part anaerobic. However, if the bursts of exercise are moderate, allowing continued participation for fifteen minutes or more without extended rest periods (i.e., the heart rate is maintained in the target zone), the activities can be considered aerobic.

Aerobic activities are exceptionally popular among adults.

Whereas activities that have a strong anaerobic component, such as sprinting, football, baseball, and sprint swimming, are very popular among youth, aerobic activities are more popular among adults. Adults report that they are most often involved in continuous swimming, jogging, cycling, walking, and calisthenics. All but vigorous calisthenics, sprint running, or sprint swimming are aerobic. When done at a slow or moderate pace, calisthenics are aerobic; when done continuously, they can be effective in producing the same benefits as jogging, swimming, and other aerobic activities.

To be effective in building all components of health-related physical fitness, aerobic exercise should be supplemented with other forms of exercise.

As already noted, aerobic exercise can be effective in aiding cardiovascular fitness, muscular endurance, and in reducing body fat. Except for some types of continuous calisthenics, aerobic exercise must be supplemented with exercises designed to build flexibility, strength, and, to a lesser extent, muscular endurance. If certain types of aerobic exercise, such as jogging, are done exclusively, they may actually reduce flexibility.

THERE ARE MANY POPULAR FORMS OF AEROBIC EXERCISE

Some of the most popular forms of aerobic exercise are discussed briefly here.

Bicycling

Bicycling, when done continuously, is a form of aerobic exercise. This activity requires only a bicycle and some safety equipment, such as a helmet and a light and reflectors if done after dark. A tall "flag" is needed if biking in traffic. To be most effective in building physical fitness, you should pedal continuously, rather than coasting for long periods of time. Maintaining a steady pace is recommended. Riding a different course pe-

riodically can increase enjoyment of the activity. Stationary bicycle ergometers can also be used to improve fitness if the exercise is done in the target zone for fitness.

Circuit Overload Training

Originally, circuit training was a type of physical training involving movement from one exercise station to another. A different type of exercise was performed at each station. In order to complete the circuit, you had to complete all the exercises at the different stations. Your goal was to perform the circuit in progressively shorter periods of time.

Recently, however, circuit training has been modified by some to include several strength overload stations. These stations may involve overload exercises with free weights or exercise machines. There is some evidence that when this type of exercise is done at a moderate and continuous pace, it can be effective in building cardiovascular fitness. In these cases, circuit training can be considered an aerobic form of exercise. When repetitions of weight training exercises are followed by a relatively long rest period (longer than the exercise time) and are done very vigorously, they are primarily anaerobic. If repetitions of the exercise are done at a slow or moderate pace, and are followed by an extended rest period, they may still be aerobic. Because they are not continuous and do not elevate the heart rate for a sustained period of time, they are not effective in building cardiovascular fitness however.

Cooper's Aerobics

Based on the needs of military personnel, Dr. Kenneth Cooper developed a physical fitness program that he calls aerobics. In fact, he popularized the term. His program includes a variety of aerobic activities having point values for the different types of exercises involved. To develop fitness, especially cardiovascular fitness, a person is expected to earn from twenty-seven and thirty-two "points" per week. Aerobic points are part of Cooper's system for helping people to know when they are exercising frequently enough, intensely enough, and long enough. Many activities Cooper includes in his program are described in this concept. Table 7.1 charts some of the point values for various activities. (For more complete details on the Cooper aerobics program, refer to his book, *The Aerobics Program for Total Well-Being.*)

Continuous Calisthenics

Survey results repeatedly indicate that calisthenics is one of the top two or three participant activities performed. Calisthenics, exercises such as sit-ups and push-ups, are designed to build flexibility, strength, or mus-

TABLE 7.1 Aerobic Points Chart

Points	Walking-Running (Time for 1 Mile)	Cycling (Speed for 2 Miles)	Swimming (300 yds.)	Handball, Basketball	Stationary Running for 5 Minutes	Stationary Running for 10 Minutes	Points
0	Over 20 min.	Less than 10 mph	Over 10 min.	Less than 10 min.	Less than 60 steps/min.	Less than 50 steps/min.	0
1	20:00–14:30 min.	10–15 mph	8:00–10:00 min.	10 min.	60–70 steps/min.	50–65 steps/min.	1
2	14:29–12:00 min.	15–20 mph	7:30–8:00 min.	20 min.	80–90 steps/min.	65–70 steps/min.	2
3	11:59–10:00 min.	Over 20 mph	6:00–7:30 min.	30 min.		70–80 steps/min.	3
4	9:59–8:00 min.			40 min.		80–90 steps/min.	4
5	7:59–6:30 min.			50 min.			5
6	Less than 6:30 min.			60 min.			6

Used by permission of K. Cooper. *The New Aerobics* (New York: M. Evans and Co., 1970.)

cular endurance in specific muscle groups. Even though most calisthenics are aerobic, they are often done intermittently. That is, calisthenic exercises are done a few at a time followed by a rest period. This type of calisthenics can build flexibility, strength, and muscular endurance, but does little for cardiovascular fitness or fat control.

Continuous calisthenics, or calisthenics that are done without stopping or with walking, jogging, rope jumping, or some other aerobic activity performed during the rest period, can develop virtually all health-related aspects of physical fitness. Fitness pioneer Dr. Thomas Cureton (1965) has long advocated the use of continuous calisthenics, or what he refers to as "continuous rhythmical endurance exercise." Almost everyone can plan a continuous calisthenic program by selecting exercises for each fitness part that will elevate the heart rate to the optimal level and sustain this intensity an adequate length of time. Continuous calisthenics can be done individually, but is also excellent for group use. A sample program and some suggestions for performing them are presented in the box on continuous calisthentics.

Cross-Country Skiing

In Europe, cross-country skiing is one of the most popular aerobic activities. Of course, this sport requires snow and a certain amount of specialized equipment. For those who can cross-country ski on a regular basis, studies show that it is one of the most effective cardiovascular fitness exercises.

Dance Aerobics

One of the fastest growing aerobic activities is dance aerobics. The activity was first popularized by Jackie Sorensen in the 1970s as "aerobic dance." Since then, the activity has been promoted as rhythmic aerobics, jazzercize, and dancercize to note but a few of the popular names. Dance aerobics is quite similar to continuous calisthenics though it does include dance steps as well as calisthenic exercises done to music. Initially dance aerobics was done principally by women, but recently it has become popular with men also. Current activity polls show that it is one of the most popular types of exercise in North America.

In most cases, dance aerobics consists of a preplanned or choreographed series of dance steps and exercises done to music. Jogging, skipping, hopping, and other cardiovascular activities are also included in many routines. A routine is preceded by a warm-up and followed by a cool down. Depending on the program, the warm-up and cool down may be separate exercises done before the actual dance session, or may be part of the routine itself. A single routine may last from three to fifteen minutes. If routines are short, they may be done one after another with brief rest periods in between.

When preceded by a warm-up, including stretching of all body parts, a well-planned program of dance aerobics can be good for building all components of health-related fitness. One problem with dance aerobics is that it is a preplanned exercise program, therefore, it requires all participants to do the same activity regardless of their fitness or activity levels. A vigorous

Some continuous calisthenic exercises are illustrated here.

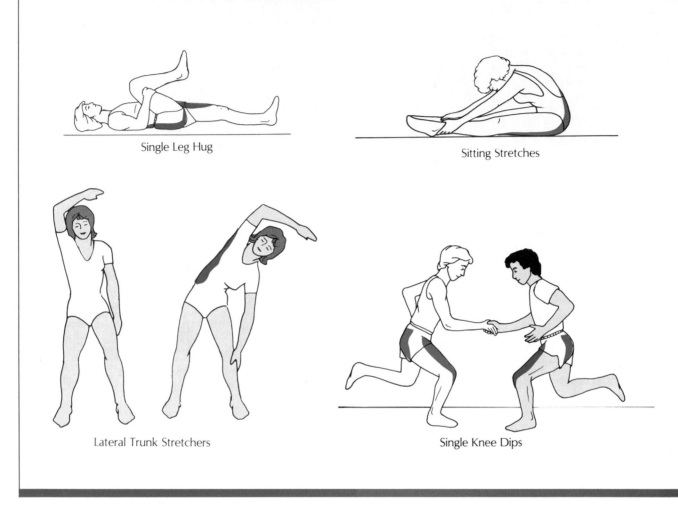

Single Leg Hug

Sitting Stretches

Lateral Trunk Stretchers

Single Knee Dips

routine could cause unfit people to overextend themselves, whereas an easy routine may not result in fitness gains for those who are already quite fit. Also, some dance aerobic routines have been known to include contraindicated exercises.

With the increased popularity of dance aerobics, there has been an increase in the number of injuries associated with the activity. In fact, one study has shown that as many as 75 percent of all instructors and 43 percent of all students injure themselves. One attempt to reduce the risk of injury with dance aerobics is commonly called "low impact aerobics." One foot stays on the floor at all times during low impact aerobic routines. Those who advocate this approach point out that the repeated jumping, kicking, and bouncing of dance aerobics cause injuries. By keeping one foot on the ground, the risk of injury is reduced. Low impact dance aerobics is probably a wise approach for those who have

a history of joint or muscle injuries and for beginners. However, a regular dance aerobic program is safe for most people if the following guidelines are adhered.

1. Wear proper shoes and exercise on a surface that "gives" rather than on a very hard floor (i.e., concrete).
2. Do static stretching before and after dance aerobics. Avoid high kicks and other exercises that cause extensive ballistic stretching until you have developed good levels of flexibility (see Concept 11).
3. Make sure that the routine you select, whether done with a live instructor or video instructor, is suited to your current level of fitness. If the routine becomes too vigorous, walk or jog in place instead of pushing to do the steps. Discontinuing arm movements can also make the exercise easier. If necessary stop and rest.

Stretching	5–Minute Circle Exercises	10–Minute Circle Exercises	15–Minute Circle Exercises
• All stretching is static and each exercise is held 5 to 6 seconds • 3 single leg hugs (each leg) • 3 lateral trunk stretches • 3 sitting trunk stretches	• Jog in a circle 1 minute • 7 bent knee sit-ups • Lateral shuffle in circle • 10 side leg-lifts (each leg) • 25 side hop-kicks • 7 push-ups • Jog in a circle	• 15 jumping jacks • 7 knee dips (each leg) • 15 jumping jacks • Jog in a circle • 5 bent knee sit-ups • Jog backward in a circle • 10 back leg-lifts (one leg at a time) • Jog in a circle	• Jog in a circle • 10 knee dips with each leg • Jog in a circle • 5 bent knee sit-ups • 5 side leg-lifts (each leg) • 220-yard jog • 220-yard walk • Repeat stretching

Some general suggestions for using this exercise program are:

1. Stretch first to establish a pattern of regular stretching and to help eliminate possible soreness associated with the regular exercise program.

2. Start "too easy" rather than "too hard." You can always increase intensity after you determine your reaction to the exercise. You may wish to start out exercising for five or ten minutes and gradually progress to fifteen minutes.

3. If you exercise in a group, you may want to select a daily leader to choose the exercises. This can help motivate group members.

4. Vary the exercises daily but make sure all body parts are exercised.

5. Walk outside the circle if you find you need a slower pace. If the exercises are too difficult, start with what you can handle, but try to exercise continuously, even if it is just walking at first.

6. Use exercises appropriate for your individual needs. The ones listed are merely examples.

*Adapted from C. B. Corbin. "An Exercise Program for Large Groups," *The Physical Educator* 30 (March, 1973):46–47. Used by permission.

4. Consider exercising with others of similar fitness so that routines can be chosen to meet the needs of all group members.

5. Like jogging and other forms of aerobic exercise, it is recommended that you not perform the activity seven days a week. Taking off at least one, and maybe two, days a week will lessen the risk of injury.

6. When an injury does occur, start slowly upon your return to exercise. Compulsive aerobic dancers may create problems for themselves by trying to dance again too soon after an injury. Low impact dance aerobics may be a good way to come back after an injury.

7. Avoid contraindicated exercises that are a part of some prechoreographed routines.

8. Avoid landing or supporting the weight on the balls of the feet. This can result in lower leg problems such as shin splints or calf pain.

9. Avoid competing or trying to perform kicks or other dance steps that are beyond your fitness capabilities. Injuries can result if you overextend yourself to prove you can do what others do.

10. You may want to create your own routines to make sure they meet your own personal needs.

An easy dance aerobic routine is presented as follows to give you an idea of how this popular activity is done. If you choose dance aerobics as part of your exercise program, you can select more difficult routines. In general, dance aerobics is most enjoyable when done to music. However, when you are learning you may want to perform the routine to a drumbeat, a metronome, or a verbal count. Sometimes dance aerobic routines are learned to a count and then done to music.

DANCE AEROBIC SKILLS

To do this routine, you will need to perform the following skills. Learn these skills first, then put them together in a routine. A routine is a series of skills done to music or to a count.

Schottische Step

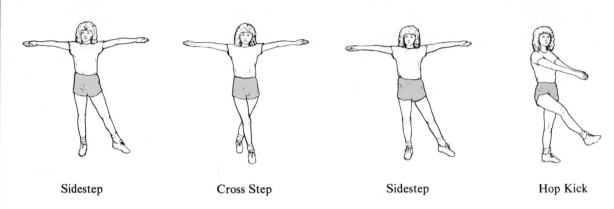

| Sidestep | Cross Step | Sidestep | Hop Kick |

The Schottische step can be done to the right or to the left. On 1, sidestep; on 2, cross-step; on 3, sidestep again; and on 4, hop-kick. Practice doing the step in each direction. Hold your arms out to your sides at shoulder level. After you have learned the Schottische step, you can add a clap of the hands on the hop-kick (count of 4).

Jesse Polka Kick

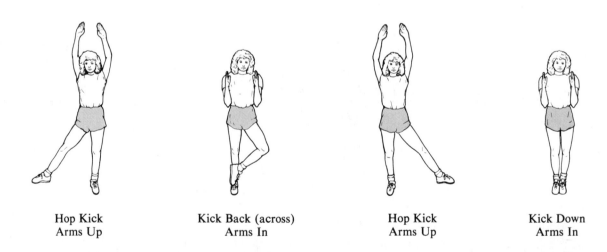

| Hop Kick
Arms Up | Kick Back (across)
Arms In | Hop Kick
Arms Up | Kick Down
Arms In |

The Jesse Polka Kick can be done while standing (hopping) on either foot. On 1, hop-kick; on 2, kick back so that your heel crosses on the opposite side of the hopping leg; on 3, hop-kick again; on 4 kick-down (return to standing position). When you have learned the step well, add the arm movements. On 1, the arms are over the head; on 2, the arms are at shoulder level; on 3 the arms are over the head; on 4, the arms are back at shoulder level. You may want to say "up, in, up, in" as you practice moving your arms. Practice the step while hopping on the right then on the left foot.

Side Lunge

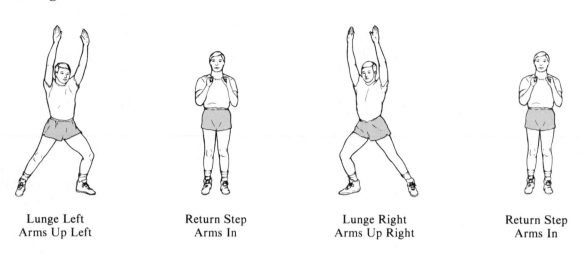

Lunge Left
Arms Up Left

Return Step
Arms In

Lunge Right
Arms Up Right

Return Step
Arms In

On 1, face left and throw your arms up above your head to the left while your right leg steps behind you; on 2, face forward, bring your arms in to your shoulders and return your right foot to the starting position; on 3, face right and throw your arms above your head to the right while your left leg steps behind you; on 4, face forward, bring your arms in to your shoulders and return your left foot to the starting position. As you get better, you can hop rather than step when doing the lunge.

Ponies

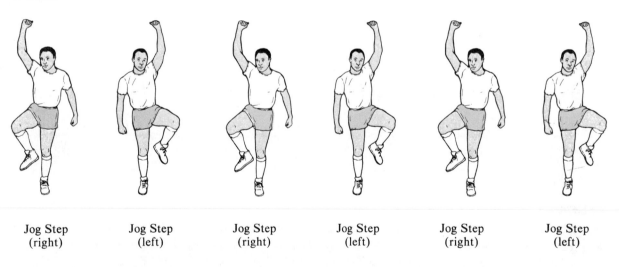

Jog Step
(right)

Jog Step
(left)

Jog Step
(right)

Jog Step
(left)

Jog Step
(right)

Jog Step
(left)

On counts 1 and 2, jog-step right, left, right (three steps in two counts); on counts 3 and 4, jog-step left, right, left (three steps in two counts). Face slightly to the right when doing the three steps starting with the right foot; and face slightly to the left when doing the three steps starting with the left foot. After you learn the step, lift the right arm with the right leg and the left arm with the left leg on each step.

Backward Lunges

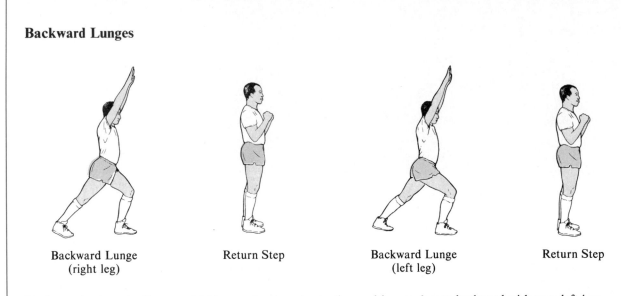

| Backward Lunge (right leg) | Return Step | Backward Lunge (left leg) | Return Step |

On 1, step backward with your right leg; on 2, return to starting position; on 3, step backward with your left leg; and on 4, return to the starting position. When you have learned the step, reach upward and forward with the arms on the back lunges and bring the arms to the shoulders when you return to the starting position.

Twists

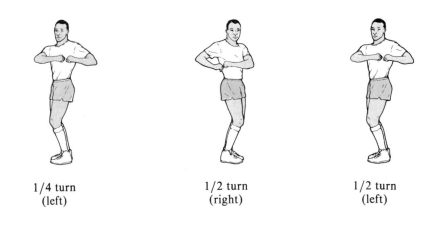

| 1/4 turn (left) | 1/2 turn (right) | 1/2 turn (left) |

On counts 1 and 2, hop in the air and make a 1/4 turn to the left; hold your arms at shoulder height with your elbows up and swing them in the opposite directions of the leg twist. On counts 3 and 4, hop in the air and make a 1/2 turn to the right; turn your arms and shoulders in the opposite direction. Repeat alternating twists to the left and right every two counts. On the last twist, a 1/4 turn is used to get back to the starting position.

DANCE AEROBICS ROUTINE

16 counts	Jog in place. Clap your hands.
32 counts	8 Schottische steps, alternate right and left.
32 counts	8 Jesse polka steps, alternate right and left.
32 counts	8 Schottische steps, alternate right and left.
32 counts	8 Jesse polka steps, alternate right and left.
32 counts	16 Side lunges, alternate left and right.
32 counts	16 Ponies.
32 counts	16 Backward lunges.
32 counts	8 Schottische steps, alternate right and left.
32 counts	8 Jesse polka steps, alternate right and left.
32 counts	16 Twists, alternate right and left.
32 counts	Jog and double-time clap.
32 counts	8 Schottische steps, alternate right and left.
32 counts	8 Jesse polka steps, alternate right and left.

GENERAL SUGGESTIONS FOR USING THIS ROUTINE

1. Warm-up before and cool down after the routine.

2. If the routine is too vigorous for you, jog in place or eliminate arm movements for several counts.

3. Learn the skills first, then try the routine.

4. Learn the foot steps first, then add arm movements.

5. Perform the routine to Lionel Richie's "Dancing on the Ceiling" or another song with four-count rhythm.

Aerobics Dance Routine choreographed by Donna Landers, Arizona State U.

Hiking and Backpacking

Like walking and jogging, hiking is an excellent form of exercise. Hiking has the advantage of an out-of-doors setting, often in a very scenic environment. It does require some equipment, such as a rucksack and good hiking shoes, but highly specialized skills are not needed.

Backpacking is a form of hiking that usually covers longer distances and involves an overnight stay, often in the mountains. When done continuously, backpacking is excellent for building muscular endurance as well as cardiovascular fitness. Like other aerobic activities, it can be helpful in controlling body fatness. In recent years, it has become a popular activity; nearly 11 million American adults report regular involvement in backpacking.

Jogging/Running

The aerobic activity that has rapidly grown in popularity in recent years among both adult men and women is jogging or running. Though there is no "official" distinction between jogging and running, those who run more than a few miles per day, who participate in races, and who are concerned about improving the time in which they run a certain distance often prefer to be called runners rather than joggers. Fifteen to 20 million American adults report that they jog or run on a regular basis.

The major advantage of jogging/running is that it requires only a good pair of running shoes, some inexpensive exercise clothing, and very little skill. With effort, almost anyone can benefit from the activity and even improve performance if that is the goal.

There are some techniques that every jogger should be familiar with before starting a jogging program.

1. *Foot Placement*—The heel of the foot hits the ground first in jogging. Your heel should strike before the rest of your foot (but not vigorously), then you should rock forward and push off with the ball of your foot. Contrary to some opinions, you should *not* jog on your toes. (A flat foot landing can be all right as long as you push off with the ball of your foot.) Your toes should point straight ahead. Your feet should stay under your knees and *not* swing out to the sides as you jog.

2. *Length of Stride*—For efficiency, you should have a relatively long stride. Your stride should be several inches longer than your walking stride. If necessary, you may have to "reach" to lengthen your stride. Most older people find it more efficient to run with a shorter stride.
3. *Arm Movement*—While you jog, you should swing your arms as well as your legs. The arms should be bent at about 90 degrees and should swing freely and alternately from front to back in the direction you are moving, not from side to side. Keep your arms and hands relaxed.
4. *Body Position*—While jogging, you should hold your upper body nearly erect and your head and chest up. There should not be a conscious effort to lean forward as is the case in sprinting or fast running.

Those just beginning a jogging program should pay careful attention to the guidelines for exercise preparation outlined in Concept 4. Of course, for jogging/running to be effective in developing cardiovascular fitness, the heart rate must be elevated above threshold levels and into the target heart rate zone (see Concept 6).

Rope Jumping

Rope jumping is aerobic if done at a slow or moderate pace, but is anaerobic if done vigorously. One study shows that typical exercisers jump very briskly, and for this reason, cannot maintain the jumping continuously. Even those who are highly trained or who jump at a moderate pace find it difficult to continue this exercise long enough to build cardiovascular fitness because of leg fatigue, high heart rate, or loss of interest in the activity. To be most effective, a continuous routine involving several different jump steps should be used in combination with other forms of exercise. For example, rope jumping could be a part of a continuous calisthenic program or a dance aerobic routine.

Sports (Continuous)

As noted earlier in this concept, some activities at least partially anaerobic are considered aerobic if they are done at a continuous pace. Many sports have extended rest periods and do not allow for continuous involvement. Some sports considered to be good aerobic activities when performed continuously are basketball, handball, racquetball, and soccer. (For more information on sports, see Concept 16.)

Swimming and Water Exercises

The most recent exercise polls rank swimming as the first or second most popular form of regular exercise among adults. Most of those who swim for exercise swim laps or do water exercises. When done at a mild or moderate pace, both of these can be aerobic. When done continuously, these are excellent forms of exercise. Another popular but more formal program for this type of exercise is Aquadynamics prepared by the President's Council for Physical Fitness and Sports (see references).

Walking

Approximately one-quarter of all adult Americans report that they walk regularly for exercise. This popularity is probably due to the fact that the activity can be done easily by people of all ages and of all ability levels. Contrary to some opinions, walking can be a very good exercise for developing and maintaining cardiovascular fitness and for helping to control body fatness. Of course, the exercise must be done in the target zone for it to be effective. Some regular walkers do not exercise often enough, hard enough, or long enough to reap optimal health benefits. Those who walk for exercise should walk briskly and continuously. They should follow the guidelines for preparing for exercise outlined in Concept 4, and vary their destination frequently to make the walk more interesting.

Different aerobic activities have different health-related benefits.

The health-related benefits of various aerobic activities are summarized in table 7.2.

THE FACTS ABOUT ANAEROBIC EXERCISE

Anaerobic exercise is useful for building cardiovascular and other aspects of physical fitness.

The advantages and disadvantages of anaerobic exercise are outlined in Concept 6 (table 6.1). Anaerobic exercise is especially useful for building cardiovascular fitness. The types of health-related fitness that can be developed into anaerobic exercise programs are rated in table 7.3.

TABLE 7.2 Achieving Fitness through Aerobic Exercise

Program Type	Cardiovascular Fitness	Strength and Muscular Endurance	Flexibility	Body and Fat Control	Skill-Related Fitness	Enjoyment or Fun[1]
Bicycling	***	**	*	***	*	**
Circuit Overload Training	**	***	*	**	*	**
Cooper's Aerobics	***	*	*	***	*	**
Continuous Calisthenics	***	**	***	***	*	**
Cross-Country Skiing	***	**	*	***	**	**
Dance Aerobics	***	**	***	***	*	**
Hiking and Backpacking	**	**	*	**	*	**
Jogging/Running	***	*	*	***	—	**
Rope Jumping	**	*	—	**	*	*
Swimming and Water Exercises	**	**	**	**	**	**
Walking	**	*	*	**	*	**

***Very Good   **Good   *Minimum   —Low

[1]Enjoyment and fun are relative, and for this reason, it is impossible to classify activities accurately. However, for the average person, some activities seem to be more enjoyable than others. The above listed classifications reflect the opinions of the typical person. *Any of the activities listed above can be fun and enjoyable for a given person in the right circumstances.*

TABLE 7.3 Achieving Fitness through Anaerobic Exercise

Program Type	Cardiovascular Fitness	Strength and Muscular Endurance	Flexibility	Body and Fat Control	Skill-Related Fitness	Enjoyment or Fun[1]
Fartlek or "Speed Play"	***	**	—	***	—	*
Interval Training	***	**	—	***	—	*

***Very Good   **Good   *Minimum   —Low

[1]Enjoyment and fun are relative and for this reason it is impossible to classify activities accurately. However, for the average person some activities seem to be more enjoyable than others. The above listed classifications reflect the opinions of the typical person. *Any of the activities listed can be fun and enjoyable for a given person in the right circumstances.*

POPULAR ANAEROBIC EXERCISE PROGRAMS

Fartlek or "Speed Play"

Fartlek is a Swedish word for speed play. This exercise was developed in Scandinavia where pinewood paths follow curves of lakes, up and down many hills, where the scenery takes your mind off the task at hand. The idea is to get away from the regimen of running on a track and to enjoy the woods, lakes, and mountains. Because of the terrain, the pace is never constant. The uphill path requires a slow pace, while a straight stretch or downhill trail allows for speed. In the "speed play," or fartlek system, you run easily for a time, at a steady hard speed for a while, walk rapidly following that, alternate short sprints with walking, go full speed uphill and perhaps at a fast pace for a while.

You can plan your own speed play program using your own course, which may include both uphill and downhill running with other variations. A sample program of moderate intensity is shown in table 7.4.

TABLE 7.4 A Sample Speed Play Program*

1. Jog easily for 3 minutes.
2. Perform brisk calisthenics—no rest between exercises.
   a. Trunk stretch—With the feet spread, reach through the legs as far as possible. Hold for 8 seconds. Repeat 3 times.
   b. Do 5 to 10 bent-knee sit-ups. (See page 81.)
   c. Run in place for 50 steps.
   d. Do 5 to 10 push-ups or modified push-ups. (See page 80.)
   e. Do 10 side leg raises with each leg. (See page 82.)
3. Run 200 yards at 3/4 speed. Run on grassy area if possible.
4. Walk 200 yards.
5. Repeat 3 and 4.
6. Jog for 2 minutes.
7. Run 100 yards at 3/4 speed.
8. Walk 100 yards.
9. Repeat 7 and 8.
10. Jog for 2 minutes.

*If this *sample* program is too vigorous for your current level of fitness, try walking instead of jogging or running.

Interval Training Program

An interval training program involves repeated fast anaerobic running or swimming for short periods of time, separated by measured intervals of slow recovery jogging or swimming. (Developed by Gerschler of Germany, the stress of anaerobic running raises the heart rate to near maximal from which it drops to a moderate level during recovery.) This program controls distance, pace, number of reptitions, and recovery interval, allowing for a wide variety of programs of various intensities. Guidelines are presented in Concept 6 (table 6.3).

Research suggests that short interval workouts should use maximum speed with rest intervals lasting from ten seconds to two minutes. These should be repeated eight to thirty times. Interval training having long intervals use 90 to 100 percent speed with rest intervals lasting from three to fifteen minutes. These should be repeated four to fifteen times. A sample short interval program and a sample long interval running program are presented in table 7.5. Using the guidelines in Concept 6, you can plan your own interval training program.

TABLE 7.5 Sample Interval Training Program (Moderate Intensity)

Short Intervals	Long Intervals
1. Do a flexibility and cardiovascular warm-up (see Concept 4).	1. Do a flexibility and cardiovascular warm-up (see Concept 4).
2. Run at 100% speed for 10 seconds (approximately 70 to 100 yards).	2. Run at 90% speed for one minute (approximately 300 to 500 yards).
3. Rest for 10 seconds by walking slowly.	3. Rest for 4 minutes by walking slowly.
4. Alternately repeat steps 2 and 3 until 20 runs have been completed.	4. Alternately repeat steps 2 and 3 until 5 runs have been completed.

REFERENCES

*Burkett, L. N. and Darst, P. W. *Cycling.* Glenview, Il., Scott Foresman, 1987.

Clement, D. B. "A Survey of Overuse Running Injuries." *Physician and Sportsmedicine* 9(1981):47.

*Cooper, K. H. *The Aerobics Program for Total Well-Being.* New York: M. Evans, 1982.

Cooper, K. H. *Running Without Fear.* New York: M. Evans, 1985.

Corbin, C. B., and R. Lindsey. *Fitness for Life.* 2d ed. Glenview, IL: Scott, Foresman and Co., 1985.

Corbin, C. B. "Profiling for Flexibility." In *Clinics in Sports Medicine: Profiling,* edited by J. Nicholas and J. Herschberger. Philadelphia: W. B. Saunders Co., 1984.

Corbin, C. B., and R. Lindsey. *The Ultimate Fitness Book.* New York: Leisure Press, 1984.

*Corbin, D. E. *Jogging.* Glenview, Il., Scott Foresman and Company, 1987.

Cureton, T. K. *Physical Fitness and Dynamic Health.* New York: Dial Press, 1965.

Fitness Canada. *Canada Fitness Survey—Highlights.* Ottawa, Ontario, Canada: Government of Canada, 1983.

*Fox, E., D. Matthews, and J. Bairstow. *Interval Training for Lifetime Fitness.* New York: Dial Press, 1980.

Garrick, J. G., et al. "The Epidemiology of Aerobic Dance," *American Journal of Sports Medicine* 14(1986):67.

Getchell, B., and P. Cleary. "The Caloric Costs of Rope Skipping and Running." *Physician and Sportsmedicine* 8(1980):56.

Hempel, L. S., and C. L. Wells. "Cardiorespiratory Cost of the Nautilus Express Circuit." *Physician and Sportsmedicine* 13(1985):83.

Hooper, P. L. "Aerobic Dance Program Improves Cardiovascular Fitness in Men." *Physician and Sportsmedicine* 12(1984):132.

Kissele, J. and K. Nazzeo. *Aerobic Dance: A Way to Fitness.* Englewood, CO, Morton Publishing Co. 1983.

Koszuta, L. E. "Low Impact Aerobics: Better Than Traditional Aerobic Dance?" *Physician and Sportsmedicine* 14(1986):156.

Mahurin, J., and T. P. Martin. "Anaerobic Threshold: A Trainable Component of CV Fitness." *Motor Skills: Theory Into Practice* 6(1982):41.

Nash, J. B. *Philosophy of Recreation and Leisure.* Dubuque, IA: Wm. C. Brown Publishers, 1960.

O'Shea, J. P., C. Novak, and F. Gaulard. "Bicycle Interval Training for Cardiovascular Fitness." *Physician and Sportsmedicine* 10(1982):156.

Powell, K. E., et al. "An Epidemiological Perspective on the Cause of Running Injuries." *Physician and Sportsmedicine.* 14(1986):100.

*President's Council on Physical Fitness and Sports. *Aquadynamics.* Washington, D.C.: U.S. Government Printing Office, publication no. 040–000–00360–6. Copies available from Superintendent of Documents.

Richie, D. H. "Aerobic Dance Injuries: A Retrospective Study of Instructors and Participants." *Physician and Sportsmedicine* 13(1985):130.

*Schultz, P. "Walking for Fitness: Slow but Sure." *Physician and Sportsmedicine* 8(1980):24.

Snyder, E. E., and E. Spreitzer. "Adult Perceptions of Physical Education in the Schools and Community Sports Programs for Youth." *The Physical Educator* 40(1983):88.

Vickery, S. R., K. J. Cureton, and J. L. Langstaff. "Heart Rate and Energy Expenditure during Aqua Dynamics." *Physician and Sportsmedicine* 17(1983):67.

*Wilmore, J. H. *Sensible Fitness.* Champaign, IL: Human Kinetics, 1986.

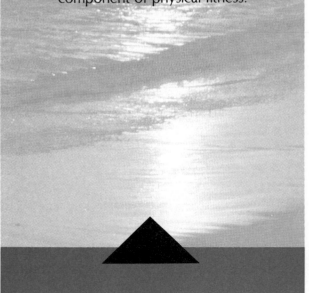

8

STRENGTH

CONCEPT 8

Strength is an important health-related component of physical fitness.

INTRODUCTION

Strength is measured by the amount of force you can produce with a single maximal effort. You need strength to increase work capacity; to decrease the chance of injury; to prevent low back pain, poor posture, and other hypokinetic diseases; to improve athletic performance; and perhaps to save life or property in an emergency situation.

TERMS

Anabolic Steroid—A synthetic hormone similar to the male sex hormone testosterone.

Antagonistic Muscles—The muscles that have the opposite action from those that are contracting (agonists); normally, antagonists reflexly relax when agonists contract.

Concentric Contraction—An isotonic muscle contraction in which the muscle gets shorter as it contracts, such as when a joint is "bent" and two body parts move closer together. An example is the biceps muscle contraction that occurs when pulling up on a chinning bar.

"Definition" of Muscle—The detailed external appearance of a muscle.

Eccentric Contraction—"Negative exercise." An isotonic muscle contraction in which the muscle gets longer as it contracts; that is, when a weight is gradually lowered and the contracting muscle gets longer as it gives up tension. Lowering the body from a pull-up on a chinning bar is an example of eccentric contraction of the biceps muscle.

Hypertrophy—Increase in the size of muscles as the result of strength training; increase in bulk.

Isokinetic Exercise—Isotonic concentric exercises done with a machine that regulates movement velocity and resistance.

Isometric Contraction—A type of muscle contraction in which the muscle remains the same length. Isometric exercises are those in which no movement takes place while a force is exerted against an immovable object (also known as "static contraction").

Isotonic Contraction—Type of muscle contraction in which the muscle changes length, either shortening (concentrically) or lengthening (eccentrically). Isotonic exercises are those in which a resistance is raised and then lowered, as in weight training and calisthenics (also called "dynamic" or "phasic").

Plyometrics—An isometric or concentric isotonic muscle contraction performed after a prestretch or eccentric contraction of a muscle.

61

PRE—Progressive resistance exercise, such as those done with free weights or weight machines.

Sticking Point—The point in the range of motion where the weight cannot be lifted any farther without extreme effort or assistance; the weakest point in the movement.

THE FACTS

There are three types of muscle tissue.

The three types of muscle tissue—smooth, cardiac, and skeletal—have different structures and functions. Smooth muscle tissue consists of long spindle-shaped fibers; each fiber usually contains only one nucleus. The fibers are involuntary and are located in the walls of the esophagus, stomach, and intestines where they function to move food and waste products through the digestive tract. Cardiac muscle tissue is also involuntary, and as its name implies, it is found only in the heart. Skeletal muscle tissues consist of long, cylindrical, multinucleated fibers. They provide the force needed to move the skeletal system and may be controlled voluntarily. Skeletal muscles are made up of slow (red), intermediate, and fast (white) twitch fibers.

Some experts suggest that strength training using high resistance exercises tends to selectively develop fast twitch *muscle fibers.*

Fast twitch fibers generate greater tension than slow twitch fibers, but they fatigue more quickly. They primarily use anaerobic metabolism. These fibers are particularly suited to fast, high-force activities such as explosive weight lifting movements, sprinting, and jumping.

An example of fast-twitch muscle fiber in animals is the white meat in the flying muscles of a chicken. The chicken is heavy and must exert a powerful force to fly a few feet up to a perch. A wild duck that flies for hundreds of miles has dark meat (slow twitch fibers) in the flying muscles for better endurance.

Strength is best developed by applying the "overload principle" so that exercise is done with a near maximum resistance with only a few repetitions.

When your primary concern is developing the ability to exert a large force with your muscles, then you should train for "pure" strength. Strength training requires an overload in the amount of the resistance, while muscular endurance training (see Concept 10) requires an overload in the number of repetitions. Therefore, according to the law of specificity, when designing a program for strength development, high resistance and low repetitions at a moderately slow speed should be used for maximum effectiveness.

There is a threshold of training and a target zone for muscular strength development.

Experts generally agree that in **progressive resistance exercise (PRE)** using a maximum load (resistance) for three to ten repetitions in one to three sets three or four times per week will develop strength. Experts do *not* agree, however, on the ideal combination of repetitions, sets, and speed.

Table 8.1 compares thresholds and target zones of **isometrics, isotonics,** and **isokinetics** that might be

TABLE 8.1 Strength Threshold of Training and Fitness Target Zones for Beginners

	Threshold of Training			Target Zone		
	Isometrics	Isotonics	Isokinetics	Isometrics	Isotonics	Isokinetics
Frequency	3 days a week	3 days a week	3 days a week	5 days a week	Every other day	Every other day
Intensity	Use 65–70% of maximum contraction	First set: lift 50% of maximum; second set: lift 75% of maximum, third set: lift 100%	90% of maximum effort at set speed	Maximum contractions	Maximum resistance (for number of repetitions) on every set	Maximum effort at set speed
Time	1 set 1 repetition held for 2–5 seconds Repeat once a day	3 sets 3 repetitions per set	2 sets 3 repetitions lasting 3–4 seconds (30–60° per second)	1 set 6 repetitions, held 6–8 seconds (or 2 sets of 3 repetitions each); rest 30 seconds between repetitions	3 sets 3–10 repetitions	3–5 sets 3–10 repetitions lasting 1–2 seconds (70–120° per second)

used by beginners who desire to improve pure strength. Note, however, if you are training for a specific skill, these target zones may not be appropriate (refer to the principle regarding specificity). If you are an advanced strength trainer, a body builder, or a competitive weight lifter, you will need special training programs to excel at these activities.

A strength training program should apply the "principle of specificity" by closely resembling the activity for which the strength is needed.

Specificity of training will enhance performance. If you want your arms to be stronger so you can carry heavy loads, or if you want finger strength to grip a heavy bowling ball, much of your strength exercise should be done isometrically, using the arm muscles the way you use them to carry loads or using the fingers the same way you hold a bowling ball. On the other hand, if the task for which you are training is performed isotonically, your strength program should be primarily isotonic use of the muscles involved in that skill.

If you are training for a particular skill that requires explosive power, such as in throwing, striking, kicking, or jumping, your strength exercises should be done with less resistance and greater speed. If you are training for a skill that uses both **concentric** and **ec-** **centric contractions** or is **plyometric,** you should perform strength exercises using these characteristics.

If you are not training for a specific skill, but merely wish to develop pure strength, then consider the advantages and disadvantages of isometrics, isotonics, and isokinetics listed in table 8.2. You may wish to use a variety of methods to avoid boredom.

Progressive resistance exercise (PRE) is the most effective type of strength training program.

Muscles adapt only to the load placed upon them; therefore, in order to continue increasing strength, you must progressively increase the stress on the muscle as it adapts to each new load. Muscle groups differ in their strength potential, so each muscle group must have an individualized program (target zone). For example, the legs and trunk can usually lift greater loads than the arms.

There are several good PRE programs for strength development, each having advantages and disadvantages.

Progressive resistance exercise can be performed in properly designed weight-training programs using free weights, constant resistance weight machines, variable (accommodating) resistance weight machines, pulleys

TABLE 8.2 Advantages and Disadvantages of Isometric, Isotonic, and Isokinetic Exercises

Isometrics	Isotonics	Isokinetics
1. Can be done in small area.	1. Develops more strength than isometrics.	1. Not good to train specifically for athletic skill. Cannot accelerate against resistance.
2. No equipment needed.	2. May aid coordination.	
3. No feedback, so lack of motivation is a problem.	3. Faster recovery from fatigue.	2. Equal to isotonics for strength.
4. Good in rehabilitation where no joint movement is desired.	4. Strengthens throughout range of motion.	3. Provides maximum resistance at all angles in the range of motion.
5. Builds strength only at the joint angle practiced.	5. Produces greater hypertrophy.	4. Less injury and soreness than isotonics.
6. Causes very little soreness.	6. Progress easy to follow.	5. Machines are very expensive; simple devices less expensive.
7. Easy to maintain strength.	7. More soreness and injury.	6. Good for rehabilitation and testing.
8. Lacks movement so does not train coordination.	8. If equipment is used, it is more expensive than isometrics.	7. Some machines and devices do not control speed and resistance accurately throughout range of motion.
9. May be hazardous for those with high blood pressure.	9. Strength occurs at weakest point in range of motion, so entire range not trained equally.	8. Only resists concentric contractions.

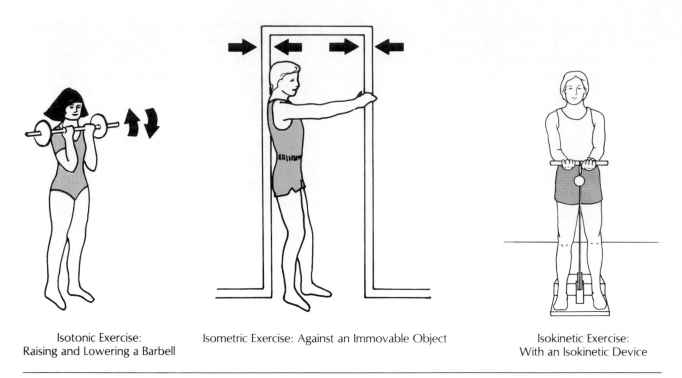

Isotonic Exercise:
Raising and Lowering a Barbell

Isometric Exercise: Against an Immovable Object

Isokinetic Exercise:
With an Isokinetic Device

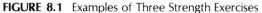

FIGURE 8.1 Examples of Three Strength Exercises

and controlled velocity isokinetic dynamometers, isometric exercises, and calisthenics. (See figure 8.1.) Concept 10 describes some sample exercises and compares some of these programs. Weight training is considered the fastest and best method of improving strength. However, properly designed calisthenics are adequate for developing strength in most people.

The most popular form of strength exercise utilizes isotonic contractions of the muscles.

As can be deduced from table 8.2, isotonic exercise refers to such activities as weight lifting, calisthenics, and pulley weights, in which the muscles alternately shorten concentrically and lengthen eccentrically. Typically, the stress on the muscle in these types of exercises varies with speed, joint position, and muscle length. Thus, the muscle may work harder at the beginning of a lift than it does near the end of the range of motion or as the weight is lowered.

Isokinetics, plyometrics, and "negative" exercises are special forms of isotonic exercise. These are discussed later in this concept.

Isometric strength exercises have advantages and disadvantages.

Isometric exercises are effective for developing strength, require no equipment and only minimal space. They have been found to be quite useful for some athletes, such as wrestlers and gymnasts, and work especially well for people in the early stages of some rehabilitation programs. Research has shown that isotonic

training can be enhanced significantly by using isometrics at the **sticking points** during isotonic lifts.

However, isometric exercises do not develop as much strength as isotonic and isokinetic exercises, nor do muscles hypertrophy as much. They work the muscle only at the angle of joint used in the exercise. Isometrics may be dangerous for those with high blood pressure or cardiovascular disease. (See table 8.2 for a comparison with other types of exercise.)

Isokinetic exercises are effective for developing strength.

Isokinetic exercises are isotonic-concentric muscle contractions performed on devices such as the Apollo, Exer-Genie, and Mini-Gym, or on electromechanical dynamometers, such as the Cybex II. These machines keep the velocity of the movement constant and match their resistance to the effort of the performer, permitting maximal tension to be exerted throughout the range of motion. For example, on the Cybex II, speeds may be preset from 0 to 300 degrees per second. This rate-limiting mechanism prevents the performer from moving faster no matter how much force is exerted.

Thus, isokinetic devices attempt to overcome the basic weakness of isotonics. On the other hand, these devices do not permit acceleration, so it is not possible to train specifically for sports skills, such as throwing or kicking, in which the limb is accelerated while applying maximum force. Some devices are more successful than others in accurately controlling the speed and resistance.

Isokinetic exercise has the advantage of being safer than most other forms of exercise and may be better for developing power (see Concept 9). It is not better for developing pure strength however. More research is needed to determine the best training regimen for isokinetic exercise.

Variable resistance machines have some advantages over constant resistance machines and free weights.

Some machines, such as Nautilus and Universal, offer what is called variable or accommodating resistance. The Nautilus, for example, uses a cam to adapt the resistance as the performer moves through the range of motion. The Universal Trainer uses a rolling pivot to do the same thing. These adaptations attempt to compensate for the weakness in isotonic constant resistance exercises, but they are only partially successful in adapting to the shape, sizes, and torque of individual human bodies. There is no evidence that variable resistance machines develop more strength than other devices, although they may strengthen a muscle through more of its range.

Free weights have some advantages and some disadvantages when compared to other methods of strength development.

Free weights include barbells and dumbbells as well as homemade weights, such as sandbags or bottles filled with water. These are compared with weight machines (for example, Nautilus, Universal, Marcy, Hydra-Gym, Dynacam, and Paramount) in table 8.3.

"Negative" exercise has no advantage over other types of exercise for strength development.

Contrary to the claims of some enthusiasts, there does not seem to be any difference between eccentric (negative) exercise, and concentric (positive) exercise (see definitions) in terms of their effectiveness in developing strength. Eccentric exercise is performed more comfortably even though more weight can be handled. It is particularly useful in rehabilitation settings, but has a tendency to cause more muscle soreness. This type of exercise also requires the assistance of another person or the use of a very large, expensive machine (except in calisthenics).

Eccentric contractions are combined with concentric contractions in most everyday activities and sports skills utilizing strength. For example, if you lift something you also lower it. Thus, to apply the law of specificity, some of the strength training for those activities should include both types of contractions.

TABLE 8.3 Advantages and Disadvantages of Free Weights and Weight Machines

Free Weights	Weight Machines
1. Requires balance and coordination; uses more muscle for stabilization.	1. Other body parts are stabilized; easier to isolate particular muscle group.
2. Truer to real-life situation, so skills transfer to daily life.	2. Controlled path of weight not true to life.
3. Creates more possibility of injury.	3. Safer because weight cannot fall on participant.
4. Requires spotters for safety.	4. No spotters required.
5. Takes more time to change weights.	5. Easy and quick to change weights.
6. Unlimited number of exercises possible.	6. Restricted to range and angle of movement permitted by the machine.
7. Less expensive.	7. Expensive; need to go to club if cannot afford; need more than one machine to get variety.
8. Loose equipment clutters area and may get lost or stolen.	8. Machines are stationary but occupy large space.

Plyometrics may be useful in athletic training for certain sports events.

A quick prestretch, or eccentric contraction of a muscle, immediately followed by an isometric or concentric contraction can produce more power. This has been called "preexertion countermovement" or "wind up" or "plyometrics." Russian Olympic coaches have pioneered in this area, developing drills for their athletes. Track and field athletes may, for example, perform a hopping drill for thirty to one hundred meters. This is called "depth jumping," "drop jumping," or "bounce loading." As the body lands, some of the major leg muscles lengthen in an eccentric contraction then follow immediately with a strong concentric contraction as the legs push off for the next jump or stride. The prestretch of the muscle during landing adds an elastic recoil that provides extra force to the push-off.

Plyometrics are used to apply the specificity principle to training for certain skills. Because eccentric exercise tends to result in more muscular soreness, it would be wise to proceed slowly with this type of training.

The "double progressive system" is an effective variation of the PRE system.

The double progressive system of progression periodically adjusts both the resistance and the number of repetitions. For example, you may begin with three repetitions for the arms. Once a week, you add one repetition. When you have progressed to ten repetitions, increase the arm weight by five pounds. Decrease the repetitions to three and begin the progression again.

Strength capacity differs with gender and age.

Because of differences in hormones and muscle mass, women have only about two-thirds of the strength of men. Women are as strong as men, however, when strength is expressed per unit of cross section of muscles. Maximum strength is usually reached in the twenties then declines with age. Regardless of age, strength can be improved.

Training for bulk (hypertrophy) and "definition" may differ from strength training.

Most body builders use three to seven sets of ten to fifteen repetitions, rather than the three sets of three to ten repetitions recommended for most weight trainers. Sometimes, "definition" is difficult to obtain because it is obscured by fat. It should be noted that those with the largest looking muscles are not always the strongest.

Strength developed in one limb can be transferred to another unexercised limb.

When the right arm is trained with biceps curls until its strength increases, the unexercised left arm will also increase in strength though not as much as the exercised arm. This phenomenon is called "transfer of training," "bilateral transfer," or "cross-education." The reason for this is not fully understood, but the phenomenon is sometimes applied to rehabilitation to prevent a limb from atrophying.

The amount of force you can exert during a strength test depends upon the speed of contraction, muscle length, warm-up, and other muscle-related factors.

If you want to score high on a strength test, consider some of the "secrets of success" used by experienced lifters and proven by research. Generally, a muscle exerts the least force as it becomes shorter (toward the end of a movement), and can exert more force during an isometric contraction than when it is shortening. The muscle exerts the most force when it is lengthening (lowering a weight). If a muscle is placed on a slight stretch immediately before it contracts, it can exert more force than it could if it started from a resting length.

Speed of contraction affects the amount of force that can be exerted. A slow contraction can lift a heavier weight than a fast contraction. If muscles are warmed up before lifting, more force can be exerted and heavier loads lifted.

There is a proper way to perform strength exercises.

The following are some guidelines for safe and effective strength training:

1. Make sure you are well prepared to begin. (See Concept 4 for details.)
2. To ensure overall development, include all body parts and balance the strength of **antagonists.** For example, the ratio of quadriceps strength to hamstring strength should be 60:40. Exercise large muscles before small muscles.
3. When beginning a weight program, start with weights that are too light so you can learn proper technique and avoid soreness and injury. Novices might, for example, start with one-fourth of their body weight for the military press; ten pounds less than the press for the curl; ten pounds more than the press for the bench press; and half of the body weight for back and leg exercises.
4. Progress gradually. For example, use one set of three repetitions with a light weight to begin; add two repetitions when it gets easy, then another, until you reach ten repetitions; then drop back to three repetitions and add a second set. Repeat until you can do three sets. After this, the double progressive system (previously described) can be used, increasing the weight and the repetitions.
5. Athletes should train muscles the way they will be used in their skill, employing similar patterns, range of motion, and speed (the principle of specificity). This applies to anyone who knows the precise skill for which he or she is training.
6. Sports participants should include some eccentric training, such as plyometrics, to prevent injury to decelerating muscles during sports events and to develop power in accelerating muscles.
7. Choose an exercise sequence that alternates muscle groups so muscles have a rest period before being used in another exercise.
8. Beginning weight trainers should probably train for endurance initially (see Concept 9). For example, a reasonable goal might be ten to fifteen repetitions at 50 to 70 percent of the maximum amount of weight they can lift for one repetition.
9. When circuit training, move from one station to another with no waste of time, allowing about forty-five seconds of rest between stations.

10. Isometric training should be done at several joint angles.
11. To avoid boredom especially when you reach a plateau or sticking point, use such motivating techniques as music, record keeping, partners, competition, and variation in routine.
12. To prevent injury:
    a. Warm up ten minutes before the workout and stay warm during the workout.
    b. Do not hold your breath while lifting. This may cause blackout or hernia.
    c. Avoid hyperventilation before lifting a weight.
    d. Avoid dangerous or high-risk exercises.
    e. Progress slowly.
    f. Use good shoes with good traction.
    g. Avoid arching your back. Keep the pelvis tipped backward.
    h. Keep the weight close to the body.
    i. Do not lift from a stoop.
    j. Do not let the hips come up before your upper body when lifting from the floor.
    k. For bent-over rowing, put the head on a table and bend the knees.
    l. Stay in a squat as short a time as possible and do not do a full squat.
    m. Be sure collars are on free weights tightly.
    n. Use a moderately slow, continuous, controlled movement and hold the final position a few seconds.
    o. Do not pause between repetitions.
    p. Try to keep a definite rhythm.
    q. Do not allow the weights to drop or bang.
    r. Do not train without medical supervision if you have a hernia, high blood pressure, fever, infection, recent surgery, or heart disease.
    s. Use chalk or a towel to keep hands dry when handling weights.
13. To avoid overtraining, take a break by resting or choosing some other activity after eight to ten weeks. Also, try varying your training days so one is light (75 to 80 percent) one is medium (85 to 90 percent) and one is heavy (100 percent).
14. Beginners should not attempt to use advanced techniques. After training for several months, you may wish to experiment with such things as supersets, split routines, and plateau systems used by advanced trainers.

There are many fallacies, myths, and superstitions associated with strength training.

Some common misconceptions about strength training have been refuted.

1. It is *not* true that you will become "muscle-bound" and lose flexibility just because you do strength training. This could happen only if you train improperly.
2. It is *not* true that women will become masculine looking if they develop strength. Contrary to popular belief, most women will not be able to develop large and bulky muscles as a result of strength training, neither will their muscles be as well defined.

    As a group, females lack muscle mass and testosterone, the hormone necessary for developing muscle bulk. The greater percentage of fat in most women prevents the muscle definition possible in leaner men. Those females who have a relatively large muscle mass without training will most likely be able to develop bulk further through training.
3. Strength training does *not* make you move more slowly or make you more uncoordinated. Up to a point, increased strength may help to increase speed.
4. The expression "no pain, no gain" is a fallacy. It may be helpful to strive for a burning sensation in the muscle, but this is not painful. If it hurts, you are probably harming yourself.
5. Supplements of wheat germ, liver, brewer's yeast, yogurt, blackstrap molasses, protein, and vitamins do *not* benefit muscle mass or strength building. You do need a balanced diet.
6. **Anabolic steroids** should *not* be used. They produce such side effects as liver damage or liver cancer and endocrine disturbances. Also, among males, side effects include testicular atrophy and impotency. Among females, masculine characteristics may develop as well as changes in the reproductive system.
7. Strength training is *not* effective for cardiovascular fitness, nor for flexibility or weight loss. Muscles will get firmer, and desirable changes may occur in girth, but other aspects of fitness are specific and so require specific training.
8. It does *not* require two hours to complete a workout in weight training—unless you are a competitive lifter or body builder. If you are training for athletics, you will need forty-five to ninety minutes; the beginner or the person training for fitness or recreation can complete a circuit in thirty to forty-five minutes.

Evaluating Isotonic Strength

Tests	Point Value

I. 1. One bent-knee push-up, keeping your body straight and rigid.   1

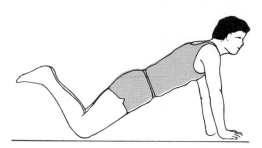

2. One straight-leg push-up, keeping your body rigid.   3

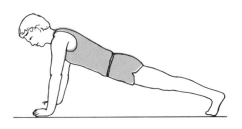

3. One straight-leg push-up, keeping your body rigid and your feet on the bench.   5

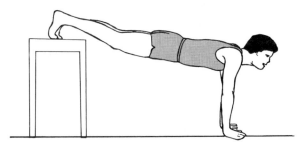

4. Same as no. 2, except have partner do a push-up on back of your shoulders at the same time.   7

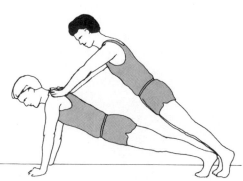

Tests	Point Value

5. Same as no. 2, except use only one arm.   10

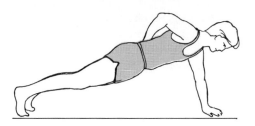

II. 1. a. Hang from a bar placed at the height of the lower end of your sternum.   1
    b. Body should be inclined at a forty-five degree angle.
    c. Have partner brace your feet.
    d. Pull up until your chin or chest touches the bar.

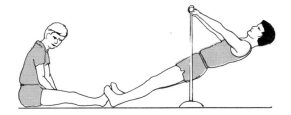

2. a. Stand on a chair and assume a position with palms facing body, elbows bent, and chin over bar.   3
    b. Remove chair.
    c. Hang in this position for ten seconds.

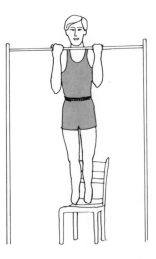

Tests	Point Value	Tests	Point Value

3. Perform one regulation chin-up (pull-up) from a hanging position with palms facing your body.   5

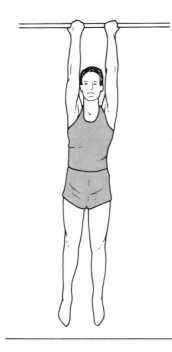

5. Climb a rope to a height of ten feet above your head, using arms only (no leg use).   10

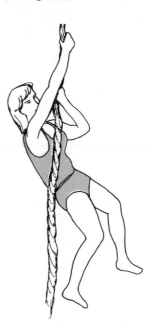

4. Same as no. 3, except pull up while two bleach bottles filled with water are suspended on the ends of a short rope across the back of your neck.   7

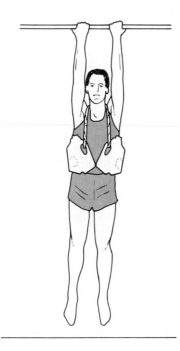

III. Squat on one leg and pick up a paper cup with one hand; return to a stand. Keep the back erect and maintain balance.
    1. Use one leg only.   4
    2. Use right leg only, then use left only.   8

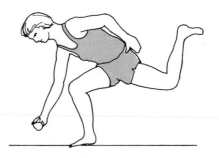

Evaluating Isotonic Strength *Continued*

Tests	Point Value
IV. Lie prone. Lift your upper trunk until the sternum leaves the floor (do not lift higher and arch the lower back) Keep your feet on the floor.	
1. Place the hands under the thighs.	3

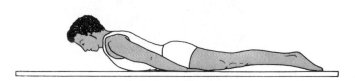

    2. Clasp the hands behind the neck.   6

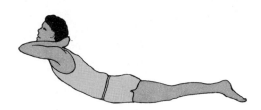

    3. Extend both arms forward and clamp them against the ears.   9

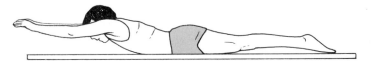

Evaluating Isometric Strength

1. *Grip Strength*
   Adjust a hand dynamometer to fit your hand size. Squeeze it as hard as possible. You may bend or straighten the arm, but do not touch the body with your hand, elbow, or arm. Perform with both right and left hands.
2. *Leg Strength*
   Use the belt provided and place it low over the hips; attach the belt to the handle. Hold the bar with both hands in the center of the handle, palms down, so it rests at the level of the hip joint. Place the feet parallel, six inches apart, with the chain centered between them. Knees should be bent 115 to 124 degrees. The arms and the back should be kept straight, the head erect, and the chest up. Pull as hard as possible on the chain by trying to straighten the legs.
3. *Back Strength*
   Stand as in no. 2 except keep the legs straight. Place hands on front of thighs. Adjust chain length so handle is just below finger tips. Bend at hips, keep head up and eyes straight ahead; grasp bars at ends of handles, one palm forward and one palm backward. Lift steadily, pulling as hard as possible on the chain as you roll your shoulders back.
4. When not being tested, perform the isometric strength exercises in Concept 10 or try to squeeze and indent a new tennis ball.

CHART 8A.1 Isotonic Strength *Rating Scale* (Men)

	Age				
Classification	17–26	27–39	40–49	50–59	60+
High Performance Zone	35+	33+	31+	29+	27+
Good Fitness Zone	30–34	28–32	26–30	24–28	23–26
Marginal Zone	25–29	23–27	21–25	19–23	17–21
Low Zone	<25	<23	<21	<19	<17

CHART 8A.2 Isotonic Strength *Rating Scale* (Women)

	Age				
Classification	17–26	27–39	40–49	50–59	60+
High Performance Zone	30+	29+	27+	25+	23+
Good Fitness Zone	26–30	25–28	24–26	22–24	20–22
Marginal Zone	20–25	19–24	18–23	17–21	15–19
Low Zone	<20	<19	<18	<17	<15

CHART 8B.1 Isometric Strength *Rating Scales*

Classification	Left Grip	Right Grip	Back Strength	Leg Strength	Total Score	Strength per/lb./wgt.
Strength *Rating Scale* for Men (Pounds)						
High Performance Zone	125+	135+	425+	450+	1150+	6.50+
Good Fitness Zone	100–124	110–134	300–424	375–449	885–1149	5.10–6.49
Marginal Zone	90–99	95–109	225–229	325–374	735–884	4.90–5.09
Low Zone	<90	<95	<225	<325	<735	<4.90

Classification	Left Grip	Right Grip	Back Strength	Leg Strength	Total Score	Strength per/lb./wgt.
Strength *Rating Scale* for Women (Pounds)						
High Performance Zone	75+	85+	235+	255+	660+	5.25+
Good Fitness Zone	60–74	70–84	175–234	185–254	490–659	4.00–5.24
Marginal Zone	45–59	50–69	100–174	120–184	315–489	2.75–3.99
Low Zone	<45	<50	<100	<120	<315	<2.75

These rating charts are suitable for use by young adults between 18 and 30 years of age. After 30, an adjustment of 0.5 of 1 percent per year is appropriate because some loss of muscle tissue typically occurs as you grow older.

REFERENCES

Basmajian, J. V. *Therapeutic Exercise*. Baltimore: Williams and Wilkins, 1984.

Buck, J. A., L. R. Amundsen, and D. H. Nielsen. "Systolic Blood Pressure Response during Isometric Contractions of Large and Small Muscle Groups." *Medicine and Science in Sports and Exercise* 12(1980):145.

Clark, D. H. "Sex Differences in Strength and Fatigue." *Research Quarterly for Exercise and Sport* 57(June 1986):144

*Cook, Brian, and G. W. Stewart. *Get Strong*. Ganges, B. C., Canada: 3S Fitness Group, 1981.

Corbin, C., and K. Lindsey. *The Ultimate Fitness Book*. New York: Leisure Press, 1984.

Coyle, E. F., et al. "Specificity of Power Improvements through Slow and Fast Isokinetic Training." *Journal of Applied Physiology* 51(1981):1437.

deVries, H. A. *Physiology of Exercise*. 3d. ed. Dubuque, IA: Wm. C. Brown Publishers, 1980.

Fardy, P. S. "Isometric Exercise and the Cardiovascular System." *Physician and Sportsmedicine* 9(September 1981):42.

*Garhammer, J. *Sports Illustrated Strength Training*. New York: Harper and Row, 1986.

Garnica, R. A. "Muscular Power in Young Women After Slow and Fast Isokinetic Training." *Journal of Orthopedic and Sports Physical Therapy* 11:1(July 1986):1.

*Gettman, L. R., and M. L. Pollock. "Circuit Weight Training: A Critical Review of its Physiological Benefits." *Physician and Sportsmedicine* 9(June 1981):44.

Hage, P. "Prescribing Exercises: More Than Just a Running Program." *Physician and Sportsmedicine* 11(May 1983):123.

Hay, J. G., J. G. Andrews, and C. L. Vaugh. "The Effect of Lifting Rate on Elbow Torques during Arm Curl Exercises." *Medicine and Science in Sports and Exercises* 15(1983):63.

Hickson, R. S., M. A. Rosen-Roetter, and M. M. Brown. "Strength Training Effects on Aerobic Power and Short-Term Endurance." *Medicine and Science in Sports and Exercise* 12(1980):336.

Jackson, A., et al. "Strength Development: Using Functional Isometrics in an Isotonic Strength Training Program." *Research Quarterly for Exercise and Sport* 56:3(1985):234.

Jackson, A. "Strength Measurement." *Journal of Physical Education, Recreation, and Dance* 57(August 1986):83.

Johnson, J. H. "Accommodating Resistance for Knee Extension." *American Corrective Therapy Journal* 39:2(March–April 1985):42.

Katch, V., et al. "Muscular Development and Lean Body Weight in Body Builders and Weight Lifters." *Medicine and Science in Sports and Exercise* 12(1980):340.

Kisner, C., and L. A. Colby. *Therapeutic Exercise: Foundations and Techniques*. Philadelphia: F. A. Davis Co., 1985.

Kottke, F. J., G. K. Stillwell, and J. F. Lehmann. *Krusen's Handbook of Physical Medicine and Rehabilitation*. 3d ed. Philadelphia: W. B. Saunders Co., 1982.

Kreighbaum, E., and K. M. Barthels. *Biomechanics*. Minneapolis: Burgess Publishing Co., 1985.

Kusinitz, I., M. Fine, and Editors of Consumer Reports Books. *Physical Fitness for Practically Everybody*. Mount Vernon, NY: Consumers Union, 1983.

Moffroid, M. T., and J. E. Kusial. "The Power Struggle—Definition and Evaluation of Power and Muscular Performance." *Physical Therapy* 55(1975):1098.

Osternig, L. R., et al. "Relative Influence of Torque and Limb Speed on Power Production in Isokinetic Exercise." *Medicine and Science in Sports and Exercise* 14(1982):178.

Perrine, J. J., and R. V. Edgerton. "Muscle Force-Velocity and Power Velocity Relationships Under Isokinetic Loading." *Medicine and Science in Sports and Exercise* 10(1978):159.

Pollock, M., J. Willmore, and S. Fox. *Health and Fitness through Physical Activity.* New York: John Wiley, 1978.

*Rasch, P. J. *Weight Training.* 4th ed. Dubuque, IA: Wm. C. Brown Publishers, 1982.

Sale, D., and D. McDougall. "Specificity in Strength Training—A Review for the Coach and Athlete." *Sports-Science Periodical On Research and Technology in Sport.* (Canada) March, 1981.

Salle, A., et al. "New Muscle Fiber Production During Compensatory Hypertrophy." *Medicine and Science in Sports and Exercise* 12(1980):268.

Schwane, J. A., et al. "Is Lactic Acid Related to Delayed-Onset Muscle Soreness?" *Physician and Sportsmedicine* 11(March 1983):124.

Stamford, B. "The Differences Between Strength and Power." *Physician and Sports Medicine* 3:7(July 1985):155.

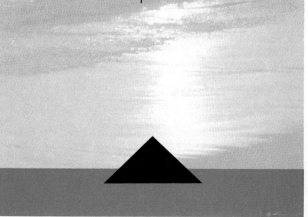

9

MUSCULAR ENDURANCE AND MUSCULAR POWER

CONCEPT 9

Muscular Endurance is an important health-related component of physical fitness, whereas power is an important combination of skill and health-related components.

INTRODUCTION

Power is usually classified as a skill-related component of fitness whereas strength and muscular endurance are classified as health-related components; yet all three are closely related. When considering training programs, it is difficult to isolate these three factors from one another because a program designed specifically to develop one component would also tend to develop the other attributes to some extent. The first part of this concept offers facts about muscular endurance and the last part gives facts about power.

TERMS (Also see Concept 8 terms)

Dynamic Endurance—A muscle's ability to contract and relax repeatedly. This is usually measured by the number of times (repetitions) you can perform a body movement in a given period of time.

Static Endurance—A muscle's ability to remain contracted for a long period of time. This is usually measured by the length of time you can hold a body position.

THE FACTS ABOUT MUSCULAR ENDURANCE

Muscular endurance is an important health-related component of physical fitness.

Muscular endurance is the capacity of a skeletal muscle or group of muscles to continue contracting over a long period of time. You have the ability to resist fatigue when you hold a position or carry something for an extended period of time. You also have the ability to repeat a movement without getting tired. Muscular endurance prevents undue fatigue from work and other daily activities, and allows greater success and enjoyment in athletic and recreational endeavors.

Muscular endurance training tends to develop the slow twitch fibers in your muscles.

As you train specifically for endurance, the slow twitch fibers will selectively adapt to the activity in such a way that the trained muscles will become more efficient and fatigue resistant.

The overload principle applies to muscular endurance.

Though strength is developed by high resistance overload with low repetitions, **dynamic muscular endurance** requires just the opposite: higher repetitions and lower resistance. The ideal combination for maximum endurance is not known at this time. One study suggests

73

TABLE 9.1 Muscular Endurance Threshold of Training and Fitness Target Zone

	Threshold of Training	Target Zone
Dynamic Endurance		
Frequency	• 3 days per week.	• Every other day.
Intensity	• Lift resistance 20%–30% of the maximum you can lift.	• Lift resistance 40%–70% of the maximum you can lift.
Time	• One set of 8 repetitions of each exercise.	• 2–5 sets of 9–25 repetitions.
Static Endurance		
Frequency	• 3 days per week.	• Every other day.
Intensity	• Hold a weight 50%–100% of the weight you ultimately will need to hold in your work or leisure activity.	• Hold a weight equal to and up to 50% greater than the amount you will need to hold in your work or leisure activity.
Time	• Hold for lengths of time 10%–50% shorter than the time you plan to do the activity. Repeat 10–20 times.	• Hold for lengths of time equal to and up to 20% greater than the time you plan to do the activity. For longer times, use fewer repetitions (5–10).

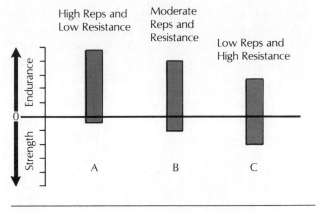

FIGURE 9.1 Comparison of Absolute Endurance and Strength Developed by Different Exercise Regimes. *Adapted from Anderson and Kearney, 1982.*

that after progressing to twenty-five repetitions, it may be more effective to increase the resistance and keep the repetitions constant.

To develop **static muscular endurance,** the overload principle is applied by progressively increasing the length of time the muscles remain contracted against an immovable resistance.

There is a threshold of training and a target zone for muscular endurance exercises.

There is a level of frequency, intensity, and time at which a training effect will begin to take place (threshold). There is also an optimal range, or target zone, where the most effective and efficient improvement will occur (see table 9.1). We do not know the optimum range, but studies suggest that it has wide limits. The intensity, or resistance (load), is less important than the number of repetitions or the length of time a muscle contracts.

Muscular endurance is slightly related to cardiovascular endurance, but it is not the same thing.

Cardiovascular endurance depends primarily upon the efficiency of the heart muscle, circulatory system, and respiratory system. It is developed with activities that stress these systems, such as running, cycling, and

swimming. Muscular endurance depends upon the efficiency of the local skeletal muscles and the nerves that control them. You might train for cardiovascular endurance by running, but if the leg muscles lack the muscular endurance to continue contracting for more than five minutes, the cardiovascular system will not be stressed, even if it is in good condition.

Muscular endurance is related to strength, but is different.

Studies show that the person who is strength-trained will fatigue as much as four times faster than the person who is endurance-trained. However, there is a slight correlation between strength and endurance because the person who trains for strength will develop some endurance, and the person who trains for muscular endurance will develop some strength.

The graph in figure 9.1 illustrates the relationship between strength and muscular endurance. In *A,* the training program calls for a high number of repetitions and light resistance. This results in a small gain in strength (the area of the bar below the line), and a large increase in endurance (the area of the bar above the line). In *B,* the training program calls for a moderate number of repetitions (less than in *A*), and a moderate resistance (more than in *A*). This results in slightly less endurance and slightly more strength than in program *A.* Program *C* results in the least gain in endurance and the most gain in strength because it uses high resistance and low repetitions. Thus, if you are primarily interested in muscular endurance, program *A* is your optimal choice.

Some endurance tests penalize the weaker person.

If you are tested on absolute endurance (the number of times you can move a designated number of pounds), a stronger person has an advantage. However, if you are tested on relative endurance (the number of times you can move a designated percentage of your maximum strength), the stronger person does not have an advantage and men and women can compete more evenly. Strength training will not help you improve your relative endurance.

There are a variety of effective programs for developing muscular endurance.

All methods used in strength development are applicable to endurance development. Weight training, calisthenics, isometrics, isokinetics, and such activities as running, swimming, and aerobic dance can all be designed to increase muscular endurance. Even games, such as rope climbing, tug-of-war, Indian wrestling, and hopping races, can contribute to muscular endurance.

A muscular endurance training program should apply the principle of specificity by closely resembling the activity for which the endurance is needed.

Muscular endurance is specific to the muscles being used, the type of muscle contraction (static or dynamic), the speed or cadence of the movement, and the amount of resistance being moved.

For example, if you want endurance in the elbow flexor muscles (e.g., biceps), you must train those muscles. Performing muscular endurance exercise for the elbow extensor (e.g., triceps) or the leg muscles will not improve the muscular endurance of the biceps. Likewise, if you are trying to develop endurance for a dynamic task, you should do isotonic exercises. If you need endurance in muscles that hold you in a static position, do isometric exercises. If the activity requires a rapid movement, it is better to train with fast movements. There may be transfer from fast practice to slow movement in a skill, but the reverse is not true.

Garhammer (1986) believes that athletes wishing to develop muscular endurance for a particular sport may benefit more from performing the sport skill repeatedly than from doing special exercises such as weight training. If injury or weather prevents practice of the sport, then weight training for endurance would be an effective alternative.

Guidelines for muscular endurance training programs are the same as those for strength development.

Performance guidelines for safety and effectiveness presented in Concept 8 should be reviewed before starting a program of exercise. It is particularly important that all muscle groups are exercised. For example, if your program for cardiovascular fitness stresses the muscles of the legs (front and back), then these might be omitted from your muscular endurance program and special attention given to the muscles on the inside and the outside of the legs and the muscles of the trunk and upper extremities.

Endurance training may have a negative effect on strength and power.

Some studies have shown that for athletes who rely primarily on strength and power in their sports event, too much endurance training can cause a loss in strength and power because of modification of different muscle fibers. Strength and power athletes need some endurance training, but not too much; just as endurance athletes need some strength and power training, but not too much.

Some training methods can interfere with athletic performance.

Some research studies have shown that certain techniques used in training may actually cause a decrease in performance. For example, when distance runners were trained with weighted wristlets, anklets, and belts, they performed worse than runners who did not wear weights in training. In another study, people who were running and bicycling for aerobic endurance six days per week combined those exercises with a strength training program five days per week. The results yielded a decrease in strength development near the upper limits.

Exercises to "slim" the figure/physique should be of the muscular endurance type.

Women in particular seem interested in exercises designed to decrease girth measurements. The high repetition, low resistance exercise is suitable for this because it usually brings about some strengthening and, therefore, some "firming" of flabby muscles, which in turn, changes body contour. Exercises do *not* "spot reduce" fat (see Concept 25). Endurance exercises do speed up metabolism so more calories are burned, but if weight or fat reduction is desired, aerobic (cardiovascular) exercises are best. To increase girth, strength exercises such as those power lifters use for hypertrophy are best (see Concept 8).

FACTS ABOUT POWER

Power is a combination of strength and speed, which is both health related and skill related.

Most experts classify power as a skill-related component of fitness (see Concept 2) because it is partially dependent on speed. On the other hand, power is also dependent on strength and can be classified as a health-related component to the extent that strength is involved. Thus, power falls somewhere in between the two distinct groups of fitness attributes. Certainly its use is not limited to sports and dance. We use power extensively in our daily activities every time we apply a force to move something quickly. Power is important in pro-

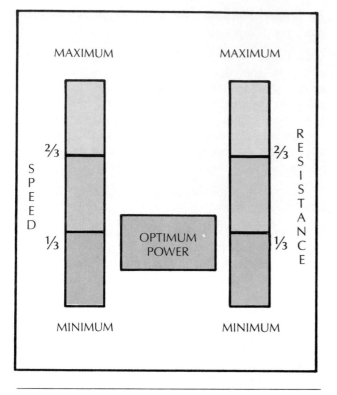

FIGURE 9.2 Optimum Power Is Produced When the Load and Speed are Each About One-Third of Maximum

"strength-related power" by working against heavy resistance at slower speeds. (See figure 9.2.) If you need to move light objects at great speed, such as in throwing a ball, you need to develop "speed-related power" by training at high speeds with relatively low resistance. There must be trade-offs between speed and power because the heavier the resistance, the slower the movement.

There is a target zone for optimum power.

Studies show that power is best developed when the force is between 30 and 60 percent of maximum. But the optimum is probably when the load and the speed are about one-third of maximum. (See figure 9.2.) Stamford (1985) uses the following illustration of the relationship between speed, strength, and power. If your maximum strength is represented by 2 and maximum speed by 2, then your power is $2 \times 2 = 4$. If you double your strength ($4 \times 2 = 8$), your power would be doubled. However, if your strength and speed were increased by only 50 percent, then even more power results ($3 \times 3 = 9$).

There are several effective techniques for developing power.

For specificity of training, as mentioned previously, much of an athlete's program should closely resemble the activity for which he or she is training, using similar speed, force, angle, range of motion, and so forth. However, if one is striving for all-round fitness or if an athlete is unable to perform the specific skill because of weather or injury or is seeking variety, then plyometrics, isokinetics, and weight training (especially with free weights or pulleys if simulating a sport skill) are effective means of developing power.

Power exercises can increase muscular endurance or strength.

Power exercises done at high speeds have been shown to increase muscular endurance. Likewise, power exercises that use heavy resistance at lower speeds will increase strength.

As explained elsewhere in Concepts 8 and 9, the exercises should resemble the activity for which you are training in speed and in every other aspect. Jumpers, for example, should jump as a part of their training programs in order to learn correct timing at the same time they are developing power.

The principle of specificity should be applied to training programs for power events.

Athletes who need explosive power to perform their events should use training that closely resembles the event. This includes Olympic weight lifters, shotputters, jumpers, ballet dancers, and others. These athletes need both strength and endurance, however, studies show that too much of either can have a negative effect on performance.

tective movements, such as a pedestrian jumping to dodge a car or a driver jerking the steering wheel to avoid a collision or jamming on the brakes to stop in an emergency. A worker heaves a heavy load from a truck to a dock and a carpenter uses force to hammer a nail.

Power is usually neglected in fitness literature and often in fitness programs as well. Garnica (1986) believes it to be the "most functional mode in which all human motion occurs." If this is true, all fitness programs should consider appropriate exercises that develop power.

The stronger person is not necessarily the more powerful.

Power is the amount of work per unit of time. To increase power, you must do more work in the same time or the same work in less time. If you extend your knee and move a 100 pound weight through a 90 degree arc in one second, you have twice as much power as a person who needs two seconds to complete the same movement. Power requires both strength and speed. Increasing one without the other limits power.

Some power athletes (for example, football players) might benefit more by trying for less strength and more speed.

There is probably no one best training program for developing power.

If you need power for an activity in which you are required to move heavy weights, then you need to develop

Evaluating Muscular Endurance

1. *Sitting Tucks*
   Sit on the floor so that your back and feet are off the floor. Interlock your fingers on top of your head. Alternately draw your legs to your chest and extend them away from your body. Keep your feet and back off the floor. Repeat as many times as possible up to thirty-five.

2. *Chins or Bent-arm Hang*
   a. *Chins*—Pull your body weight above the horizontal bar, gripping the bar with palms facing the bar. Repeat as many times as possible.
   b. *Bent-arm Hang*—(For men and women who cannot perform one chin.) Hang from a horizontal bar with palms facing the bar. Count the number of seconds that your chin can be held above the bar. *This test is only for people who cannot do one chin.* A separate rating chart is provided for this measure of muscular endurance.

CHART 9.1 *Rating Scale* for Muscular Endurance (Men)

Age	17–26		27–39		40–49		50–59		60+	
Classification	Tucks	Chins	Tucks	Chins	Tucks	Chins	Tucks	Chins	Tucks	Chins
High Performance Zone	35+	25+	34+	20+	33+	15+	32+	13+	31+	12+
Good Fitness Zone	20–34	10–24	19–33	9–19	18–32	8–14	15–31	7–12	12–30	6–11
Marginal Zone	15–19	7–9	13–18	5–8	12–17	4–8	10–14	3–6	8–11	2–5
Low Zone	<15	<7	13	<5	<12	<4	<10	<3	<8	<2

Age	17–26		27–39		40–49		50–59		60+	
Classification	Tucks	Chins	Tucks	Chins	Tucks	Chins	Tucks	Chins	Tucks	Chins
High Performance Zone	25+	3+	24+	2+	23+	2+	22+	1+	21+	1+
Good Fitness Zone	20–24	1–2	19–23	1	18–22	1	17–21	1	10–20	1
Marginal Zone	10–19	—	9–18	—	8–17		7–14	—	6–9	—
Low Zone	<10	—	<9	—	<8		<7	—	<6	

CHART 9.3 *Rating Scale* for Flexed Arm Hang (For people who cannot do one chin)

Classification	Score in Seconds
Making progress toward chin-up	25 +
Need more exercise	<24

Evaluating Leg Muscle Power

Lie on a mat and have your partner mark your body length (height) from head to toe on the mat. Perform a standing long jump the distance of your body height if possible. Make two jumps and measure the better of the two.

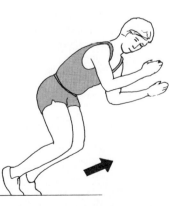

CHART 9.4 *Rating Scale* of Leg Power (Men)

Age	17–26	27–39	40–49	50–59	60+
Classification	**Length of Jump (by height)**				
High Performance Zone	ht. +	ht. +	¾ht. +	¾ht. +	½ht. +
Good Performance Zone*	¾ht.	¾ht.	½ht.	½ht.	½ht.
Marginal Zone	½ht.	½ht.	⅓ht.	⅓ht.	⅓ht.
Low Zone	<½ht.	<½ht.	<⅔ht.	<⅓ht.	<⅓ht.

Because power is a skill-related fitness component and relates more to performance than to health, "good performance zone" is used rather than "good fitness zone."

CHART 9.5 *Rating Scale* of Leg Power (Women)

Age	17–26	27–39	40–49	50–59	60+
Classification	**Length of Jump (by height)**				
High Performance Zone	¾ht. +	¾ht. +	¾ht. +	⅔ht. +	½ht. +
Good Performance Zone*	⅔ht.	⅔ht.	½ht.	½ht.	⅓ht
Marginal Zone	½ht.	½ht.	⅓ht.	⅓ht.	¼ht.
Low Zone	<½ht.	<½ht.	<⅓ht.	<⅓ht.	<¼ht.

Because power is a skill-related fitness component and relates more to performance than to health, "good performance zone" is used rather than "good fitness zone."

REFERENCES

Anderson, T., and J. T. Kearney. "Effects of Three Resistance Training Programs on Muscular Strength and Absolute and Relative Endurance." *Research Quarterly for Exercise and Sport* 53(1982):1.

Barnes, W. S. "The Relationship Between Maximum Isokinetic Strength and Isokinetic Endurance." *Research Quarterly for Exercise and Sport* 51(1980):714.

Basmajian, J. V. *Therapeutic Exercise.* Baltimore: Williams and Wilkins, 1984.

Cook, B., and G. W. Stewart. *Get Strong.* Ganges, B. C., Canada: 3S Fitness Group, 1981.

Coyle, E. F., et al. "Specificity of Power Improvements through Slow and Fast Isokinetic Training." *Journal of Applied Physiology* 51(1981):1437.

*Garhammer, J. *Sports Illustrated Strength Training.* New York: Harper and Row, 1986.

Garnica, R. A. "Muscular Power in Young Women After Slow and Fast Isokinetic Training." *Journal of Orthopedic and Sports Physical Therapy* 11:1(July 1986):1.

Hickson, R. C. "Interference of Strength Development by Simultaneously Training for Strength and Endurance." *European Journal of Applied Physiology* 45(1980):255.

Kottke, F. J., G. K. Stillwell, and J. F. Lehmann. *Krusen's Handbook of Physical Medicine and Rehabilitation.* 3d ed. Philadelphia: W. B. Saunders Co., 1982.

Kreighbaum, E., and K. M. Barthels. *Biomechanics.* Minneapolis: Burgess Publishing Co., 1985.

Kroll, W., P. M. Clarkson, G. Kamen, and J. Lambert. "Muscle Fiber Type Composition and Knee Extension Isometric Strength Fatigue Patterns in Power and Endurance Trained Males." *Research Quarterly for Exercise and Sport* 51(1980):323.

Kusinitz, I., M. Fine, and Editors of Consumer Reports Books. *Physical Fitness for Practically Everybody.* Mount Vernon, NY: Consumers Union, 1983.

Lamb, D. R. *Physiology of Exercise.* New York: MacMillan Publishers, 1978.

*Lindsey, R., B. Jones, and A. V. Whitley. *Fitness.* 5th ed. Dubuque, IA: Wm. C. Brown Publishers, 1983.

Moffroid, M. T., and E. Kusial. "The Power Struggle—Definition and Evaluation of Power and Muscular Performance." *Physical Therapy* 55(1975):1098.

*Rasch, P. J. *Weight Training.* 4th ed. Dubuque, IA: Wm. C. Brown Publishers, 1982.

*Stamford, B. "The Difference Between Strength and Power." *Physician and Sportsmedicine* 3:7(July 1985):155.

Tesch, P. A., and J. Karlsson. "Muscle Fiber Types and Sizes in Trained and Untrained Elite Athletes." *Journal of Applied Physiology* 59(December 1985):1716.

10

STRENGTH AND MUSCULAR ENDURANCE EXERCISES

CONCEPT 10

Strength exercises should be
performed against a near maximum
resistance using
only a few repetitions.
Endurance exercises
require only a moderate resistance,
but a high number of repetitions.

INTRODUCTION

There are several kinds of strength and endurance exercises. Among the most popular are *isotonic calisthenics,* which require little or no special equipment; *isometric exercises,* which can be done in a small space; and *progressive resistance exercises (PRE),* which can be performed isotonically or isokinetically. The "Stations" mentioned in parentheses throughout this concept refer to Universal stations pictured on page 90. The muscles used in each exercise may be developed on the Universal machine. Other exercise machines can also be effective in developing strength and muscular endurance.

TERMS

Detailed descriptions of important strength and muscular endurance terms are presented in Concept 8.

THE FACTS

Isotonic calisthenic exercises are among the most popular forms of exercise among adults.

Isotonic calisthenics, such as sit-ups and push-ups, are suitable for people of different ability levels, and can be used to improve both strength and muscular endurance. One disadvantage is that this type of exercise does little to increase strength unless more resistance is added. For example, doing a push-up will build strength to a point. However, once you can do several, adding more repetitions will only build muscular endurance, NOT strength. To develop additional strength, you can add more weights to increase the resistance or change the body position so there is a greater gravitational effect or more torque. For example, you can elevate your feet or wear a weighted vest while doing push-ups. Some isotonic calisthenics that you can do at home are illustrated on pages 80–83.

SAMPLE ISOTONIC EXERCISES FOR MUSCULAR ENDURANCE AND MILD STRENGTHENING

The exercises suggested here should be performed as described until you are able to increase the repetitions to approximately twenty-five. Additional weight should then be added. Muscles depicted in color are those primarily involved in the exercises.

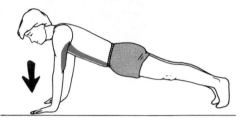

1. Full-length Push-ups

Purpose

Develop muscles of arms, shoulders, and chest.

Position

Take front-leaning rest position, arms straight.

Movement

Lower chest to floor. Press to beginning position in same manner. Repeat. (See stations 3, 7, and 9.)

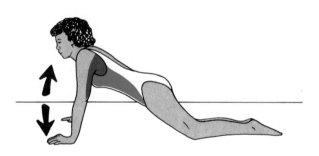

2. Bent-knee Push-ups

For those who cannot do full-length push-ups.

Purpose

Develop muscles of the arms, shoulders, and chest.

Position

Assume the push-up position, but rest the weight on the knees, not the feet.

Movement

Lower the body until the chest touches the floor; return to the starting position keeping the body straight. Repeat. (See stations 2 and 9.)

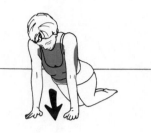

3. Bent-knee Let-downs

For those who cannot do bent-knee push-ups.

Purpose

Develop muscles of the arms, shoulders, and chest.

Position

Same as a bent-knee push-up position.

Movement

Slowly lower the body to the floor, keeping the body line straight; return to the starting position in any manner. Repeat. (See stations 2 and 9.)

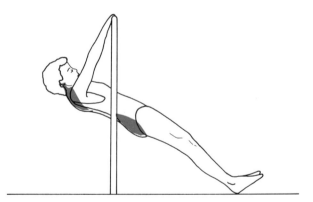

4. Modified Pull-ups

Purpose

Develop muscles of the arms and shoulders.

Position

Hang (palms forward and shoulder width apart) from a low bar (may be placed across two chairs), heels on floor, with the body straight from feet to head.

Movement

Pull up, keeping the body straight, touch the chest to the bar, then lower to the starting position. (Stronger persons may hang from a bar vertically and pull up.) Repeat. (See stations 4, 6, and 12.)

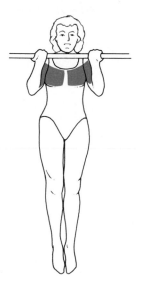

5. Pull-ups (Chinning)

Purpose

Develop muscles of arms and shoulders.

Position

Hang from bar, palms forward, body and arms straight.

Movement

Pull up until chin is over bar. Repeat. (See station 6.)

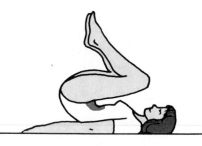

6. Reverse Sit-ups

Purpose

Develop the lower abdominal muscles and correct abdominal ptosis.

Position

Lie on the floor. Bend the knees, place the feet flat on the floor, and place arms at sides.

Movement

Lift the knees to the chest raising the hips off the floor; do not let the knees go past the shoulders. Return to the starting position. Repeat. (See stations 8 and 9.)

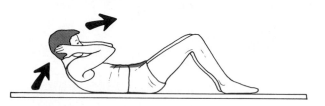

7. Bent-knee Sit-ups

Purpose

Develop the upper abdominal muscles and correct abdominal ptosis.

Position

Assume a hook-lying position with arms crossed and hands on shoulders.

Movement

Curl up until shoulder blades leave floor then roll down to the starting position. Repeat. For less resistance, place hands at side of body (do not put hands behind neck and do not anchor feet). (See station 9.)

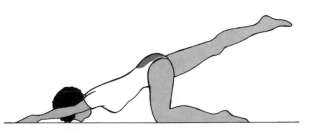

8. Leg Extension Exercise

Purpose

Develop muscles of the hips.

Position

Assume a knee-chest position, hands on floor with arms extended as far as possible.

Movement

Extend right leg upward in line with trunk, then lower. Continue repetitions. Repeat with other leg. (See stations 5 and 16.)

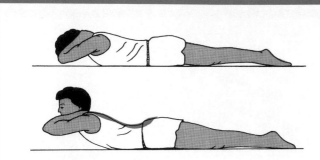

9. Upper Back Lift

Purpose

Develop muscles of the upper back. Correct kyphosis and round shoulders.

Position

Lie prone (face down) with hands clasped behind the neck.

Movement

Pull the shoulder blades together, raising the elbows off the floor. Slowly raise the head and chest off the floor by arching the upper back. Return to the starting position; repeat. *Caution:* Do not arch the lower back; lift only until the sternum (breast bone) clears the floor. (See station 11.)

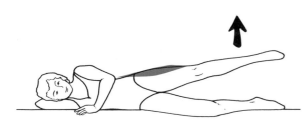

10. Side Leg Raises

Purpose

Develop muscles on outside of thighs.

Position

Lie on the side.

Movement

Raise the top leg toward the ceiling, then return. Do the same number of repetitions with each leg.

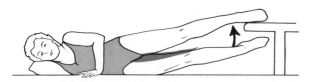

11. Lower Leg-lift

Purpose

Develop muscles on the inside of thighs.

Position

Lie on the side with the upper leg (foot) supported on a bench.

Movement

Raise the lower leg toward the ceiling; repeat. Roll to opposite side and repeat.

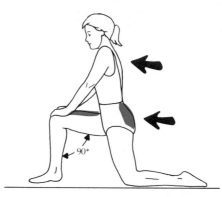

90°

12. Forward Lunge

Purpose

Develop muscles of the legs and hips.

Position

Stand tall, feet together.

Movement

Take a step forward with the left foot, touching the right knee to the floor. The knees should be bent only to a 90° angle. Return to the starting position and step out with the other foot. Repeat, alternating left and right. (See stations 1, 10, and 16.)

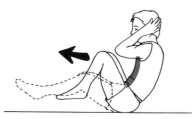

13. Sitting Tucks or "V Sit"

Purpose

Develop muscles of abdomen and legs.

Position

Sit on the floor so that the back and feet are off the floor. Interlock fingers on top of the head or extend arms forward for balance. Do not put hands behind neck.

Movement

Alternately draw the legs into the chest and extend the feet away from the body. Keep feet and back off the floor. Continue repeating. (See stations 8 and 9.)

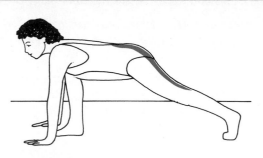

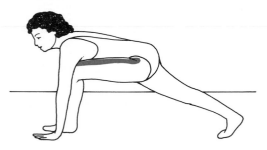

14. Stationary Leg Change

Purpose

Develop muscles of the legs and hips.

Position

Crouch on the floor with weight on hands, left leg bent under the chest, right leg extended behind.

Movement

Alternate legs; bring right leg up while left leg goes back. Repeat. (See station 16.)

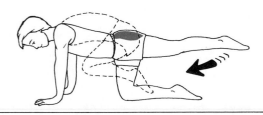

15. Knee-to-Nose Touch/Kneeling Leg Extensions

Purpose

Strength or endurance of gluteal muscles; stretch low back.

Position

Kneel on "all fours."

Movement

Pull knee to nose, then extend leg horizontally (do not go higher). Alternate legs; repeat. (See stations 1 and 16.)

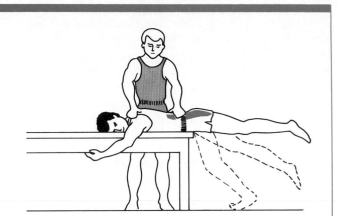

16. Lower Trunk Lift

Purpose

Develop low back and hip strength.

Position

Lie prone on bench or table with legs hanging over the edge.

Movement

Have a partner stabilize the upper back or grasp the edges of the table with hands. Raise the legs parallel to the floor and lower them. Do not raise past the horizontal or arch the back. (See station 11.)

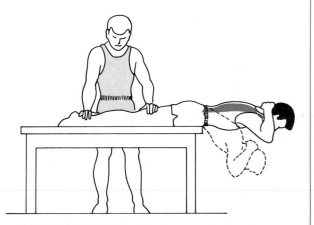

17. Upper Trunk Lift

Purpose

Develop upper back strength.

Position

Lie on a table or bench with the upper half of the body hanging over the edge.

Movement

Have a partner stabilize the feet while the trunk is raised parallel to the floor, then lower the trunk to the starting position. Place hands behind neck. Do not raise past the horizontal or arch the back. (See station 11.)

Weight training with "free weights" is a popular form of isotonic progressive resistance exercise.

Free weights are weights that are not attached to a machine or exercise device. They can be put on a bar so that the weight can be adjusted as necessary for different exercises to provide optimal resistance. Weight training with free weights is very popular because it can be done in the home with inexpensive equipment. Homemade weights can even be constructed from pieces of pipe and plastic bottles filled with water. Some exercises that are best for developing strength and muscular endurance are illustrated on pages 84–86.

Strength and Muscular Endurance Exercises can be performed for all of the major muscle groups in the body.

Figure P.1 in the Preface illustrates the major muscle groups. The names of the muscles and the common "nicknames" are also included.

SAMPLE FREE WEIGHT TRAINING EXERCISES

The exercises suggested here should be performed as described until you are able to increase repetitions. Muscles depicted in color are those primarily involved in the exercises.

1. Shoulder Shrug

Purpose

Strengthen the muscles of the shoulders.

Position

Stand with palms toward body, bar touching thighs, legs straight, and feet together.

Movement

Lift shoulders (try to touch ears) then roll shoulders smoothly backward, down, and forward. Repeat maximum number of times. (See stations 3 and 5.)

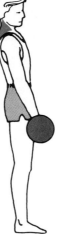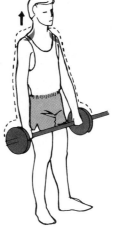

2. Military Press

Purpose

Strengthen the muscles of the shoulders and arms.

Position

Stand erect, bend elbows, palms forward at chest level, hands spread (slightly more than shoulder width). Have bar touching chest, spread feet (comfortable distance), keep legs straight.

Movement

Move bar to overhead position (arms straight). Lower to chest position. Repeat. (See station 3.)

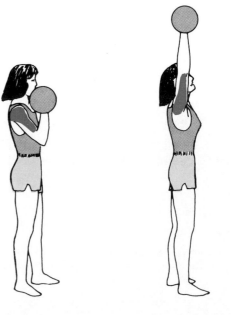

3. Half Squat

Purpose

Strengthen the muscles of the thighs and hips.

Position

Stand erect, feet turned out 45°. Rest bar behind neck on shoulders. Spread hands in a comfortable position.

Movement

Squat slowly, keeping back straight, eyes ahead. Bend knees to 90°; keep knees over feet. Pause, then stand. Repeat. (See stations 1, 10, and 16.)

4. Biceps Curl

Purpose

Strengthen the muscles of the upper front part of the arms (biceps).

Position

Stand erect, palms forward; arms spread in order not to touch body; bar touching thighs. Spread feet in comfortable position.

Movement

Move bar to chin, keeping body straight and elbows forward of center line of body. Do not allow elbows to touch body. Lower to original position. Repeat. (See station 5.)

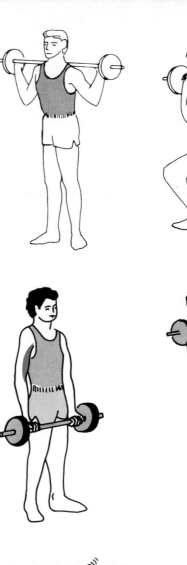

5. Triceps Curl

Purpose

Strengthen the muscles of the back part of the upper arms (triceps).

Position

Stand erect, elbows up, palms up. Rest bar behind neck on shoulders, hands near center of bar, feet spread.

Movement

Keep upper arms stationary. Raise weight overhead, return bar to original position. Repeat. (See stations 6 and 7.)

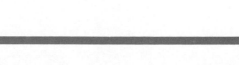

6. Toe Raise

Purpose

Strengthen muscles of the legs (calf).

Position

Stand erect with front grip, hands wider than shoulder width apart, bar resting behind neck on shoulders. Rest balls of feet on two-inch block with heels on floor. Toes together, heels apart.

Movement

Rise on toes quickly, hold for one second. Lower heels to floor. Repeat. Keep toes in and heels out. (See stations 1 and 5.)

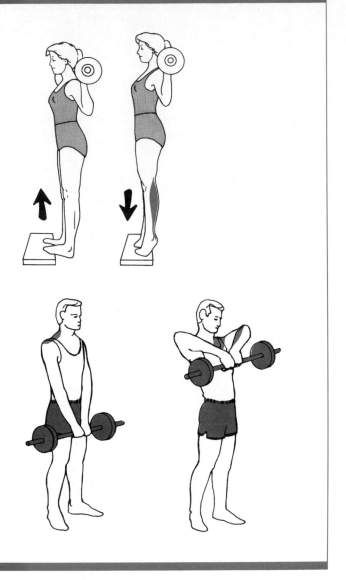

7. Pull to Chin

Purpose

Strengthen muscles of the shoulders and arms.

Position

Stand erect with a front grip (loose), hands together at center of bar, bar touching thighs, feet spread, head erect, eyes straight ahead.

Movement

Pull bar to chin. Keep bar close to body and elbows well above bar. Lower to extended position. Repeat. (See station 3.)

Exercise with "weight training machines" or "pulley exercisers" has become more popular and more accessible in recent years.

Weight training can be done on exercise machines and pulley devices. These have become more popular in recent years as lower priced machines have been developed and exercise clubs have made them accessible to more people. These machines can be effective in developing strength and muscular endurance if used properly. They can save time because unlike free weights, the weight to be lifted can be changed easily and quickly. They are also safer because you are less likely to drop weights on machines. The kinds of exercises that can be done on these machines are more limited than those for free weights. Some good exercises using weight training machines and pulley exercisers are illustrated on pages 87–89.

SAMPLE WEIGHT TRAINING MACHINE/PULLEY EXERCISES

The exercises suggested here should be performed as described until you are able to increase repetitions. Muscles depicted in color are those primarily involved in the exercises. (See universal weight machine stations p. 90.)

1. Biceps Curl (Low Pulley)

Purpose

Strengthen elbow flexor muscles on front of arm.

Position

Stand erect, arms at sides, palms up. Grasp bar.

Movement

Flex elbows, bringing bar to chest. Keep elbows pressed against sides. Lower; repeat. (See station 12.)

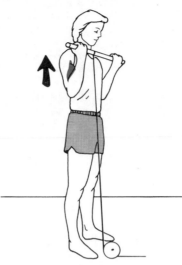

2. Seated Rowing (Low Pulley)

Purpose

Develop upper arms and shoulders.

Position

Sit facing pulley, feet braced and knees slightly bent. Grasp bar, palms up with hands shoulder width apart.

Movement

Pull bar to chest and return; repeat. (See station 12.)

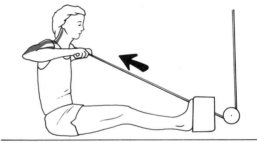

3. Leg Press

Purpose

Develop thigh and hip muscles.

Position

Sit on chair with feet on pedals, knees bent to right angle. Grasp handles.

Movement

Extend legs and return; repeat. Do not lock knees when legs straighten. (See station 1.)

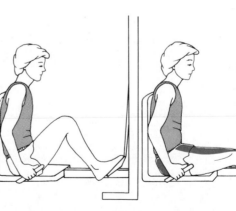

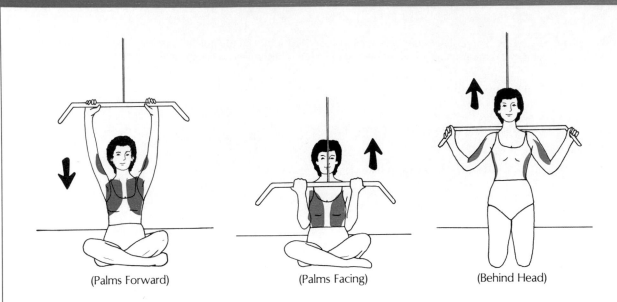

(Palms Forward)   (Palms Facing)   (Behind Head)

4. Lat Pull-down (High Pulley)

Purpose

Develop latissimus ("lats"), biceps, and pectorals ("pecs").

Position

Tailor sit or kneel on both knees. Grasp bar with palms facing away from you, hands shoulder distance apart.

Movement

Pull bar down to chest and return; repeat.

Variations

Turn palms toward face; move hands out to ends of bar; pull bar behind head. (See station 4.)

5. Triceps Curl

Purpose

Develop triceps and other muscles on back of arm.

Position

Stand erect. Grasp bar near center; palms down.

Movement

With elbows clamped against sides, pull bar down to thighs and return to chest height without moving elbows; repeat. (See station 4.)

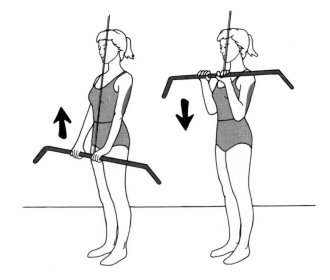

6. Bench Press

Purpose

Develop chest (pectoral) and triceps muscles.

Position

Lie supine on bench with feet on floor, or knees bent and feet flat on bench. Grasp handles at shoulder level.

Movement

Push bar up until arms are straight. Return; repeat; do not arch lower back. (See station 2.)

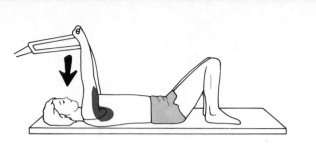

7. Ankle Press

Purpose

Develop the calf muscles.

Position

Sit at leg press station with legs straight. Grasp handles. Put ball of foot at lower edge of pedal.

Movement

Keeping legs straight, point toes by extending (plantar flexing) ankles. Return; repeat. (See station 1.)

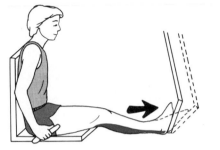

8. Knee Extension

Purpose

Develop thigh (quadriceps) muscles.

Position

Sit on end of bench with ankles hooked under padded bar. Grasp edge of table.

Movement

Extend knees. Return; repeat. (See station 10.)

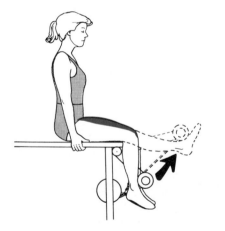

9. Hamstring Curl

Purpose

Develop hamstrings (muscles on back of thigh) and other knee flexors.

Position

Lie prone on bench with ankles hooked under padded bar. Rest chin on hands or grasp bench.

Movement

Flex knees as far as possible without allowing hips to raise. Return; repeat. (See station 10.)

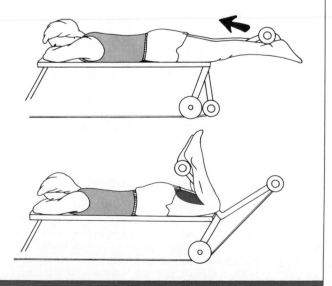

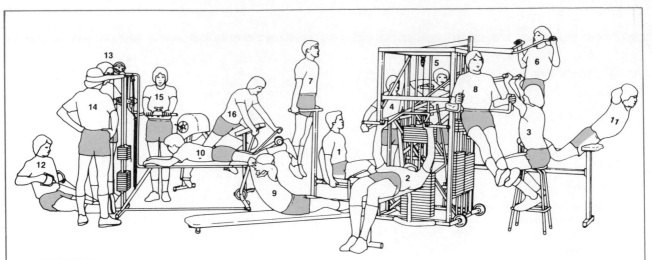

STATIONS

1. **Leg Press** – Push the pedal, extending the hips and knees; to strengthen the thigh (quadriceps) muscles.

*2. **Chest Press (Bench Press)**—Push upward on the handles, extending the elbows and bringing the upper arms toward the chest; to strengthen the chest muscles (pectorals) and the triceps on the back of the arms. Note: It is better if the feet are placed on the bench with knees and hips flexed and lower back flattened.

*3. **Shoulder Press (Military Press)**—Push upward on the handles, extending the elbows, bringing the arms toward the ears; to strengthen the shoulder (deltoids) and the back of the arm (triceps). NOTE: The stool should be closer to the machine than shown to prevent arching of the back.

4. **Lat Pull Down Bar or High Pulley** – Kneel or stand and pull the bar down behind your neck, alternating with a pull to the chest; to strengthen the biceps and the latissimus. To strengthen the triceps, perform a "triceps curl" by pulling the bar from chest height to waist or thigh level. Extend the elbows while keeping them hugged against your sides.

5. **Low Pulley and Dead Lift** – Perform "biceps curls" by standing and pulling the handle from thigh level to chest level, flexing the elbows while keeping elbows hugged close to the sides. Note: The Dead Lift is not recommended, but a sitting "Rowing" exercise (shown at station 12) may be substituted to strengthen the upper back muscles and biceps.

6. **Chinning** – Grasp handles and pull up until the chin is at hand level; to strengthen biceps, latissimus and upper back muscles.

7. **Dipping** – Support your weight on the handles then lower the body by bending the elbows 90°, then push-up to a straight-arm position again; to strengthen triceps and upper pectorals (chest muscles).

*8. **Hip Flexors**—Support your weight on the forearms. Either with knees bent or knees straight, flex at the hip joint and lift one or both legs. Keep pelvis tilted backward and abdominals contracted; to strengthen hip flexors and lower abdominals. NOTE: This exercise may be hazardous to the back. Single and/or bent knee lifts are less hazardous than the exercise shown. Most people do not need to strengthen the hip flexors.

*9. **Abdominal (Tilt) Board**—Tilt the board at an angle appropriate for your ability. Perform sit-ups with knees bent (rather than as shown), to strengthen upper abdominals.

10. **Thigh and Knee** – "Hamstring Curl": lie prone with heels under pads and flex knees through a full range of motion; to strengthen the knee flexors (including hamstrings); "Knee Extensions": sit on end of bench with ankles under the lower set of pads. Extend the knees through a full range of motion to strengthen the knee extensors, including the quadriceps.

11. **Back Extension** – Adjust the apparatus so the feet can be braced while the pelvic bones rest on the pad. Let the trunk hang relaxed toward the floor. Extend the back until the trunk is parallel with the floor (Caution: do not arch the back); to strengthen the lower back muscles.

12. **Low Pulleys** – Sit with the feet braced, legs straight; grasp handles and keeping elbows out at chest level, pull handles to chest; to strengthen upper back muscles, including trapezius. To strengthen lower back muscles, lean the trunk backward at the hip joint during the pull.

13. **Wrist Conditioner** – Adjust the resistance then grasp the handles, palm down, and rotate the handles by hyperextending the wrists; to strengthen the extensors. Reverse the direction of rotation to strengthen the wrist flexors.

14. **Neck Conditioner** – Place the strap around the forehead and flex the neck, or place the strap around the back or the side of the head and pull backward or sideward to strengthen the neck muscles. Caution: use only light resistance to avoid neck injury.

15. **Hand Gripper** – Adjust the resistance and grasp the handles, palm down. Alternate squeezing the right and the left; to improve grip strength.

16. **Real Runner** – Adjust the resistance; place the feet in the stirrups, the hands on the grips and the chest on the pad. Push and pull with the legs in a running motion; to strengthen the leg muscles.

Centurion 16 – Station Machine
Source: Figure furnished courtesy of Universal Gym Equipment, Inc., Cedar Rapids, Iowa.

Isometric exercise is an effective and inexpensive way to build strength and muscular endurance.

Isometric exercise is an attractive form of exercise because it is effective in building strength and muscular endurance and can be done in the home, office, or car, in a limited space and with no costly equipment. All that is necessary to do many isometric exercises is a piece of rope or a towel and a doorway. It may be hard for some people to motivate themselves when performing isometrics because of the lack of movement involved. Also, isometric exercises may elevate blood pressure, and for that reason, those who have known cardiovascular problems should be under the supervision of a physician when involved in them. Recent evidence indicates that for normal, healthy individuals, isometrics do not cause cardiovascular problems. Some good isometric exercises that can be done in the home are illustrated on pages 91–97.

SAMPLE ISOMETRIC EXERCISES

Isometric exercises are intended primarily to develop muscular strength and endurance. Eighteen different exercises for different body parts are presented here. You should select exercises for your program (if you choose isometric exercise) that meet your own personal needs. All of the following exercises should be held for five to eight seconds and should be repeated several times a day. Muscles depicted in red are those primarily involved in the exercises.

1. Chest Push

Purpose

Develop muscles of the chest and upper arms.

Position

Place left fist in palm of right hand. Keep hands close to chest, forearms parallel to floor.

Movement

Push hands together with maximum strength. (See station 2.)

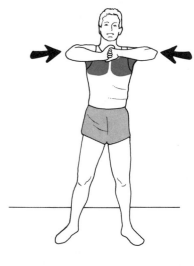

2. Fist Squeeze

Purpose

Develop muscles of the lower arm.

Position

Arms extended at side.

Movement

Clench fists as hard as possible. Repeat. (See stations 13 and 15.)

3. Shoulder Pull

Purpose

Develop muscles of the upper back and arms.

Position

Cup hands and interlock fingers. Keep hands close to chest, forearms parallel to floor.

Movement

Attempt to pull hands apart with maximum force. (See station 12.)

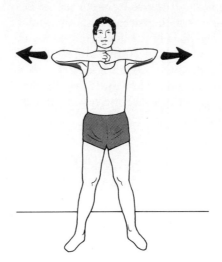

4. Neck Pull

Purpose

Develop muscles of the neck, upper back, and arms.

Position

Interlock fingers behind head, elbows pointing forward.

Movement

Force head backward. Pull hands forward with maximum strength. (See station 14.)

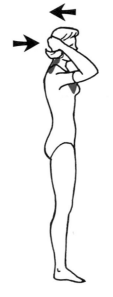

5. Leg Extension

Purpose

Develop muscles of shoulders, legs, and hips.

Position

Loop rope under feet. Stand on rope, feet spread shoulder width. Keep back straight. Bend knees, grasp both ends of rope, back erect, arms straight, and buttocks low.

Movement

Try to straighten legs by lifting upward with maximum strength. (See stations 1 and 16.)

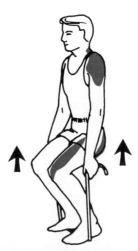

6. Overhead Pull

Purpose

Develop muscles of the arms.

Position

Fold rope in a double loop. Grasp rope overhead, palms outward. Extend arms.

Movement

Push outward at maximum force. Repeat with palms in. (See stations 4, 6, and 12.)

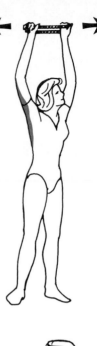

7. Curls

Purpose

Develop muscles on the front of the arms.

Position

Place rope loop behind thighs while standing in a half squat position. Grasp loop, palms up, shoulder width.

Movement

Lift upward with maximum strength. For reverse curls, repeat gripping with palms down. (See stations 5 and 12.)

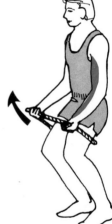

8. Foot Lift

Purpose

Develop muscles of legs.

Position

Stand on loop with left foot. Place loop around right ankle. Flex knee until taut.

Movement

Apply maximum strength upward. Repeat forward and to side with both feet. (See station 10.)

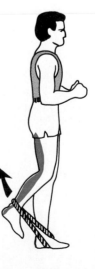

9. Military Press in Doorway

Purpose

Develop muscles of the arms and shoulders.

Position

Stand in doorway, face straight ahead, hands shoulder width apart, elbows bent.

Movement

Tighten leg, hip, and back muscles. Push upward as hard as possible. (See station 3.)

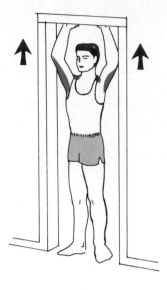

10. Arm Press in Doorway

Purpose

Develop muscles of the arms.

Position

Stand in doorway, back flat on one side of doorway, hands placed on other side.

Movement

Push with maximum strength. (See stations 2 and 3.)

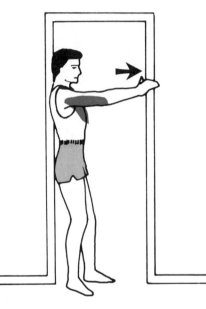

11. Leg Press in Doorway

Purpose

Develop muscles of the legs and hips.

Position

Sit in doorway facing side of door frame. Grasp molding behind head. Keep back flat on side of doorway, feet against other side.

Movement

Push legs with maximum strength. (See stations 4 and 16.)

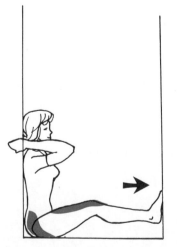

12. Wall Seat

Purpose

Develop muscles of the leg and hips.

Position

Assume half-sit position, back flat against wall, knees bent to 90°.

Movement

Push back against wall with maximum strength. (See stations 4 and 16.)

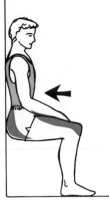

13. Triceps Extension

Purpose

Develop muscles of upper arm.

Position

Grasp towel at both ends. Hold left hand at small of neck, right hand over shoulder.

Movement

Pull towel with maximum force; repeat exercise, changing position of hands. (See stations 2, 3 and 7.)

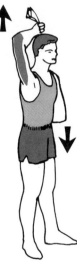

14. Knee Extension

Purpose

Develop muscles of top of upper leg.

Position

Place towel around right ankle, knee bent to 90° angle.

Movement

Grasp towel with both hands behind back, extend leg downward with maximum force. Repeat exercise, changing legs. (See station 10.)

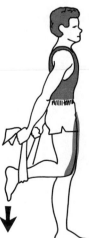

15. Waist Pull

Purpose

Develop muscles of the abdomen, chest, and arms.

Position

Grasp ends of towel, palms in, towel around back of waist, elbows flexed to right angle.

Movement

Pull forward on towel with maximum strength while contracting abdomen and flattening back. (See stations 2 and 9.)

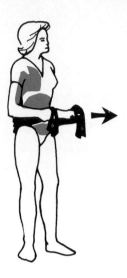

16. Bow Exercise

Purpose

Develop muscles of shoulders and upper back.

Position

Take archer's position with bow (towel) drawn, left elbow partially extended, right hand at chin, right arm parallel to floor.

Movement

Grasp towel and pull arms away from each other. Exchange positions of hands and repeat. (See stations 7 and 12.)

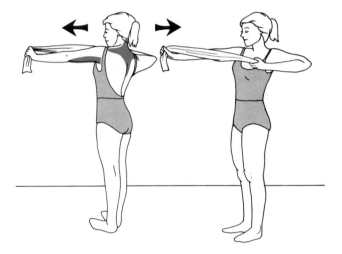

17. Gluteal Pinch

Purpose

Develop muscles of the buttocks.

Position

Lie prone, heels apart and big toes touching.

Movement

Pinch the buttocks together. Hold several seconds. Slowly relax; repeat several times. (See station 1.)

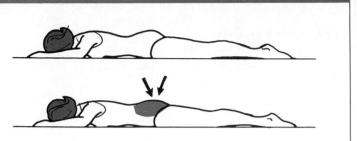

18. Pelvic Tilt

Purpose

Develop muscles of the abdomen and buttocks.

Position

Assume a supine position with the knees bent and slightly apart.

Movement

Press the spine down on the floor and hold for several seconds. Keep abdominals and gluteals tightened. (See stations 1 and 9.)

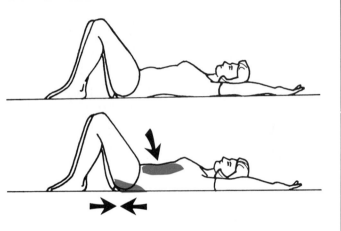

Exer-Genie Exercises

Examples of some of the isokinetic exercises that can be performed on the Exer-Genie (figure 10.1) are described below:

A. **Back Extension**—Keep the arms straight and bend the knees and hips until the handle can be grasped. Pull on the rope by extending knees, hips and back, rolling the shoulders backward; strengthens hip, knee and back extensors.

B. **Straight-Leg Position**—Stand erect and grasp handles with hands either palm-down or palm-up; perform "biceps curls" by hugging elbows to the sides while flexing elbows and pulling the handle to the chest; strengthens elbow flexors (biceps).

C. **Curling and Abduction Position**—Perform an "Upright Rowing" exercise by starting as in Position B with palms down, then pull the rope upward, bending the elbows out to the side and pulling the shoulders back until the handle reaches chin level; strengthens elbow flexor (including biceps), shoulder rotators and deltoids and upper back (including trapezius).

D. **Press Overhead**—Start with the handle at chin level, elbows bent and at the sides of the chest. Push the handle overhead by extending the elbows as in a "military press"; strengthens shoulders and arms (including deltoids and triceps).

E. **Big Four**—All of the muscle groups described above could be strengthened in one exercise by combining movements through the four positions into one continuous movement as shown in figure 10.1. Note: The first portion (A) of this exercise is potentially harmful to the back.

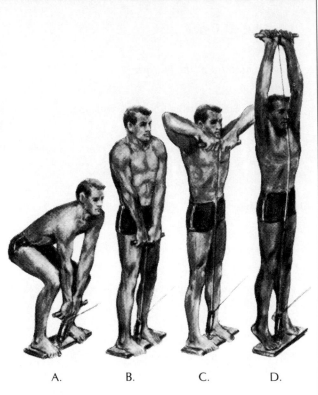

A.   B.   C.   D.

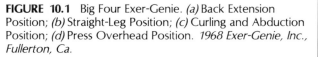

FIGURE 10.1 Big Four Exer-Genie. *(a)* Back Extension Position; *(b)* Straight-Leg Position; *(c)* Curling and Abduction Position; *(d)* Press Overhead Position. *1968 Exer-Genie, Inc., Fullerton, Ca.*

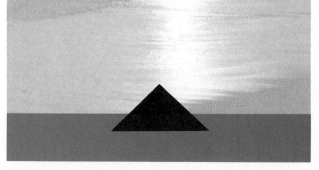

11

FLEXIBILITY

CONCEPT 11

Adequate flexibility permits
freedom of movement and may contribute
to ease and economy of muscular effort,
success in certain activities,
and less susceptibility to
some types of injuries
or musculoskeletal problems.

INTRODUCTION

Flexibility* is a measure of the range of motion available at a joint or group of joints. It is determined by the shape of the bones and cartilage in the joint, and by the length of muscles and ligaments that cross the joint. Traditionally, body flexibility has been the most neglected of the five health-related components of physical fitness. However, there has been a recent surge of interest in "stretching exercises" by athletes, fitness buffs, and researchers.

The range of movement at a joint may vary. It may be restricted so that it will not bend or straighten, and is said to be "tight," "stiff," or have "contractures." The deformed hand of an arthritic is an example of this extreme. At the other end of the spectrum is a high degree of flexibility referred to as "loose jointed," "hypermobility," or erroneously, "double-jointedness." An example of this extreme is the contortionist seen at the circus. Each person, depending upon his or her individual needs, must have a reasonable amount of flexibility to perform efficiently and effectively in daily life.

*The classifications of the types of flexibility exercises described in this concept are consistent with those currently being used in the clinical setting.

TERMS

Active Stretch (formerly called antagonist stretch)—
Muscles are stretched by the active force of the contraction of the opposing, or antagonist, muscle. For example, when doing a toe-touch exercise, the muscles on the front of the thigh (quadriceps) contract to cause a stretch of the muscles on the back of the thigh (hamstrings). (See figure 11.1A.)

Ballistic Stretch (Dynamic)—Muscles are stretched by the force of momentum of a body part that is bounced, swung, or jerked, as in the toe-touch exercise shown in figure 9.1D and E. The trunk is bounced forward either by antagonist muscle force or by an assist from another person or another body part.

Flexibility—Range of motion (ROM) in a joint or group of joints. Because muscle length is a major factor limiting the range of motion, those having long muscles that allow for good joint mobility are considered to have good flexibility.

Hamstrings—Muscles that cross the back of the hip joint and the back of the knee joint causing hip extension and knee flexion. They make up the bulk on the back of the thigh.

Laxity—Looseness or slackness of the muscles and ligaments (soft tissue) surrounding a joint.

Ligaments—Bands of tissue that connect bones.

Lumbar Muscles—Erector spinae and other muscles of the lower back (lumbar region of the spine); the muscles in the "small of the back." These muscles are used to arch (hyperextend) the lower back.

Passive Stretch (formerly called assisted stretch)— Stretch imposed on a muscle by another person or another body part, or something other than the opposing muscle. For example, when doing the toe-touch exercise, the force causing the stretch is provided by an assist from another person pushing gently on your back (figure 11.1B); or you may grasp your ankles and pull with your arms (figure 11.1C); or you could use gravity; or you could use an extra weight to provide the assist.

PNF Exercise (Proprioceptive Neuromuscular Facilitation)—Special exercise techniques to increase the contraction or the relaxation of muscles through reflex mechanisms (figure 11.1F and G).

Reciprocal Innervation—When a muscle (agonist) contracts, its opposing muscle (antagonist) will reflexly relax.

Static Stretch—A muscle is slowly stretched and then held in that stretched position for several seconds. For example, if you lie on your back, pull one knee to your chest and hold it there with your arms for a count of ten, you are placing a static stretch on your back muscles.

Trigger Point—An especially irritable spot, usually a tight band or "knot" in a muscle or fascia. This often refers pain to another area of the body. For example, a trigger point in the shoulder might cause a headache. This condition is referred to as "myofascial pain syndrome" and is often caused by muscle tension, fatigue, or strain.

THE FACTS

To increase the length of a muscle, you must stretch it (overload) more than its normal length.

There is much that is not known about **flexibility,** but the best evidence suggests that muscles should be stretched to about 10 percent beyond their normal length to bring about an improvement in flexibility. Exercises that do not cause an overload by stretching beyond normal will not increase flexibility.

There are several effective methods of exercising to develop flexibility.

Three commonly used types of stretching exercises are **static, ballistic,** and **PNF.** Each of these can be performed as an **active stretch** or as a **passive stretch.** All are effective in developing flexibility.

Static stretching is widely recommended because it is less apt to cause injury and soreness.

Because static stretching is done slowly and held for a period of time, there is less probability of tearing the soft tissue, particularly if the force comes from your own muscles.

Active stretch is safer and more effective than passive stretch.

When active stretch is used, the opposing muscles contract. This makes the muscles you are trying to stretch relax (reflexly) so that they can be stretched farther. When stretching is done passively by something other than the antagonist muscle, the reflex relaxation does not occur, so there is more potential for injury. For this reason passive stretching is not as effective as the active stretch. Because it is difficult to get an overload by using only the opposing muscles, most people will need to combine the active stretch with a passive assist. This gives the advantage of a relaxed muscle and a greater stretch. (See figure 11.1, exercises A, B, and C, for further clarification.)

Ballistic stretching may be an important technique for active people.

A ballistic stretch uses momentum to produce the stretch. Momentum is produced by vigorous motion, such as flinging a body part or rocking it back and forth to create a bouncing movement. Because this produces a sudden stretch on the muscle, and may stretch it farther than other methods, there is the potential for injury. Most people avoid this type of stretching, but everyone does not agree that its disadvantages outweigh its advantages.

Since many athletic activities are ballistic in nature, some experts recommend the use of predominantly static stretching in early training, with an increasing amount of ballistic exercise as flexibility improves. The principle of specificity of training implies that one should use the type of stretching movements that are most apt to occur in the activity for which one is training. Ballistic exercises are illustrated in figure 11.1D and E. Passive ballistic stretching is particularly risky and is not recommended for use outside of the clinic.

Some PNF (Proprioceptive Neuromuscular Facilitation) techniques have proven to be effective methods of improving flexibility.

PNF has been popular for rehabilitation since the 1960s. It consists of dozens of techniques to stimulate muscles to contract more strongly or to relax more fully so that they can be stretched. Two techniques have become popular in fitness programs to improve the flexibility of healthy people: "contract-relax-contract," and "contract-relax."

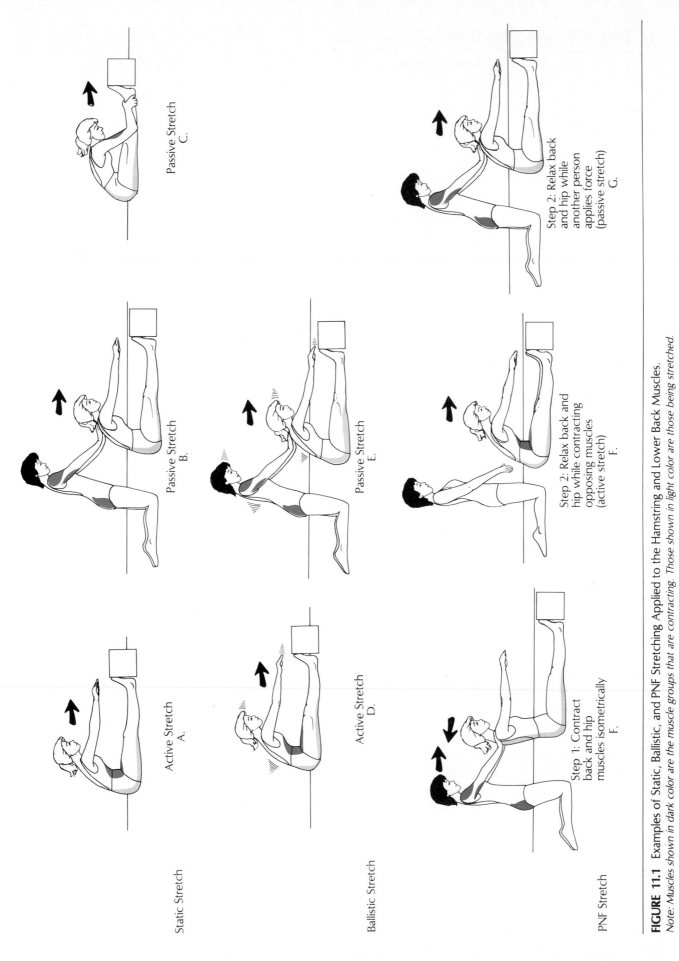

FIGURE 11.1 Examples of Static, Ballistic, and PNF Stretching Applied to the Hamstring and Lower Back Muscles.
Note: Muscles shown in dark color are the muscle groups that are contracting. Those shown in light color are those being stretched.

Static Stretch

Active Stretch
A.

Passive Stretch
B.

Passive Stretch
C.

Ballistic Stretch

Active Stretch
D.

Passive Stretch
E.

PNF Stretch

Step 1: Contract back and hip muscles isometrically
F.

Step 2: Relax back and hip while contracting opposing muscles (active stretch)
F.

Step 2: Relax back and hip while another person applies force (passive stretch)
G.

TABLE 11.1 Flexibility Threshold of Training and Fitness Target Zones

	Threshold of Training			Target Zones		
	Static	Ballistic	PNF	Static	Ballistic	PNF
Frequency	• 3 days per week for all methods.			• 3 to 7 days per week for all methods.		
Intensity	• Stretch as far as you can go without pain; with slow movement, hold at the end of the range of motion.	• Stretch muscle beyond normal length with gentle bounce or swing, but do not exceed 10% of active-static range of motion.	• Same as static except use a maximum isometric contraction of the muscle prior to stretch.	• When *active stretch* is used, the muscle should be stretched as far as possible using only the antagonist muscles. • When *passive stretch* is used, the muscle should not be stretched more than 10% beyond its normal range of motion, and it should not reach the point of pain. Care should be taken to avoid overstretch.		
Time (Duration)	• Hold the stretch for 10 seconds.	• 1 set of 5–10 repetitions.	• Hold isometric contraction 6 seconds; hold stretch 20 seconds; repeat 3 times.	• Hold 10–60 seconds; 1–3 repetitions.	• 1–5 sets of 5–10 repetitions; 10 seconds rest between sets.	• Hold isometric contraction 6 seconds. • Hold stretch 20–60 seconds for 1–3 sets. • 30-second rest between sets.

The contract-relax-contract technique involves three steps: (1) move the limb so the muscle to be stretched is elongated initially, then contract it isometrically against an immovable object or the resistance of a partner for six seconds; (2) relax the muscle; (3) stretch the muscle immediately by contracting the antagonist for twenty to sixty seconds. Recent research suggests that this type of PNF stretch is more effective than a simple static stretch without the preceding isometric contraction. An example of the contract-relax-contract PNF exercise is shown in figure 11.1F.

A variation of this PNF procedure is contract-relax. This is the same procedure as the contract-relax-contract technique except that the static stretch is done passively (with an assist). Following the isometric contraction, another person applies force to stretch the muscles. There is no contraction of the opposing muscles during the stretch.

It is possible to combine these two techniques so that the opposing muscles contract while another person assists in applying the stretch. Theoretically, the muscle would be elongated more by this procedure, but any time assistance is provided by another person or a machine, there is danger of overstretching the muscle. This modification is shown in figure 11.1G.

There is a minimum amount of exercise (threshold of training) and an optimal amount of exercise (target zone) necessary for developing flexibility.

The threshold of training and target zones for static, ballistic, and PNF stretching are presented in table 11.1. The time required to stretch tissue varies inversely with the force used. Low force requires more time, whereas high force requires less time.

Each form of flexibility exercise has its advantages and disadvantages.

The advantages and disadvantages of ballistic, static, and PNF exercises using both active stretch and passive stretch methods are summarized in table 11.2. The best method or methods for you may depend upon your physical condition, and whether you wish to increase your range of motion, or just maintain it.

The temperature of the muscle being stretched influences the effectiveness of the stretch.

Studies show that tendons can be stretched farther when warmed to 104° F or more. This can be done with warm-up exercises or the application of heat. It has also been found that cooling the muscle with two to three minutes of ice massage before the tension is released can aid in retaining the lengthening effect and may also help to reduce soreness and stiffness.

TABLE 11.2 Comparison of Advantages and Disadvantages of Six Types of Flexibility Exercises

A. Active Stretch

Static-Active Stretch	Ballistic-Active Stretch	PNF with Active Stretch (Contract-Relax-Contract)
1. Will not overstretch tissue.	1. If done vigorously, can overstretch tissue, especially in presence of scar tissue or pathology.	1. Will not overstretch tissue; therapists use PNF in treatment of arthritics.
2. May be ineffective in producing enough stretch to increase muscle length. It can be used to maintain current flexibility levels or in combination with *passive stretch* to improve flexibility.	2. Is effective for increasing flexibility because momentum produces overload.	2. More effective than static and ballistic for increasing flexibility, especially if combined with *passive stretch*.
3. Useful if combined with *passive stretch* to relieve muscle cramps.	3. Not recommended for cramps.	3. Useful if combined with *passive stretch* to relieve muscle cramps.
4. Useful if combined with *passive stretch* for some types of muscle soreness.	4. If done vigorously, may cause soreness.	4. Useful if combined with *passive stretch* for some types of muscle soreness.
5. Does not develop strength.	5. Does not develop strength.	5. Strength is developed in muscle being stretched.
6. Stretched muscle relaxes through reciprocal innervation with contracting antagonist.	6. Stretched muscle relaxes through reciprocal innervation with contracting antagonist.	6. Stretched muscle relaxes because of reciprocal innervation and previous isometric contraction.
7. Stretch will elicit mild reflex contraction that will gradually subside as stretch is held.	7. Stretch reflex will be elicited more strongly, but muscle will not strengthen because it is not overloaded during contraction.	7. Stretch will elicit mild reflex contraction that will gradually subside as stretch is held.
8. May become boring.	8. More nearly resembles movements needed in some athletics and daily activities.	8. Easier to do if another person applies resistance.

B. Passive Stretch

Static-Passive Stretch	Ballistic-Passive Stretch	PNF with Passive Stretch (Contract-Relax)
1. May overstretch tissue.	1. Most apt to overstretch tissue.	1. May overstretch tissue.
2. Effective for increasing flexibility, but better if combined with *active stretch* or if muscle is consciously relaxed.	2. Effective for increasing flexibility, but better if combined with *active stretch*, or if muscle is consciously relaxed.	2. Not as effective as *active static* or PNF with *active stretch*, but would be better if combined with *active stretch* or if muscle was consciously relaxed.
3. Can aid in relief of soreness, but more effective if combined with *active stretch* or if the muscle is consciously relaxed.	3. More apt to cause soreness.	3. Can aid in relief of soreness, but more effective if combined with *active stretch* or if the muscle is consciously relaxed.
4. Can aid in relief of muscle cramps, but more effective if combined with *active stretch* or if the muscle is consciously relaxed.	4. Not recommended for muscle cramps.	4. Can aid in muscle cramps, but more effective if combined with *active stretch* or if the muscle is consciously relaxed.
5. Does not develop strength.	5. Does not develop strength.	5. Develops strength in muscle being stretched.
6. Muscle being stretched does not relax unless combined with *active stretch* or with conscious relaxation.	6. Muscle being stretched does not relax unless combined with *active stretch* or with conscious relaxation.	6. Muscle being stretched will relax because of previous isometric contraction, especially if conscious relaxation is used.
7. Will elicit mild stretch reflex that is lessened if combined with *active stretch* or with conscious relaxation.	7. Will elicit mild stretch reflex that is lessened if combined with *active stretch* or with conscious relaxation.	7. Will elicit mild stretch reflex that is lessened if combined with *active stretch* or with conscious relaxation.
8. Requires outside force: another person, other body parts, or gravity.	8. Requires outside force: another person, other body parts, or gravity.	8. Easier to do if another person applies stretch, but any outside force may be used.

For maximal effectiveness and minimal harm, there are guidelines that should be followed in performing flexibility exercises.

There is a correct and an incorrect way to exercise, and some exercises can even be harmful. Concept 12 presents guidelines for flexibility exercises and some samples of the exercises defined in this concept.

Lack of use, injury, or disease can decrease joint mobility.

Arthritis and calcium deposits can damage a joint, and inflammation can cause pain that prevents movement. Failure to move a joint regularly through its full range of motion can lead to a shortening of muscles and ligaments. Static positions held for longer periods of time, such as in poor posture, working postures, and when a body part is immobilized by a cast, lead to shortened tissue and loss of mobility. Improper exercise that overdevelops one muscle group while neglecting the opposing group results in an imbalance that restricts flexibility.

Flexibility is specific to each joint of the body.

No one flexibility test will give an indication of your overall flexibility. For example, "tight" **hamstrings** and back muscles might be revealed by a toe-touch test, but the range of motion in other joints may be quite different.

Flexibility is influenced by age and sex.

As children grow older, their flexibility increases until adolescence when they become progressively less flexible. As a general rule, girls tend to be more flexible than boys. This is probably due to anatomical differences in the joints, as well as to differences in the type and extent of activities the two sexes tend to choose. In adults, there is less difference between the sexes.

Scores on flexibility tests may be influenced by several factors.

Range of motion may be influenced by your motivation to exert maximum effort, your warm-up preparation, the presence of muscular soreness, your tolerance for pain, the room temperature, and your ability to relax. Contrary to popular opinion, there is very little relationship between leg or trunk length and the scores made on flexibility tests.

Stretching exercises are useful in preventing and remediating some cases of dysmenorrhea in women.

Painful menstruation (dysmenorrhea) of some types can be prevented or reduced by stretching the pelvic and hip joint fascia. Billig's exercise is an example of an effective exercise (see p. 111).

Static muscle stretching appears to be effective in relieving muscle soreness and "shin splints."

One theory suggests that local muscle soreness may be caused by slight reflex contractions. There is the belief that a static stretch of the affected muscle may relieve these slight contractions and thus relieve the pain. Even some cases of nonpathological shin splints may be relieved by such exercise.

Adequate flexibility may help prevent muscle strain and such orthopedic problems as backache.

Short, tight muscles are more apt to be injured by overstretching than are long muscles. One common cause of backache is shortened **lumbar** and hip flexor muscles. (See Concept 17 for more discussion on back problems.) Stretching exercises may help prevent or alleviate some backaches, muscle cramps, and muscle strains.

***Trigger points** may sometimes be prevented or inactivated by static, or PNF stretching, of the muscles involved.*

When body parts are held in static positions for long periods of time, or when muscles are chronically overloaded, fatigued, or chilled, myofascial trigger points may cause stiffness and local or referred pain. Often the trigger point can be deactivated and the pain relieved by gentle but persistent stretching of the muscle, especially if accompanied or followed by the application of heat or cold.

*Passive stretching may exceed the limits of extensibility of the muscles, tendons, and **ligaments** and cause injury.*

When force that is not under the control of the exerciser is applied to stretch the soft tissue around a joint, it may result in torn tissue. A partner or machine cannot "feel" how much stretch is being applied and so may cause injury especially with ballistic-passive exercises.

Too much flexibility in certain joints may make a person more susceptible to injury or hamper performance.

Muscles and tendons have both extensibility and elasticity. Ligaments and the joint capsule are extensible but lack elasticity. When stretched, they remain in the lengthened state. If this occurs, the joint may lack stability and is susceptible to chronic dislocation or movement in an undesirable plane. This is particularly true of weight-bearing joints, such as the hip, knee, and ankle. Loose ligaments may allow the joint to twist abnormally, tearing the cartilage and other soft tissue.

On the other hand, joint **laxity** does not necessarily mean instability. Though most studies show no relationship between laxity and subsequent injury, there is some evidence that loose knees are detrimental in football and in ballet. Dancers seem to have a decreased ability to judge how much movement has taken place in the knee and, therefore, may be more susceptible to injury.

In the fifth century, Hippocrates noted the disadvantage of hyperextension of the elbow in archery. The hyperextended position for elbows and knees is not an efficient position from which to move because of a poor angle of muscle pull. For example, it is difficult to perform push-ups when the elbows lock into hyperextension because extra effort is required to "unlock" the joint.

Good flexibility may bring about improved athletic performance.

A hurdler must have good hip joint mobility to clear the hurdle. A swimmer requires shoulder and ankle flexibility for powerful strokes. A diver must be able to reach his or her toes in order to perform a good jackknife. Low back flexibility allows a runner to lengthen the stride. The fencer needs long hamstrings and hip adductors in order to lunge a long distance.

It is not necessary to sacrifice flexibility in order to develop strength.

A person with bulging muscles may become muscle-bound, or have a restricted range of motion, if strength training is done improperly. In any progressive resistance program, both agonists and antagonists should receive equal training and all movements should be carried through the full range of motion. Properly conducted strength training does not cause a person to be muscle-bound. Furthermore, there is no evidence that a long muscle is any weaker than a short one.

There is no ideal standard for flexibility.

It is not known how much flexibility any one person should have in a joint. There are test "norms" available that list how hundreds of subjects of various ages, from both sexes, and in many walks of life have performed. But there is little scientific evidence to indicate why a person who can reach two inches past his or her toes on a sit-and-reach test is no less fit than a person who can reach eight inches past the toes. Too much flexibility could be as detrimental as too little.

▶ LAB RESOURCE MATERIALS (FOR USE WITH LAB 11, PAGE 243)

Flexibility Tests

Because it is impractical to test the flexibility of all joints, perform these tests for the joints used most frequently in movement performance.

1. *Flexibility Test of Lower Back and Hamstrings*
   a. Sit on the floor with your knees together and your feet flat against a bench turned on its side.
   b. With a partner holding your knees straight, reach forward with your arms fully extended.
   c. Measure the distance your fingertips reach on the measuring stick fixed on the bench. (The six-inch mark of the measuring stick should be flush with the end of the bench.)

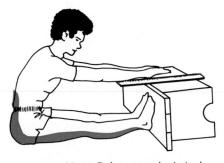

Note: Ruler extends six inches over the end of the bench

2. *Shoulder Flexibility*
   a. Raise your right arm, bend your elbow, and reach down across your back as far as possible.
   b. At the same time, extend your left arm down and behind your back, bend your elbow up across your back, and try to cross your fingers over those of your right hand as shown in the accompanying illustration.
   c. Measure the distance to the nearest half-inch. If your fingers overlap, score as a plus; if they fail to meet, score as a minus; use a zero if your fingertips just touch.
   d. Repeat with your arms crossed in the opposite direction (left arm up). Most people will find that they are more flexible on one side than the other.

3. *Hamstring and Hip Flexor Flexibility*
   a. Lie on your back on the floor beside a wall.
   b. Slowly lift one leg off the floor. Keep the other leg flat on the floor.
   c. Keep both legs straight.
   d. Continue to lift the leg until either leg begins to bend or the lower leg begins to lift off the floor.
   e. Place a yardstick against the wall and underneath the lifted leg.
   f. Hold the yardstick against the wall after the leg is lowered.
   g. Measure the angle created by the floor and the yardstick using a protractor. The greater the angle, the better your score.
   h. Repeat with the other leg.

Note: For ease of testing, you may want to draw angles on a piece of posterboard as illustrated.

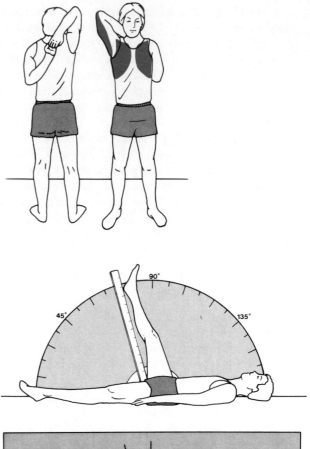

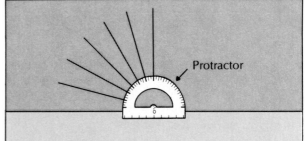

CHART 11.1 Flexibility *Rating Scale*

Classification	Men				Women			
	Test 1	Test 2		Test 3	Test 1	Test 2		Test 3
		Right Up	Left Up			Right Up	Left Up	
High Performance Zone	14+	7+	7+	111+	15+	8+	8+	111+
Good Fitness Zone	10–13	6	3–6	80–110	10–14	6–7	3–7	80–110
Marginal Zone	6–9	4–5	0–2	60–79	6–9	4–5	0–2	60–79
Low Zone	<6	<4	<0	<60	<6	<4	<0	<60

Though many people become less flexible as they grow older, for optimal health, it is recommended that you attempt to maintain adequate levels of flexibility indicated on the chart throughout life.

REFERENCES

Barrack, R. L., H. B. Skinner, M. E. Brunet, and S. D. Cook. "Joint Laxity and Proprioception in the Knee." *Physician and Sportsmedicine* 11(1983):130.

Beaulieu, J. E. "Developing a Stretching Program." *Physician and Sportsmedicine* 9(1981):59.

Brodie, D. A., H. A. Bird, and V. Wright. "Joint Laxity in Selected Athletic Populations." *Medicine and Science in Sports and Exercise* 14(1980):190.

*Corbin, C. B. "Profiling for Flexibility." In Nicholas, J. A. and J. Herschberger, *Clinics in Sports Medicine: Profiling*. Philadelphia: W. B. Saunders Co., 1984.

Cornelius, W. L., and M. M. Hinson. "The Relationship between Isometric Contractions of Hip Extensors and Subsequent Flexibility in Males." *Journal of Sports Medicine and Physical Fitness* 20(1980):75.

*Dominguez, R. H., and R. S. Gajda. *Total Body Conditioning*. New York: Charles Scribners Sons, 1982.

Gordon, G. A. "PNF Prorioceptive Neuromuscular Facilitation, 'The Super Stretch'." *National Strength and Conditioning Association Journal* 4(April–May 1982):26.

Grahame, R., and J. M. Jenkins. "Joint Hypermobility—Asset or Liability." *Annals of Rheumatic Disease* 31(1972):109.

Grossman, M. R., et al. "Review of Length Associated Changes in Muscle." *Physical Therapy* 62(1982):1799.

Hardy, L. "Improving Active Range of Hip Flexion." *Research Quarterly for Exercise and Sport* 56(June 1985):111.

Hardy, L., and D. Jones. "Dynamic Flexibility and Proprioceptive Neuromuscular Facilitation." *Research Quarterly for Exercise and Sport* 57(June 1986):150.

Hartley-O'Brien, S. J. "Six Mobilization Exercises for Active Range of Hip Flexion." *Research Quarterly of Exercise and Sport* 51(1980):625.

Holt, L. E., T. M. Travis, and T. Okita. "Comparative Study of Three Stretching Techniques." *Perceptual and Motor Skills* 31(1970):611.

Kendall, H., and E. McCreary. *Muscle Testing and Function*. Baltimore: Williams and Wilkins, 1983.

Kisner, C., and L. A. Colby. *Therapeutic Exercises. Foundations and Techniques*. Philadelphia: F. A. Davis, Co., 1985.

Kreighbaum, E., and K. M. Barthels. *Biomechanics: A Qualitative Approach for Studying Human Movement*. Minneapolis: Burgess Publishing Co., 1985.

Kuprian, W., ed. *Physical Therapy For Sports*. Philadelphia: W. B. Saunders, Co., 1982.

Lindsey, R., B. Jones, and A. Whitley. *Fitness for Health, Figure/Physique, Posture*. 5th ed. Dubuque, Iowa: Wm. C. Brown Publishers, 1983.

Luttgens, K., and K. Wells. *Kinesiology: Scientific Basis of Human Movement*. Philadelphia: Saunders College Publishing, 1982.

Millar, A. P. "An Early Stretching for Calf Muscle Strains." *Medicine and Science in Sports* 8(1976):39.

Millar, A. P. "Strains of the Posterior Calf Musculature (Tennis Leg)." *American Journal of Sports Medicine* 7(1979):172.

Moore, M. A., and R. S. Hutton. "Electromyographic Investigation of Muscle Stretching Techniques." *Medicine and Science in Sports and Exercise* 12(1980):322.

Nicholas, J. A. "Injuries to the Knee Ligaments." *Journal of the American Medical Association* 212(1970):2236.

O'Neil, R. "Prevention of Hamstring and Groin Strain." *Athletic Training* 11(1976):27.

Parry, C. W. "Stretching." In *Manipulation, Traction and Massage*, edited by J. V. Basmajian. Baltimore: Williams and Wilkins, 1985, 157.

Perez, H., and S. Famasoli. "Benefit of Proprioceptive Neuromuscular Facilitation on the Joint Mobility of Youth-Aged Female Gymnasts with Correlations for Rehabilitation." *American Corrective Therapy Journal* 38:6(November–December 1984):142.

Rivera, M. L. "Effects of Static, Ballistic, and Modified Proprioceptive Neuromuscular Stretching Exercises on the Flexibility and Retention of Flexibility in Selected Joints." Master's thesis, University of Kansas, 1979.

Rogers, J. L. "PNF: A New Way to Improve Flexibility." *Track Technique* 12(1978):2345.

Sady, S. P., M. Wortman, and D. Blank. "Flexibility Training: Ballistic, Static or Proprioceptive Neuromuscular Facilitation." *Archives of Physical Medicine and Rehabilitation* 63(June 1982):261.

Sapega, A. A., T. C. Quedenfeld, R. A. Moyer, and R. A. Butler. "Biophysical Factors in Range of Motion Exercise." *Physician and Sportsmedicine* 9(1981):57.

Schultz, P. "Flexibility: Day of the Static Stretch." *Physician and Sportsmedicine* 7(1979):109.

Shyne, K. "Richard H. Dominguez, M.D.: To Stretch or Not To Stretch." *Physician and Sportsmedicine* 10(September 1982):137.

Stevenson, E. "Stretches." *CAHPERD Journal Times* 48(January 1986):16.

Stevenson, E. "Hamstring Stretches." *CAHPERD Journal Times* 48(March 1986):6.

Surburg, P. R. "Neuromuscular Facilitation Techniques in Sports Medicine." *Physician and Sportsmedicine* 9(1981):115.

Tanigawa, M. C. "Mobilization on Increasing Muscle Length." *Physical Therapy* 52(1972):725.

Time-Life Books. *Staying Flexible: The Full Range of Motion*. Alexandria, Va.: Time-Life Books, 1987.

Travell, J. G., and D. G. Simons. *Myofascial Pain and Dysfunction: The Trigger Point Manual*. Baltimore: Williams and Wilkins, 1983.

Wathen, D. "Flexibility, Strength and Conditioning." *Strength and Conditioning Association Journal* 6(August–September 1984):71.

Wilford, H. N., and J. F. Smith. "A Comparison of Proprioceptive Neuromuscular Facilitation and Static Stretching Techniques." *American Corrective Therapy Journal* 39:2(March–April 1985):30.

12

STRETCHING EXERCISES

CONCEPT 12

Stretching exercises
are designed to maintain
or increase flexibility
by stretching the muscles
and other soft tissue around the joints.
This stretch may, in turn,
prevent or alleviate
some musculoskeletal problems.

INTRODUCTION

There are many ways to stretch muscles and improve flexibility through exercise (see Concept 11). The major types of muscle stretching exercises are static stretching, ballistic stretching, and PNF. These exercises can be done by yourself, using only your own muscles to stretch; they can be done with the aid of gravity (body weight); or they can be done with the assistance of someone else. To develop flexibility, the muscles must be stretched beyond their normal range.

TERMS

Detailed descriptions of important stretching and flexibility terms are presented in Concept 11.

THE FACTS

There is a correct way to perform stretching exercises.

Remember that while stretching may help to alleviate muscular soreness, it can also *cause* soreness, so "easy does it." Start below your threshold if you are unaccustomed to stretching a given muscle group, then work up to your target zone. The guidelines that follow will help you to gain the most benefit from your exercises.

- Warm the muscles *before you attempt to stretch them.*
- Exercises that do not cause a muscle to lengthen beyond normal may maintain, but will not increase, flexibility.
- To increase flexibility, the muscle must be overloaded (stretched beyond its normal length), but not to the point of pain. Remember, you want to stretch muscles, not joints!
- Exercises must be performed for each muscle group and at each joint where flexibility is desired.
- If ballistic stretching is used, precede it with static or PNF exercise.
- Avoid ballistic exercises on previously injured muscles or joints, especially the lower back muscles.
- Avoid passive ballistic stretches unless you are under the supervision of a therapist or trainer.
- If ballistic stretches are used, the bounces should be gentle and probably not exceed 10 percent of the normal static stretch range of motion. Avoid high risk stretching exercises (see Concept 19).
- For static stretches, stretch until you begin to feel pain, "back off" slightly and hold the position several seconds, then gradually try to stretch a little farther. The stretch should feel slightly uncomfortable but should *not* be painful.

There are certain areas of the body that especially need to be stretched for good health and fitness.

Areas of the body that are most apt to need stretching include the muscles on the back of the legs (hamstrings) in order to prevent soreness, injury in sports, and referred back pain; the muscles on the inside of the thigh in order to prevent back, leg, and foot strain; the calf muscles in order to prevent soreness and Achilles tendon injuries in jogging/running; the muscles on the front of the hip joint in order to prevent lordosis and backache; the low back muscles in order to help prevent back soreness and pain, as well as back injuries; and the muscles on the front of the chest and shoulders in order to prevent rounded shoulders and limited range of movement in the shoulder joint. The exercises pictured in this concept focus on these body areas.

Certain stretching exercises are good for therapeutic purposes, as well as for fitness.

Stretching exercises can be prescribed specifically to alleviate pain. Usually, the same exercise, if done regularly, can prevent the condition that originally caused the pain. Examples of "therapeutic" exercises include exercise 1 (or some variation of it) to stretch the calf muscle. This will relieve muscle cramps in the lower leg. Exercise 6, Billig's exercise, can be used to relieve menstrual cramps (dysmenorrhea). The shin stretcher (exercise 11) will relieve soreness in the front of the lower leg (shin splints).

SAMPLE FLEXIBILITY EXERCISES

These stretching exercises are intended primarily to develop flexibility. Fifteen exercises for different body parts are presented here. They include static and PNF type exercises that do require a partner. These exercises should be held for twenty to sixty seconds. Muscles depicted in color are those primarily involved in the exercises.

1. Lower Leg Stretcher

Purpose

To stretch the calf muscles and Achilles tendon.

Position

Stand with the toes on a thick book or lower rung of a stall bar. Hold on to a support with hands.

Movement

Rise up on toes as far as possible and hold for several seconds. Relax and lower heels to floor as far as possible; hold. If ballistic stretch is desired, bounce gently.

Note

Static stretch may alleviate sore calf muscles.

2. Sitting Stretcher

Purpose

To stretch muscles on inside of thighs.

Position

Sit with soles of feet together; place hands on knees or ankles and lean forearms against knees; resist while attempting to raise knees.

Movement

Hold several seconds then relax and press the knees toward the floor as far as possible; hold.

Note

Useful for pregnant women or anyone whose thighs tend to rotate inward causing backache, knock-knees and flat feet.

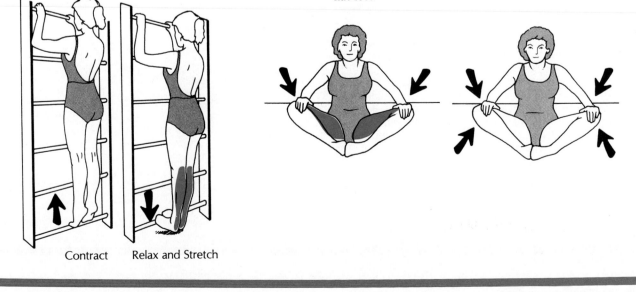

Contract   Relax and Stretch

3. One-Leg Stretcher

Purpose

To stretch lower back and hamstring muscles.

Position

Stand with one foot on a bench; keeping both legs straight.

Movement

Press down on bench with heel for several seconds, then relax and bend the trunk forward, trying to touch the head to the knee. Hold for a few seconds. Return to starting position and repeat with opposite leg. As flexibility improves, the arms can be used to pull the chest toward the legs. Do not allow either knee to lock.

Note

This is useful in relief of backache and correction of lordosis. If desired, bounce the trunk gently.

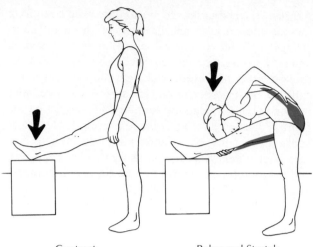

Contract   Relax and Stretch

4. Leg Hug

Purpose

To stretch lower back and gluteals.

Position

Hook-lying position.

Movement

Arch back and lift hips. Hold several seconds. Relax and pull knees to chest as hard as possible; hold.

Note

Useful for backache and lordosis (also see Concept 18).

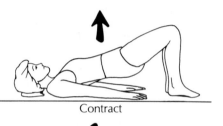

Contract

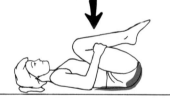

Relax and Stretch

5. Pectoral Stretch

Purpose

To stretch pectorals.

Position

Stand erect in doorway with arms raised shoulder height, elbows bent, and hands grasping doorjambs; feet in front stride position.

Movement

Press forward on door frame, contracting the arms maximally for several seconds. Relax and shift weight forward on legs so muscles on front of shoulder joint and chest are stretched; hold.

Note

Useful to prevent or correct round shoulders and sunken chest.

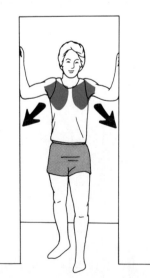

6. Billig's Exercise

Purpose

To stretch pelvic fascia, hip flexors, and inside of thigh.

Position

Stand with side to a wall and place the elbow and forearm against the wall at shoulder height. Tilt the pelvis backward tightening the gluteal and abdominal muscles.

Movement

Place opposite hand on hip and push the hips toward the wall. Push forward and sideward (45°) with the hips. Do not twist the hips. Hold. Repeat on opposite side.

Note

Useful for preventing some cases of dysmenorrhea.

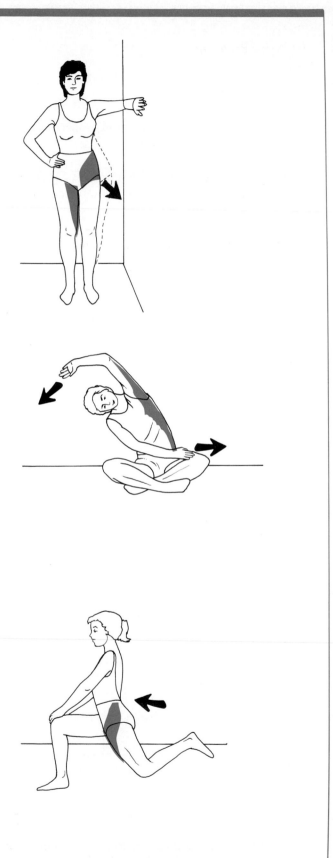

7. Lateral Trunk Stretcher

Purpose

To stretch trunk muscles.

Position

Sit on the floor.

Movement

Stretch left arm over head to right. Bend to right at waist reaching as far to right as possible with left arm and as far as possible to the left with right arm; hold. Do not let trunk rotate. Repeat on opposite side. For less stretch, overhead arm may be bent at elbow.

Note

This exercise can be done in the standing position but is less effective.

8. Hip and Thigh Stretcher

Purpose

To stretch iliopsoas and quadriceps.

Position

Place right knee directly above right ankle and stretch left leg backward so knee touches floor. If necessary, place hands on floor for balance.

Movement

Press pelvis forward and downward; hold. Repeat on opposite side. *Caution:* Do not bend front knee more than 90°.

Note

Useful for those who have lordosis or lower back problems.

9. Neck Rotation

Purpose

To stretch neck rotators.

Position

Place palm of left hand against left cheek; point fingers toward ear and point elbow forward.

Movement

Try to turn head and neck left while resisting with left hand. Hold several seconds. Relax and turn head to right as far as possible; hold. Repeat.

Note

Useful for trigger points in neck and trapezius muscles.

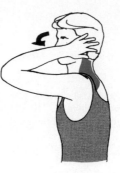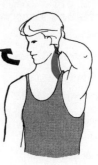

10. Arm Stretcher

Purpose

To stretch arm and chest muscles.

Position

Cross arms and turn palms of hands together. Raise arms overhead behind ears. Extend elbows.

Movement

Stretch as high as possible. Hold.

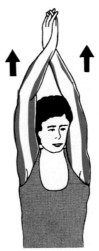

11. Shin Stretcher

Purpose

Relieve "shin" muscle soreness by stretching muscles on front of shin.

Position

Kneel on both knees, turn to right, and press down on right ankle with right hand.

Movement

Move pelvis forward. Hold. Repeat on opposite side.

Note

Except when they are sore, most people need to strengthen rather than stretch these muscles.

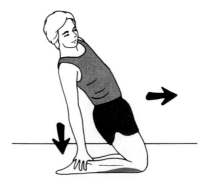

12. Wand Exercise

Purpose

To stretch front of shoulder and chest.

Position

Sit with wand grasped at ends. Raise wand overhead.

Movement

Bring it down behind shoulder blades. Keep spine erect. Hold. Hands may be moved closer together to increase stretch on chest muscles.

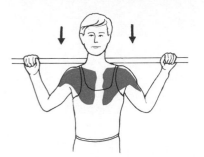

13. Hamstring Stretcher

Purpose

To stretch the muscles on the back of the thigh and behind the knee joint.

Position

Start in a hook-lying position. Bend right knee and grasp toes with right hand.

Movement

Place left hand on back of right thigh and bring knee toward chest; push heel toward ceiling. Repeat on left side.

Note

Also see Concept 4, warm-up routine (p. 32) for a sitting hamstring stretcher.

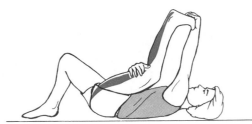

14. Calf Stretcher

Purpose

To stretch the calf muscles and Achilles tendon.

Note

This exercise is part of the sample warm-up included in Concept 4, and is described and illustrated on page 32.

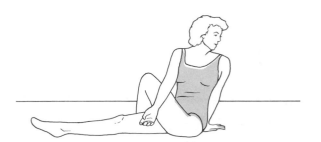

15. Sitting Toe Touch

Purpose

To stretch the muscles of the lower back and the muscles of the back of the thigh (hamstrings).

Note

Several variations of this exercise are described and illustrated in figure 11.1. Another variation is shown in the warm-up in Concept 4, page 32.

16. Trunk Twister

Purpose

Stretch the trunk muscles and muscles on outside of hip.

Position

Sit with right leg extended, left leg bent and crossed over the right knee.

Movement

Place right arm on the left side of the left leg and push against that leg while turning the trunk as far as possible to the left; place left hand on floor behind buttocks. Reverse position and repeat on opposite side.

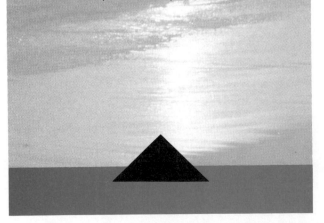

13

BODY COMPOSITION/ WEIGHT CONTROL

CONCEPT 13

Obesity is a significant health problem that
can be controlled, in most cases,
with a proper balance between caloric
consumption (diet) and
caloric expenditure (physical activity).

INTRODUCTION

Appearance is probably the major reason why most people are concerned about weight control. However, proper body composition is also very important to total health and fitness. The following discussion presents facts about weight control, including information about diet and physical activity. Special consideration is given to the use of exercise as an effective means of maintaining ideal body weight.

TERMS

Calorie—A unit of energy supplied by food; the quantity of heat necessary to raise the temperature of a kilogram of water one degree centigrade (actually a kilocalorie but usually called a calorie for weight control programs).

Caloric Balance—Consuming calories in amounts equal to the number of calories expended.

Diet—The usual food and drink for a person or animal.

MET—MET is an acronym for the basic amount of energy expended at rest. As you work, your metabolism increases. METs are multiples of the amount of energy expended at rest.

Obesity—Extreme weight, often considered as 20 to 35 percent above "normal"; probably best defined as an extreme overfat condition.

Overfat—Having too much body composition as fat; for men, having more than 25 percent of the total body composition as fat; for women, 30 percent.

Overweight—Having weight in excess of normal; not harmful unless it is accompanied by overfatness.

Percent Body Fat—The percentage of total body weight that is comprised of fat.

Somatotype—Inherent body build: ectomorph (thin); mesomorph (muscular); and endomorph (fat).

THE FACTS

There are standards that can be used to determine how much body fat an individual should possess.

Every person should possess at least a minimal amount of body fat for good health. This fat is called "essential fat" and is necessary as a source of stored energy for body temperature regulation, for shock absorption, and for regulation of essential body nutrients including vitamins. When body fat becomes too great a proportion of total body weight, overfatness occurs. For good health, an individual should not allow the body fat levels

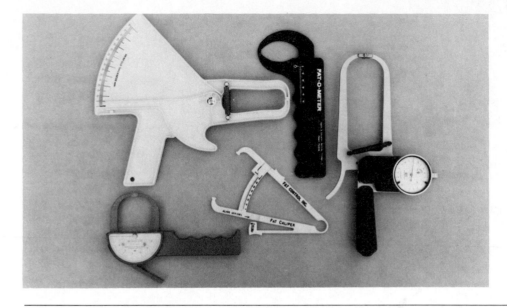

FIGURE 13.1 Skinfold Calipers

TABLE 13.1 Standards for Fatness of Men and Women (Percent Body Fat)

Classification	Men	Women
Essential fat	no less than 5%	no less than 8%
Desirable fatness for good performance	5%–13%	12%–22%
Desirable fatness for good health	10%–25%	18%–30%
Overfatness	more than 25%	more than 30%

Adapted from J. H. Wilmore, et al., "Body Composition: A Round Table," Physician and Sports Medicine 14(1986):152.

to drop too low or to become too high. There is a desirable range of fatness for good health, different from the range suggested for those who have optimal performance in athletic events as a goal. Even for athletes, especially low levels of body fat are not desirable. Table 13.1 provides standards of body fatness for both men and women.

Overfat *rather than* overweight *is more important in determining health.*

Individuals who are interested in controlling their weight usually consult a height-weight chart to determine "desirable" weight. Being 20 percent or more above the ideal chart weight is the commonly accepted criterion of obesity. Though proper height-weight charts give good general guidelines, they are not as accurate an indication of health for most people as is the **percentage of body fat.**

It is possible to estimate the percentage of the body that is fat. Some individuals having muscular body types are considered overweight and even obese in terms of height-weight charts, yet they possess very little body fat. Because the amount of body fat, not the amount of weight, is the important factor in living a healthy life, it is wise to use "overfat" rather than "overweight" as the measure. See table 13.1 for standards.

There are many ways to assess body fatness and leanness.

Underwater weighing is one of the better methods for determining the amount of fat in your body. Because this procedure takes considerable time, equipment, and specialized training, it is not practical for use except in well-equipped laboratories. Other ways of estimating body fatness are X-rays, ultrasound, impedance measurements, body girth, and skinfold measurements. Skinfold measurements are often used because they can be taken fairly easily with a caliper (see figure 13.1). This is not nearly as costly as underwater weighing or X rays. The better, more accurate calipers cost several hundred dollars. However, considerably less expensive calipers are now available. When used by a trained person, these calipers give a good estimate of fatness (see Lab Resource Materials on page 121). An expert's estimate of your body fatness determined by skinfold measurements is informative. It will also be useful for you to learn to use calipers correctly so that you can take your own measurements throughout your life.

Body fat is distributed throughout the body. About one-half of the body's fat is located around the

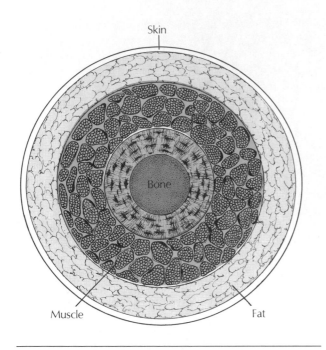

FIGURE 13.2 Location of Body Fat

various body organs and in the muscles. The other half of the body's fat is located just under the skin, or in skinfolds (figure 13.2). A skinfold is two thicknesses of skin and the amount of fat that lies just under the skin. At certain locations in the body, the thickness of the skinfolds can be used to obtain a good estimate of total body fatness (figure 13.3).

Body girth measurements, especially those using only one or two body points, are less accurate than skinfolds but they are easy to do. As the sole measure of fatness, they should be used with caution. They can provide a useful second or third source of information about body fatness, however.

***Obesity** is a problem experienced by too many Americans.*

Some experts indicate that as many as 60 million people, or half of all the adults, in the United States are overweight. Others suggest that at least one-third of adult Americans are overfat. In addition to the problem of adult obesity, statistics indicate that as many as 10 million schoolchildren can be classified as overfat or obese.

In some cases, glandular problems cause an obese condition. However, these conditions are quite rare. Obesity is usually a result of an imbalance between caloric intake and output. Crash diets, spot reducing, and passive exercise "gimmick" machines are *not* effective in producing lasting fat loss.

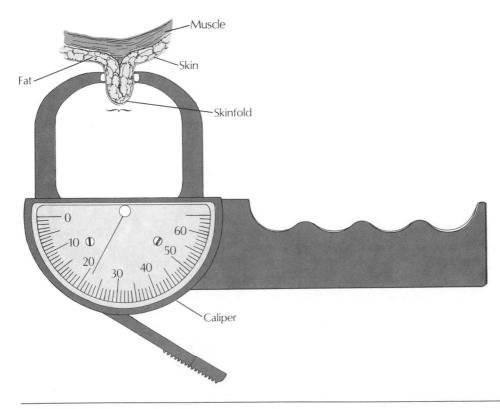

FIGURE 13.3 Measuring Body Fat

Overfatness or obesity can contribute to degenerative diseases, health problems, and even shortened life.

Some diseases and health problems associated with overfatness and obesity are presented in Concept 3. In addition to the higher incidence of certain diseases and health problems, there is evidence that people who are moderately overfat have a 40 percent higher than normal risk of shortening their lifespan. More severe obesity results in a 70 percent higher than normal death rate. This is evidenced by the exorbitant life insurance premiums paid by obese individuals.

Recent statistics indicating that underweight people had a higher than normal risk of premature death are very deceptive. Many people included in the data were underweight because of terminal illnesses. Most experts agree that those people who are free from disease and who have lower than average amounts of body fat have a lower than average risk of premature death.

Excessive concern about being thin or low in body fat can result in health problems.

More and more Americans are becoming aware of the dangers of obesity. Though this awareness is good, excessive concern for thinness can also become a problem. For example, several medical conditions are particularly prevalent among children and teenagers, especially anorexia nervosa, bulimia, and "fear of obesity." All conditions are, to a large extent, modern-day and Western-world disorders. Anorexia, which means "loss of appetite," is a condition associated with an extreme desire to be lean and thin. It can result in dramatic and dangerous losses in body weight from failure to eat, regurgitation of food to prevent digestion, and compulsive exercise to prevent weight gain. This is a serious medical-psychological disorder that can be fatal. Those suffering from bulimia are also overly conscious of gaining weight, so they eat erratically and regurgitate to prevent digestion.

"Fear of obesity" is a newly discovered condition that is not as severe as anorexia nervosa, but it can still have negative health consequences. This condition is most common among achievement-oriented teenagers who impose a self-restriction on caloric intake because they fear obesity. Consequences include stunting of growth, delayed puberty and sexual development, and decreased physical attractiveness. It is important to avoid excessive eating and inactivity to prevent the problems associated with overfatness and obesity, however, an overconcern for leanness can result in serious health problems, too.

To lose body fat, decreased caloric intake, increased caloric expenditure, or combine the two for best results.

The threshold of training and a target zone for exercise are not the only determinants of minimal and optimal body fatness. Exercise is one effective way to reduce body fat levels. Decreasing caloric intake (dieting) is another. Of course, a combination of the two is preferable (figure 13.4). Threshold of training and target zones for body fat reduction, including information for both exercise and diet, are presented in table 13.2.

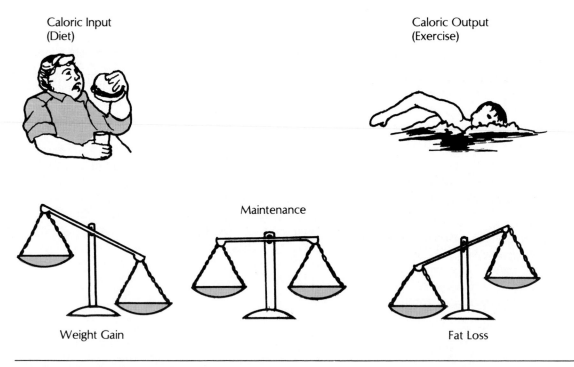

Caloric Input (Diet)

Caloric Output (Exercise)

Maintenance

Weight Gain

Fat Loss

FIGURE 13.4 Balancing Calorie Input and Output

TABLE 13.2 Threshold of Training and Target Zones for Body Fat Reduction

	Threshold of Training*		Target Zones*	
	Exercise	Diet	Exercise	Diet
Frequency	• To be effective, exercise must be regular, preferably daily, though fat can be lost over the long haul with almost any frequency that results in increased caloric expenditure.	• It is best to reduce caloric intake consistently and daily. To restrict calories only on certain days is *not* best, though fat can be lost over a period of time by reducing caloric intake at any time.	• Daily moderate exercise is recommended. For those who do regular vigorous activity, 5 or 6 days per week may be best.	• It is best to diet consistently and daily.
Intensity	• To lose 1 pound of fat, you must expend 3,500 calories more than you normally expend.	• To lose 1 pound of fat, you must eat 3,500 calories fewer than you normally eat.	• Slow, low-intensity aerobic exercise that results in no more than 1–2 pounds of fat loss per week is best.	• Modest caloric restriction resulting in no more than 1–2 pounds of fat loss per week is best.
Time	• To be effective, exercise must be sustained long enough to expend a considerable number of calories. At least 15 minutes per exercise bout is necessary to result in consistent fat loss.	• Eating moderate meals is best. Skipping meals is *not* most effective.	• Exercise durations similar to those for achieving aerobic cardiovascular fitness seem best. An exercise duration of 30–60 minutes is recommended.	• Eating moderate meals is best. Skipping meals or fasting is *not* most effective.

Note: It is best to combine exercise and diet to achieve the 3,500 caloric imbalance necessary to lose a pound of fat. Using both exercise and diet in the target zone is most effective.

Exercise is one effective means of controlling body fat.

Though physical activity or exercise will not result in immediate and large decreases in body fat levels, there is increasing evidence that fat loss resulting from exercise may be more lasting than fat loss from dieting. Vigorous exercise can increase the resting energy expenditure up to thirteen times (13 **METs**).

If a person exercises moderately for an extra fifteen minutes a day (all other things being equal), he or she may lose more than ten pounds in a year's time. Regular walking, jogging, swimming, or any type of sustained exercise can be effective in producing losses in body fat.

Exercise that can be sustained for relatively long periods of time is probably the most effective for losing body fat.

Table 13.3 shows the caloric expenditures for one hour of involvement in various recreational physical activities. The heavier the person, the more **calories** expended because more work is required to move larger bodies. Activities that are extremely vigorous can help

in losing body fatness if done regularly. For many people, these may not be as effective as some less vigorous activities. For example, running at ten miles per hour (a six-minute mile) will cause a 150-pound person to expend 900 calories in one hour. Jogging about one-half as fast, or at five and one-half miles per hour (approximately an eleven-minute mile), will result in an expenditure of about 650 calories in the same amount of time. At first glance, the more vigorous exercise seems to be a better choice. But how many people can continue to run at a ten-mile-per-hour pace for a full hour? Each mile run at ten miles per hour results in an expenditure of 90 calories, while each mile run at five and one-half miles per hour results in an expenditure of 118 calories. Per mile, you expend more calories in slow running. It takes longer to run a mile, but by the same token, you can also persist longer. The key is to expend as many calories as possible during each regular exercise period. Doing less vigorous activity for longer periods of time is better for fat control than doing very vigorous activities that can be done only for short periods of time.

TABLE 13.3 Calories Expended Per Hour in Various Physical Activities

	Calories Used per Hour				
Activity	100 lbs.	120 lbs.	150 lbs.	180 lbs.	200 lbs.
Archery	180	204	240	276	300
Backpacking (40-lb. pack)	307	348	410	472	513
Badminton	255	289	340	391	425
Baseball	210	238	280	322	350
Basketball (halfcourt)	225	255	300	345	375
Bicycling (normal speed)	157	178	210	242	263
Bowling	155	176	208	240	261
Canoeing (4 mph)	276	344	414	504	558
Circuit Training*	247	280	330	380	413
Dance, Ballet (choreographed)	240	300	360	432	480
Dance, Exercise	315	357	420	483	525
Dance, Modern (choreographed)	240	300	360	432	480
Dance, Social	174	222	264	318	348
Fencing	225	255	300	345	375
Fitness Calisthenics	232	263	310	357	388
Football	225	255	300	345	375
Golf (walking)	187	212	250	288	313
Gymnastics	232	263	310	357	388
Handball	450	510	600	690	750
Hiking	225	255	300	345	375
Horseback Riding	180	204	240	276	300
Interval Training*	487	552	650	748	833
Jogging (5½ mph)	487	552	650	748	833
Judo/Karate	232	263	310	357	388
Mountain Climbing	450	510	600	690	750
Pool; Billiards	97	110	130	150	163
Racquetball; Paddleball	450	510	600	690	750
Rope Jumping (continuous)	525	595	700	805	875
Rowing, Crew	615	697	820	943	1025
Running (10 mph)	625	765	900	1035	1125
Sailing (pleasure)	135	153	180	207	225
Skating, Ice	262	297	350	403	438
Skating, Roller	262	297	350	403	438
Skiing, Cross-Country	525	595	700	805	875
Skiing, Downhill	450	510	600	690	750
Soccer	405	459	540	621	775
Softball (fast)	210	238	280	322	350
Softball (slow)	217	246	290	334	363
Surfing	416	467	550	633	684
Swimming (slow laps)	240	272	320	368	400
Swimming (fast laps)	420	530	630	768	846
Table Tennis	180	204	240	276	300
Tennis	315	357	420	483	525
Volleyball	262	297	350	403	483
Walking	204	258	318	372	426
Waterskiing	306	390	468	564	636
Weight Training	352	399	470	541	558

*Note: Locate your weight to determine the calories expended per hour in each of the activities shown in the table based on recreational involvement. More vigorous activity, as occurs in competitive athletics, may result in greater caloric expenditures.
From C. B. Corbin and R. Lindsey, Fitness for Life, 2d ed., Glenview, IL: Scott, Foresman, Inc., 1985, 105. Used by permission.

*The only satisfactory way to control **diet** is to count caloric content of foods commonly eaten.*

When accurate records are not kept, most people greatly underestimate the amount they eat. A calorie table (Appendix B) shows the caloric content of the most commonly eaten foods. Use this table and the diet recall procedure from Lab 14A (nutrition) to help keep accurate records of your own caloric intake.

A combination of regular exercise and dietary restriction is the most effective means of losing body fat.

Recent studies indicate that exercise combined with dietary restriction may be the *most* effective method of losing fat. One study of adult women indicated that diet alone resulted in loss of weight, but much of this loss was lean body tissue. Those studied who were dieting as well as exercising experienced similar weight losses, but this loss included more body fat. On the basis of this research, all weight loss programs should combine a lower caloric intake with a good physical exercise program.

Good exercise and diet habits can be useful in maintaining desirable body composition.

Table 13.2 illustrates how fat can be lost through regular exercise and proper dieting. However, not all people want to lose fat. For those who wish to maintain their current body composition, a **balance** between **caloric** intake and expenditure is effective. For those who want to increase their lean body weight, increased caloric intake with increased exercise can result in the desired changes.

Appetite is not necessarily increased through exercise.

The human animal was intended to be an active animal. For this reason, man's "appetite thermostat" (called the appestat by some) is set as if all people are active. Those who are inactive do not have a decreased appetite. Likewise, if one is sedentary, then begins regular exercise, the appetite does not necessarily increase because this "appetite thermostat" expects activity. Very vigorous activity does not necessarily cause an appetite increase that is proportional to the calories expended in the vigorous exercise.

Fat children may become fat adults.

Retention of "baby fat" is not a sign of good health. On the contrary, excess body fat in the early years is a health problem of considerable concern. As many as 25 percent of American schoolchildren are overfat. Of these children, four of five will become overfat adults. Twenty-eight of twenty-nine teenagers who are too fat will become overfat adults. There is evidence that children who are obese may actually increase the number as well as the size of their fat cells, thus making them predisposed to obesity in later life.

Inactivity contributes to childhood obesity.

Studies of fat children show that activity restriction is more often a cause of obesity than is overeating. Many fat children eat less but are considerably less active than their nonfat peers. Research suggests that increased television viewing is associated with inactivity, and their overfatness among children.

"Creeping obesity" often accompanies an increase in age.

Many of the "too fat Americans" are between the ages of thirty and sixty. As you grow older, changes in metabolism cause a decrease in caloric expenditure necessary to sustain life. Unless activity is increased or diet is restricted, a gain in weight will occur. Activity usually decreases while eating habits remain fairly constant with age. Thus, obesity creeps up on an individual. To prevent creeping obesity, it is suggested that the average person cut caloric intake 3 percent each decade after twenty-five, so that by age sixty-five, caloric intake is at least 10 percent less than it was at age twenty-five.

The "set point" theory offers a biological basis for obesity.

Some people have suggested that every individual is born with a "set" body weight. Advocates of this set point theory feel that it will be difficult for people to deviate from their "set point weight," which is predetermined by heredity. Though many experts question the validity of set point theory for humans, they agree that there is such a thing as a familial predisposition to obesity. For years researchers have suggested that your body type, or **somatotype,** is inherited. Clearly, some people will have more difficulty than others controlling fatness because of their body types and because they come from families with a history of obesity. Scientists caution those from families with a history of obesity *not to conclude that nothing can be done to prevent obesity.* In fact, one important recent study indicates that *among those with a predisposition to obesity,* weight reduction programs can be effective. Further conclusions show that regular exercise is especially effective in the control of genetically determined overfatness.

Evaluating Body Fatness

Skinfold Measurements

Skinfold measurements are made with skinfold calipers. Some of the more accurate and expensive calipers are the Harpenden, the Lange, and the Lafayette calipers. Some of the less expensive calipers include the Slimguide, the Fat-O-Meter, and the Adipometer. Regardless of the type employed, it is important to use a consistent procedure for "drawing up" or "pinching up" a skinfold and making the measurement with the caliper. The following procedures should be used for each skinfold site.

1. Lay the caliper down on a nearby table. Use the thumbs and index fingers of both hands to "draw up" a skinfold or layer of skin and fat. The fingers and thumbs of the two hands should be about one inch apart or half an inch on either side of the location where the measurement is to be made.
2. The skinfolds are normally "drawn up" in a vertical line rather than in a horizontal line. However, if the natural tendency of the skin aligns itself less than vertical, the measurement should be done on the natural line of the skinfold, rather than on the vertical.
3. Do not "pinch" the skinfold too hard. Draw it up so that your thumbs and fingers are not compressing the skinfold.
4. Once the skinfold is "drawn up," let go with your right hand and pick up the caliper. Open the jaws of the caliper and place them over the location of the skinfold to be measured and one-half inch from your left index finger and thumb. Allow the tips, or jaw faces, of the caliper to close on the skinfold at a level about where the skin would be normally.
5. Let the reading on the caliper "settle" for two or three seconds, then note the thickness of the skinfold in millimeters.
6. Three measurements should be taken at each location. Use the middle of the three values to determine your measurement. For example, if you had values of 10, 11, and 9, your measurement for that location would be 10. If the three measures vary by more than 3 millimeters from the lowest to the highest, you may want to take additional measurements.

Skinfold Locations for Women
A. *Triceps Skinfold*—Make a mark on the back of the right arm one-half the distance between the tip of the shoulder and the tip of the elbow. Make the measurement at this location.
B. *Iliac Crest Skinfold*—Make a mark at the top front of the iliac crest. This skinfold is taken slightly diagonally because of the natural line of the skin.
C. *Thigh Skinfold*—Make a mark on the front of the thigh midway between the hip and the knee. Make the measurement vertically at this location.

Skinfold Locations for Men
A. *Chest Skinfold*—Make a mark above and to the right of the right nipple (one-half the distance from the midline of the side and the nipple). The measurement at this location is often done on the diagonal because of the natural line of the skin.
B. *Abdominal Skinfold*—Make a mark on the skin approximately one inch to the right of the navel. Make a vertical measurement at that location.
C. *Thigh Skinfold*—Make a mark on the front of the thigh midway between the hip and the knee. Make a vertical measurement at this location.

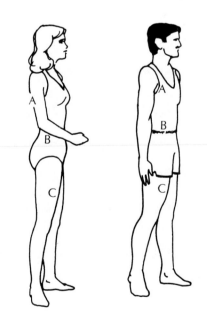

CHART 13A.1* Percent Fat Estimates for Men, Sum of Chest, Abdominal, and Thigh Skinfolds**

Sum of Skin Folds (mm)	Age to the Last Year								
	22 and under	23 to 27	28 to 32	33 to 37	38 to 42	43 to 47	48 to 52	53 to 57	Over 58
8–10	1.3	1.8	2.3	2.9	3.4	3.9	4.5	5.0	5.5
11–13	2.2	2.8	3.3	3.9	4.4	4.9	5.5	6.0	6.5
14–16	3.2	3.8	4.3	4.8	5.4	5.9	6.4	7.0	7.5
17–19	4.2	4.7	5.3	5.8	6.3	6.9	7.4	8.0	8.5
20–22	5.1	5.7	6.2	6.8	7.3	7.9	8.4	8.9	9.5
23–25	6.1	6.6	7.2	7.7	8.3	8.8	9.4	9.9	10.5
26–28	7.0	7.6	8.1	8.7	9.2	9.8	10.3	10.9	11.4
29–31	8.0	8.5	9.1	9.6	10.2	10.7	11.3	11.8	12.4
32–34	8.9	9.4	10.0	10.5	11.1	11.6	12.2	12.8	13.3
35–37	9.8	10.4	10.9	11.5	12.0	12.6	13.1	13.7	14.3
38–40	10.7	11.3	11.8	12.4	12.9	13.5	14.1	14.6	15.2
41–43	11.6	12.2	12.7	13.3	13.8	14.4	15.0	15.5	16.1
44–46	12.5	13.1	13.6	14.2	14.7	15.3	15.9	16.4	17.0
47–49	13.4	13.9	14.5	15.1	15.6	16.2	16.8	17.3	17.9
50–52	14.3	14.8	15.4	15.9	16.5	17.1	17.6	18.2	18.8
53–55	15.1	15.7	16.2	16.8	17.4	17.9	18.5	18.1	19.7
56–58	16.0	16.5	17.1	17.7	18.2	18.8	19.4	20.0	20.5
59–61	16.9	17.4	17.9	18.5	19.1	19.7	20.2	20.8	21.4
62–64	17.6	18.2	18.8	19.4	19.9	20.5	21.1	21.7	22.2
65–67	18.5	19.0	19.6	20.2	20.8	21.3	21.9	22.5	23.1
68–70	19.3	19.9	20.4	21.0	21.6	22.2	22.7	23.3	23.9
71–73	20.1	20.7	21.2	21.8	22.4	23.0	23.6	24.1	24.7
74–76	20.9	21.5	22.0	22.6	23.2	23.8	24.4	25.0	25.5
77–79	21.7	22.2	22.8	23.4	24.0	24.6	25.2	25.8	26.3
80–82	22.4	23.0	23.6	24.2	24.8	25.4	25.9	26.5	27.1
83–85	23.2	23.8	24.4	25.0	25.5	26.1	26.7	27.3	27.9
86–88	24.0	24.5	25.1	25.7	26.3	26.9	27.5	28.1	28.7
89–91	24.7	25.3	25.9	25.5	27.1	27.6	28.2	28.8	29.4
92–94	25.4	26.0	26.6	27.2	27.8	28.4	29.0	29.6	30.2
95–97	26.1	16.7	27.3	27.9	28.5	29.1	29.7	30.3	30.9
98–100	26.9	27.4	28.0	28.6	29.2	29.8	30.4	31.0	31.6
101–103	27.5	28.1	28.7	29.3	29.9	30.5	31.1	31.7	32.3
104–106	28.2	28.8	29.4	30.0	30.6	31.2	31.8	32.4	33.0
107–109	28.9	29.5	30.1	30.7	31.3	31.9	32.5	33.1	33.7
110–112	29.6	30.2	30.8	31.4	32.0	32.6	33.2	33.8	34.4
113–115	30.2	30.8	31.4	32.0	32.6	33.2	33.8	34.5	35.1
116–118	30.9	31.5	32.1	32.7	33.3	33.9	34.5	35.1	35.7
119–121	31.5	32.1	32.7	33.3	33.9	34.5	35.1	35.7	36.4
122–124	32.1	32.7	33.3	33.9	34.5	35.1	35.8	36.4	37.0
125–127	32.7	33.3	33.9	34.5	35.1	35.8	36.4	37.0	37.6

*Percent fat calculated by the formula by Siri.[39] Percent fat = $[4.95/BD] - 4.5] \times 100$, where BD = body density.

**Taken from M. L. Pollock, D. H. Schmidt, and A. S. Jackson, "Measurement of Cardiorespiration Fitness and Body Composition in the Clinical Setting," Comprehensive Therapy 6(September 1980):12–27.

CHART 13A.2* Percent Fat Estimates for Women, Sum of Triceps, Iliac Crest, and Thigh Skinfolds**

	Age to the Last Year								
Sum of Skinfolds (mm)	**22 and under**	**23 to 27**	**28 to 32**	**33 to 37**	**38 to 42**	**43 to 47**	**48 to 52**	**53 to 57**	**Over 58**
23–25	9.7	9.9	10.2	10.4	10.7	10.9	11.2	11.4	11.7
26–28	11.0	11.2	11.5	11.7	12.0	12.3	12.5	12.7	13.0
29–31	12.3	12.5	12.8	13.0	13.3	13.5	13.8	14.0	14.3
32–34	13.6	13.8	14.0	14.3	14.5	14.8	15.0	15.3	15.5
35–37	14.8	15.0	15.3	15.5	15.8	16.0	16.3	16.5	16.8
38–40	16.0	16.3	16.5	16.7	17.0	17.2	17.5	17.7	18.0
41–43	17.2	17.4	17.7	17.9	18.2	18.4	18.7	18.9	19.2
44–46	18.3	18.6	18.8	19.1	19.3	19.6	19.8	20.1	20.3
47–49	19.5	19.7	20.0	20.2	20.5	20.7	21.0	21.2	21.5
50–52	20.6	20.8	21.1	21.3	21.6	21.8	22.1	22.3	22.6
53–55	21.7	21.9	22.1	22.4	22.6	22.9	23.1	23.4	23.6
56–58	22.7	23.0	23.2	23.4	23.7	23.9	24.2	24.4	24.7
59–61	23.7	24.0	24.2	24.5	24.7	25.0	25.2	25.5	25.7
62–64	24.7	25.0	25.2	25.5	35.7	26.0	26.7	26.4	26.7
65–67	25.7	25.9	26.2	26.4	26.7	26.9	27.2	27.4	27.7
68–70	26.6	26.9	27.1	27.4	27.6	27.9	28.1	28.4	28.6
71–73	27.5	27.8	28.0	28.3	28.5	28.8	28.0	29.3	29.5
74–76	28.4	28.7	28.9	29.2	29.4	29.7	29.9	30.2	30.4
77–79	29.3	29.5	29.8	30.0	30.3	30.5	30.8	31.0	31.3
80–82	30.1	30.4	30.6	30.9	31.1	31.4	31.6	31.9	32.1
83–85	30.9	31.2	31.4	31.7	31.9	32.2	32.4	32.7	32.9
86–88	31.7	32.0	32.2	32.5	32.7	32.9	33.2	33.4	33.7
89–91	32.5	32.7	33.0	33.2	33.5	33.7	33.9	34.2	34.4
92–94	33.2	33.4	33.7	33.9	34.2	34.4	34.7	34.9	35.2
95–97	33.9	34.1	34.4	34.6	34.9	35.1	35.4	35.6	35.9
98–100	34.6	34.8	35.1	35.3	35.5	35.8	36.0	36.3	36.5
101–103	35.3	35.4	35.7	35.9	36.2	36.4	36.7	36.9	37.2
104–106	35.8	36.1	36.3	36.6	36.8	37.1	37.3	37.5	37.8
107–109	36.4	36.7	36.9	37.1	37.4	37.6	37.9	38.1	38.4
110–112	37.0	37.2	37.5	37.7	38.0	38.2	38.5	38.7	38.9
113–115	37.5	37.8	38.0	38.2	38.5	38.7	39.0	39.2	39.5
116–118	38.0	38.3	38.5	38.8	39.0	39.3	39.5	39.7	40.0
119–121	38.5	38.7	39.0	39.2	39.5	39.7	40.0	40.2	40.5
122–124	39.0	39.2	39.4	39.7	39.9	40.2	40.4	40.7	40.9
125–127	39.4	39.6	39.9	40.1	40.4	40.6	40.9	41.1	41.4
128–130	39.8	40.0	40.3	40.5	40.8	41.0	41.3	41.5	41.8

*Percent fat calculated by the formula of Siri.[39] Percent fat = $[(4.95/BD) - 4.5] \times 100$, where BD = body density.

***Taken from M. L. Pollock, D. H. Schmidt, and A. S. Jackson, "Measurement of Cardiorespiration Fitness and Body Composition in the Clinical Setting," Comprehensive Therapy 6(September 1980):12–27.*

Body Girth Measures (Circumferences)

As noted earlier, body girth measures are not as accurate as other measures of body fatness. However, they can be done easily in the home with a tape measure. If possible, this technique should be used *in addition* to the more accurate skinfold measurements. Together with other methods, this simple method can be quite useful in monitoring your body fatness. Use the following procedure:

1. Men should measure the circumference of the waist at the navel and women should measure the circumference of the hips at the widest point. Pull the tape so that it is snug but does not cause an indentation in the natural line of the skin.
2. Women should measure their height without shoes. Men should measure their weight without clothes or shoes.
3. Use charts 13A.3 and 13A.4. With a straight edge, connect weight and waist circumference for men. The point at which the straight edge crosses the body fat line will indicate your amount of body fat by percent. For women, use the straight edge to connect height and hip circumference. The point at which the straight edge crosses the body fat line will indicate the percent of your body fatness.

CHART 13A.3 Circumference Chart for Men*

Nonograms developed by Jack Wilmore, University of Texas. Used by permission.

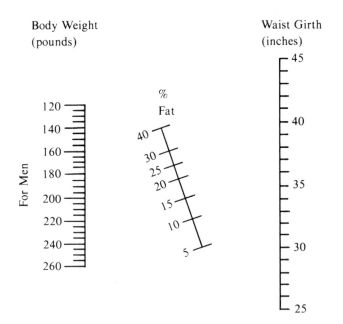

CHART 13A.4 Circumference Chart for Women*

Nonograms developed by Jack Wilmore, University of Texas. Used by permission.

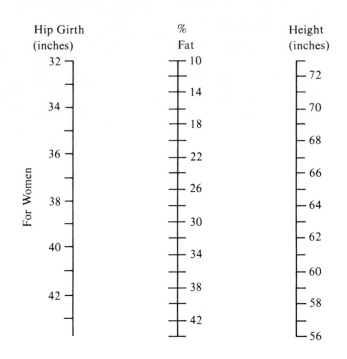

CHART 13A.5 Fatness *Rating Scale*

Classification	Men	Women
Excessively lean	Less than 5%	Less than 8%
High performance zone	5%–9%	8%–17%*
Good fitness zone	10%–20%	18%–25%
Marginal zone	21%–25%	26%–30%
Obese zone	>25%	>30%

It is recommended that these standards be maintained throughout life regardless of age.
**Experts believe that less than 12% is not best for females doing most types of athletic performance.*

Height-Weight Measurements

1. Measure your height without shoes and weight with indoor clothing.
2. Determine your frame size. First measure your wrist at its smallest point just above the styloid process (bony bump on wrist). Pull tape snugly but not tight enough to indent the wrist. (See figure 13B.1) Look up your frame size on chart 13B.1.
3. Determine your desirable weight. Locate your height in inches on the left and your frame size across the top of chart 13B.2 (Men) or 13B.3 (Women).

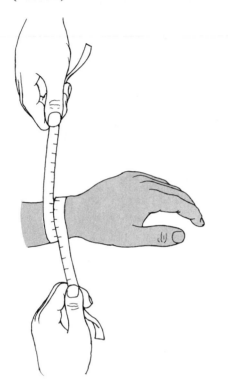

FIGURE 13B.1 Measuring Wrist Circumference

CHART 13B.1 Determining Frame Size Using Wrist Size in Inches

	Men	Women
Small frame	6½" or less	5½" or less
Medium frame	6¾"–7¼"	5¾"
Large frame	7½" or more	6" or more

CHART 13B.2 Determination of "Desirable" Weight for Men

Height		Small Frame	Medium Frame	Large Frame
Feet	Inches			
5	2	128–134	131–141	138–150
5	3	130–136	133–143	140–153
5	4	132–138	135–145	142–156
5	5	134–140	137–148	144–160
5	6	136–142	139–151	146–164
5	7	138–145	142–154	149–168
5	8	140–148	145–157	152–172
5	9	142–151	148–160	155–176
5	10	144–154	151–163	158–180
5	11	146–157	154–166	161–184
6	0	149–160	157–170	164–188
6	1	152–164	160–174	168–192
6	2	155–168	164–178	172–197
6	3	158–172	167–182	176–202
6	4	162–176	171–187	181–207

Weights at ages 25–59 based on lowest mortality. Weight in pounds according to frame (in indoor clothing weighing 3 lbs., shoes with 1" heels). *Adapted from tables provided courtesy of Metropolitan Life Insurance Co.*

CHART 13B.3 Determination of "Desirable" Weight for Women

Height		Small Frame	Medium Frame	Large Frame
Feet	Inches			
4	10	102–111	109–121	118–131
4	11	103–113	111–123	120–134
5	0	104–115	113–126	122–137
5	1	106–118	115–129	125–140
5	2	108–121	118–132	128–143
5	3	111–124	121–135	131–147
5	4	114–127	124–138	134–151
5	5	117–130	127–141	137–155
5	6	120–133	130–144	140–159
5	7	123–136	133–147	143–163
5	8	126–139	136–150	146–167
5	9	129–142	139–153	149–170
5	10	132–145	142–156	152–173
5	11	135–148	145–159	155–176
6	0	138–151	148–162	158–179

Weights at ages 25–59 based on lowest mortality. Weight in pounds according to frame (in indoor clothing weighing 3 lbs., shoes with 1" heels). *Adapted from tables provided courtesy of Metropolitan Life Insurance Co.*

CHART 13B.4 Determination of Desirable Body Weight for Men

Actual Body Weight	Percent Fat																	
	6	8	10	12	14	16	18	20	22	24	26	28	30	32	34	36	38	40
240	263	258	254	249	244	240	234	230	225	220	215	210	206	201	196	191	186	182
235	257	253	248	243	239	235	266	225	220	215	210	206	201	196	192	187	182	178
230	252	247	243	238	233	230	224	220	215	210	206	201	197	192	187	183	178	174
225	247	243	238	234	229	225	220	216	211	207	202	198	193	189	184	180	175	171
220	241	237	233	228	223	221	215	211	206	202	197	193	189	184	180	175	171	167
215	236	231	227	223	218	215	210	206	201	197	193	188	184	180	175	171	167	163
210	230	226	222	217	215	210	205	202	200	192	188	184	180	175	171	167	163	159
205	224	220	216	212	208	205	200	197	191	187	183	179	175	171	167	163	159	155
200	220	216	212	208	204	200	196	192	188	184	180	176	172	168	164	160	156	152
195	214	210	206	202	198	195	190	187	183	179	175	171	167	163	159	155	151	148
190	208	204	201	197	193	190	185	182	178	174	170	166	163	159	155	151	147	144
185	202	199	195	191	187	185	180	177	173	169	165	162	158	154	151	147	143	140
180	197	193	190	186	182	180	175	172	168	164	161	157	154	150	146	143	139	136
175	192	189	185	182	178	175	171	168	164	161	157	154	150	147	143	140	136	133
170	186	183	180	176	173	170	166	163	159	156	152	149	146	142	139	135	132	129
165	181	177	174	171	167	165	161	158	154	151	148	144	141	138	134	131	128	125
160	175	172	169	165	162	160	157	153	149	146	143	140	137	133	130	127	124	121
155	169	166	163	160	157	155	151	148	144	141	138	135	132	129	126	123	120	117
150	165	162	159	156	153	150	147	144	141	138	135	132	129	126	123	120	117	114
145	159	156	153	150	147	145	141	139	136	133	130	127	124	121	118	115	112	110
140	153	150	148	145	142	140	136	134	131	128	125	122	120	117	114	111	108	100
135	147	145	142	139	137	135	131	129	126	123	120	118	115	112	110	107	104	102
130	142	139	137	134	131	130	126	124	121	118	116	113	111	108	105	103	102	98
125	137	135	132	130	127	125	122	120	117	115	112	110	107	105	102	100	97	95
120	131	129	121	129	122	120	117	115	112	110	107	105	103	100	98	95	93	91

Along the side, locate your actual body weight; across the top, locate your estimated percent fat. The intersection of the two entries is your desirable weight (fat-free body weight plus 16 percent fat). Example: 175 pounds is the desirable weight for a man who weighs 195 pounds and currently has a total body fat of 26 percent.

Note: This chart uses 16 percent as a "desirable" fat level for males. If you weigh less than the "desirable" weight in the chart, it does not necessarily mean that you should try to gain weight.

REFERENCES

Blair, S. N., H. B. Falls, and R. R. Pate. "A New Physical Fitness Test." *Physician and Sportsmedicine* 11(1983):87.

Corbin, C. B., and R. Pate. "The AAHPERD Health-Related Fitness Test: Implications for Physical Education Curriculum." *Journal of Physical Education and Recreation* 52(1981):36.

Corbin, C. B., and W. B. Zuti. "Body Density and Skinfold Thickness of Children." *American Corrective Therapy Journal* 36(1982):50.

Corbin, C. B., and R. Lindsey. *The Ultimate Fitness Book.* New York: Leisure Press, 1984.

Hafen, B. Q. *Nutrition, Food, and Weight Control.* Boston: Allyn and Bacon, 1981.

Hagen, R. D. "The Effects of Aerobic Conditioning and/or Caloric Restriction in Overweight Men and Women." *Medicine and Science in Sport and Exercise* 18(1986): 87–94.

Hawkins, J. D. "An Analysis of Selected Skinfold Measuring Instruments." *JOPERD* 54(1983):25.

Jackson, A. S., M. L. Pollock, and A. Ward. "Generalized Equations for Predicting Body Density of Women." *Medicine and Science in Sports and Exercise* 12(1980):175.

Katch, F. I., and V. L. Katch. "Measurement and Prediction Errors in Body Composition Assessment and the Search for the Perfect Prediction Equation." *Research Quarterly of Exercise and Sport* 51(1980):249.

Kemnitz, J. W. "Body Weight Set Point Theory." *Contemporary Nutrition* 10(1985):2.

Lindsey, R., B. Jones, and A. Whitley. *Fitness for Health, Figure/Physique, Posture.* 5th ed. Dubuque, Iowa: Wm. C. Brown Publishers, 1983.

CHART 13B.5 Determination of Desirable Body Weight for Women

Actual Body Weight	Percent Fat																	
	6	8	10	12	14	16	18	20	22	24	26	28	30	32	34	36	38	40
200	228	224	220	216	212	208	204	200	196	192	188	184	180	176	172	168	164	160
195	222	218	214	210	206	202	198	195	191	187	183	179	175	171	167	163	159	156
190	216	212	209	205	201	197	193	190	186	182	178	174	171	167	163	159	155	152
185	210	207	203	199	196	192	188	185	181	177	173	170	166	162	159	155	151	148
180	205	201	198	194	190	187	183	180	176	172	169	165	162	158	154	151	147	144
175	199	196	192	189	185	182	178	175	171	168	164	161	157	154	150	147	143	140
170	193	180	177	173	170	166	163	170	166	163	159	156	153	149	146	142	139	136
165	188	184	181	178	174	171	168	165	161	158	155	151	148	145	141	138	135	132
160	182	179	176	172	169	166	163	160	156	153	150	147	144	140	137	134	131	128
155	176	173	170	167	164	161	158	155	151	148	145	142	139	136	133	130	127	124
150	171	168	165	162	159	156	153	150	147	144	141	138	135	132	129	126	123	120
145	165	162	159	156	153	150	147	145	142	139	136	133	130	127	124	121	118	116
140	159	156	154	151	148	145	142	140	137	134	131	128	126	123	120	117	114	112
135	153	151	148	145	143	140	137	135	132	129	126	124	121	118	116	113	110	108
130	148	145	143	140	137	135	132	130	127	124	122	119	117	114	111	109	106	104
125	142	140	137	135	132	130	127	125	122	120	117	115	112	110	107	105	102	100
120	136	134	132	129	127	124	122	120	117	115	112	110	108	105	103	100	98	96
115	131	128	126	124	121	119	117	115	112	110	108	105	103	101	98	96	94	92
110	125	123	121	118	116	114	112	110	107	105	103	101	99	96	94	92	90	88
105	119	117	115	113	111	109	107	105	102	100	98	96	94	92	90	88	86	84
100	114	112	110	108	106	104	102	100	98	96	94	92	90	88	86	84	82	80
95	108	106	104	102	100	98	96	95	93	91	89	87	85	83	81	79	77	76
90	102	100	99	97	95	93	91	90	88	86	84	82	81	79	77	75	73	72

Along the side, locate your actual body weight; across the top locate your estimated percent fat. The intersection of the two entries is your desirable weight (fat-free body weight plus 20 percent fat). Example: 150 pounds is the desirable weight for a woman who weighs 160 pounds and currently has a body fat amount of 26 percent.

Note: This chart uses 20 percent as a "desirable" fat level for females. If you weigh less than the "desirable" weight in this chart, it does not necessarily mean you should try to gain weight.

*Lohman, T. G. "Skinfolds and Body Density and Their Relation to Body Fatness: A Review." *Human Biology* 53(1981):181.

Lohman, T. G., and M. L. Pollock. "Skinfold Measurements: Which Caliper?" *Journal of Physical Education and Recreation* 52(1981):27.

*Lohman, T. G. "Body Composition Methodology in Sports Medicine." *Physician and Sportsmedicine* 10(1982):46.

National Institutes of Health. "Health Implications of Obesity." *Contemporary Nutrition* 10(1985):9.

Oscai, L. B. "Exercise or Food Restriction: Effect of Adipose Cellularity." *American Journal of Physiology* 27(1974):902.

Pate, R. R. "A New Definition of Youth Fitness." *Physician and Sportsmedicine* 11(1983):77.

Pollock, M. L., D. H. Schmidt, and A. S. Jackson. "Measurement of Cardiorespiratory Fitness and Body Composition in the Clinical Setting." *Comprehensive Therapy* 6(1980):12.

*Pugliese, M. T., et al. "Fear of Obesity: A Cause of Short Stature and Delayed Puberty." *New England Journal of Medicine* 309(1983):513.

Roche, A. F., ed. *Body-Composition Assessments in Youth and Adults.* Columbus, Ohio: Ross Laboratories, 1985.

Stunkard, A. J. "An Adoption Study of Human Obesity." *The New England Journal of Medicine* 314(1986):193.

*Svoboda, M. "Addressing Weight Management in Physical Education." *Journal of Physical Education and Recreation* 51(1980):49.

Williams, M. H. *Nutrition for Fitness and Sports.* Dubuque, Iowa: Wm. C. Brown Publishers, 1983.

*Wilmore, J. H., et al. "Body Composition: A Round Table." *Physician and Sportsmedicine* 14(1986):144.

14

EXERCISE AND NUTRITION

CONCEPT 14

The basic nutritional needs
of exercisers or athletes compared to those
of sedentary people
do not differ except for caloric
requirements.
Although there are special considerations
for athletes/exercisers,
many of their dietary practices are faddish,
unsound, and even dangerous.

INTRODUCTION

In spite of the fact that nutrition is an advanced science, many myths and misconceptions prevail. These are propagated by commercial interests. Product sales are advanced by the public's, and even the physicians' and educators', superstition and ignorance of the true facts. Superstition seems to thrive particularly among athletes and coaches. Such misconceptions can lead to unbalanced diets, high cost, and disappointment over the influence on performance.

Some current theories and practices are discussed in this concept, and an attempt is made to dispel some myths about the diets of athletes and others who engage in regular physical activity.

Because nutrition affects us all, it is important that we are knowledgeable about the subject. It is far too complicated to cover even the fundamentals in these pages; therefore, the reader is encouraged to enroll in a nutrition course taught by a registered dietitian, or to study reliable books on the subject, such as those listed in the references at the end of this concept.

TERMS (Also see Concept 13 terms)

Basal Metabolic Rate—Metabolic rate at rest.
Cellulose—Indigestible fiber (bulk) in foods.
Dehydration—Excessive loss of body fluids (e.g., through perspiration, diarrhea, or urination).
Kilogram—A metric unit of weight equaling 2.2046 pounds.
"Making Weight"—Quick loss or gain in weight so an athlete (usually a wrestler) can compete in a given weight category.
Metabolic Rate (MR)—The rate at which the body produces heat, which is measured in calories; an indication of the body's activities, including exercise and normal body functions.
Saturated Fat—Dietary fat that is usually solid at room temperature and comes primarily from an animal source.
Unsaturated Fat—Monosaturated or polysaturated dietary fat that is usually liquid at room temperature and comes primarily from a vegetable source.

THE FACTS

The amount and kind of food you eat affects your health and well-being.

There are about forty-five to fifty nutrients in food that are believed to be essential for the body's growth, maintenance, and repair. These are classified into six categories: carbohydrates (and fiber), fats, proteins, vitamins, minerals, and water. The first three provide energy, which is measured in calories.

The Food and Nutrition Board of the National Academy of Sciences—National Research Council has established a "recommended daily allowances" (RDA) for each nutrient. To help assure that you select foods containing the essential elements, the board has classified foods into groups, each of which should be included in the daily diet. The quantity of nutrients recommended varies with age and other considerations; for example, a young, growing child needs more calcium than an adult, and a pregnant woman needs more calcium than other women.

Some foods contain some of all six classes of nutrients (e.g., whole wheat bread) while others (e.g., sugar) contain only one. No food is a "complete" food because none contains all the specific essential nutrients.

There are ten "key nutrients" central to human nutrition. They are usually accompanied by other nutrients when obtained through plant and animal sources.

If an adequate supply of the ten key nutrients shown in table 14.1 are included in the diet, you will probably receive an ample supply of all the other essential nutrients. Some of the better plant and animal sources of each of the ten is also shown in table 14.1.

It is important to choose foods that have a high "nutrient density."

A nutritionally dense food gives you more nutrients per calorie than a low density food. It is like "getting more for your money (calorie)." For example, a 200 calorie piece of Boston cream pie has very few vitamins and minerals and is high in fat and refined carbohydrates, while 200 calories of tuna has very little

TABLE 14.1 Ten Key Nutrients and Significant Food Sources from Plants and Animals

Nutrient	Plant Source	Animal Source
Carbohydrate	Breads Cereals Fruits and vegetables	
Fat	Margarine Salad dressings	Fat in meats Butter
Protein	Dried beans and peas Nuts	Meat Poultry Fish Cheese Milk
Vitamin A	Dark green leafy vegetables Yellow vegetables Margarine	Butter Fortified milk Liver
Vitamin C	Citrus fruits Broccoli, potatoes Strawberries, tomatoes Cabbage, dark green leafy vegetables	Liver
Vitamin B$_1$ (thiamin)	Breads Cereals Nuts	Pork Ham
Vitamin B$_2$ (riboflavin)	Breads Cereals	Milk Cheese Liver
Niacin	Breads Cereals Nuts	Meat Fish Poultry
Iron	Dried peas and beans Spinach, asparagus Prune juice	Meat Liver
Calcium	Turnip greens, okra Broccoli, spinach	Milk Cheese Mackerel Salmon

From Williams, Melvin H. *Nutrition for Fitness and Sport* (Dubuque, Iowa: Wm. C. Brown Publishers, 1983), 5.

fat, 100 percent of the RDA for protein, niacin, vitamin B$_{12}$, and substantial B$_6$ and phospherous.

Eating nutritionally dense food is particularly important for one who is on a low calorie diet. It is difficult to get all the essential nutrients in a 1,000 to 1,200 calorie diet, for example, unless foods are chosen carefully.

TABLE 14.2 Recommended Food Selections for Good Health

Food Group	Amount for Adults	Special Role in Diet
1. Milk, cheese, ice cream, and other dairy products	• 2 or more servings	• Protein, calcium and other minerals, vitamins
2. Meat, poultry, fish, eggs (alternates: nuts, dried beans, peas)	• 2 or more servings	• Protein, iron and other minerals, B vitamins

3. All vegetables and fruits, including potatoes
   a. Green and yellow vegetables
   b. Citrus fruits, tomatoes, raw cabbage, etc.
	• 4 or more servings	• Minerals, vitamins, fiber, iron, vitamin A, folacin, vitamin C

4. Grain products—bread, flour, cereals, baked goods (perferably whole-grain or enriched)	• 4 or more servings	• Inexpensive source of energy, iron, vitamin B

An adequate intake of the four food groups on a daily basis will provide the ten key nutrients and a well-balanced diet for most people, including exercisers/athletes.

See table 14.2, "Recommended Food Selections for Good Health," for information on the four food groups and the recommended number of daily servings.

The number of calories needed per day depends upon one's **metabolic rate (MR)**, *which, in turn, depends upon such factors as age, sex, size, muscle mass, glandular function, emotional state, climate, and exercise.*

Your **basal metabolic rate** (**BMR**) is the basis for your caloric needs. The higher the BMR, the more calories you burn at rest. Your MR is a combination of your BMR and calories expended in normal daily activities. The MR is usually higher in males, the young, the large, the lean and muscular, the excited; in cold and hot weather; and during exercise.

A moderately active college-age woman needs about 2,000 calories per day, while a moderately active man of the same age needs about 2,800 calories. A female athlete in training might burn 2,600 to 4,500 calories; a male athlete in training may expend 3,500 to 6,000. If weight remains at the optimum, the caloric content of the diet is correct. If weight varies from optimal, the caloric content of the diet may need to be altered. (See Concept 13 regarding weight control.)

Complex carbohydrates should make up about 55 to 60 percent of the calories for an adult.

Complex carbohydrates are known as starches and include whole grain breads and cereals, fruits, and vegetables. These foods are nutritionally dense and also contain **cellulose** (popularly known as fiber). Cellulose does not provide nutrition and is not digested, but is considered essential for the bulk it provides to prevent constipation and possibly colon cancer. Carbohydrates are a primary energy source during exercise, particularly during intense exercise.

Simple carbohydrates are sugars (sucrose, lactose, maltose, glucose, and fructose). These nutritionally low density carbohydrates should be limited to 15 percent or less of the total caloric intake of most normal adults, which will help decrease the incidence of tooth decay, obesity, and perhaps coronary heart disease.

Athletes and active people do not need relatively more protein than nonathletes or inactive people.

Protein needs vary with age, size, and other factors, such as pregnancy, but the well-balanced diet includes about sixty grams of protein per day. This is well over the minimum needed and is adequate for most people. The recommended protein intake is about one gram per **kilogram** of body weight, or 10 to 15 percent of the total calories per day.

Athletes or active people frequently consume more calories than nonathletes or inactive people, and for this reason, consume more protein (assuming that they eat a balanced diet). Because protein is not an important source of energy, and because high quality protein is provided by all meats, milk, eggs, and cheese, there is no need to supplement the athlete's or active person's diet with protein. Consequently, there is no reason for athletes to gorge themselves on beefsteak or to take supplemental proteins, such as "protein energizers" or "protein powerizers," if they eat a balanced diet.

Fat should be eaten only in moderate to low amounts.

Humans need some fat in their diet because fats are carriers of vitamins E, K, D, and A; are a source of essential linoleic acid; make food taste better; and provide a concentrated form of calories, which serves as an important source of energy during mild to moderate exercise.

Fat has twice the calories per gram as carbohydrates. To use fat for energy requires more oxygen than using carbohydrates for energy. High fat diets provide no special benefits for the athlete. Most popular weight loss diets are high in protein; unfortunately, this usually means lots of meat and, therefore, lots of fat. Red meat is high in **saturated fat,** which is considered to be more likely to contribute to heart disease than **unsaturated fat.** Most Americans consume about 40 percent of their calories in fats. This amount should probably be reduced to about 25 to 30 percent.

High fat intake has been associated with increased incidence of breast, prostate, and colon cancer. High fat also means high cholesterol, a coronary heart disease risk factor (see Concepts 6 and 13). To reduce dietary fat, eat less beef and pork and more poultry and fish (not fried!) and use skimmed milk.

The American Heart Association recommends that cholesterol intake be limited to 250 to 300 milligrams per day for normal adults. To meet this standard, no more than 10 percent of the fat in the diet should be **saturated.** As discussed in Concept 6, aerobic exercise is believed to reduce levels of blood lipids.

A person who has trained and achieved good cardiovascular endurance will be a good "fat burner" (burn more energy derived from fat) with mild to moderate exercise than a person who has not trained. When this occurs, it "spares glycogen" (a carbohydrate source) in your muscles.

Sodium intake should not exceed three grams per day.

The American Heart Association recommends that sodium (which is found in table salt) be restricted to 1 gram per 1,000 calories consumed, and not to exceed 3 grams per day. Three grams is the amount of sodium found in 1 teaspoon of table salt. Typically, an adult will use 6 to 12 grams of salt per day! In addition, sodium occurs naturally in a wide variety of foods, and some people ingest even more by drinking "soft" water.

Too much sodium contributes to medical problems such as heart attacks, high blood pressure, strokes, and kidney disorders. (Also see Concept 19 regarding dehydration and salt tablets.)

There is no scientific basis for eliminating milk from the athlete's diet.

Milk does *not* cause "cotton mouth." A dry mouth is due to decreased saliva flow caused by dehydration or an emotional state. Milk does *not* decrease speed, "cut wind," produce sour stomach, or interfere with performance unless the individual has a milk intolerance. Milk is a good source of protein and calcium.

Breakfast is an important meal.

Numerous studies have shown that skipping breakfast impedes performance because blood sugar drops in the long period between dinner the night before and lunch the following day. About one-fourth of the day's calories should be consumed at breakfast.

For the athlete or active person, food should be taken at four-to-six-hour intervals throughout the day for good performance. Skipping meals or snacking during the day and eating one big meal in the evening may adversely affect performance.

"Quick energy" foods eaten just before events of short duration do not enhance performance.

Ingesting honey, glucose, or other sweets just prior to short-term performance does not provide the athlete with a burst of energy. The body will use its own energy reserves. The carbohydrates eaten will help replace the energy used in the performance.

No carbohydrates should be eaten one and one-half to two hours before an endurance event because this may produce a physiological effect leading to premature exhaustion of the glycogen stores.

"Carbohydrate loading" may improve performance in long endurance events, but is not without hazard.

The normal recommended daily allowance of carbohydrate is 55 to 60 percent of the total caloric intake. Carbohydrates provide most of the energy used in heavy exercise and endurance events exceeding thirty to sixty minutes, such as in marathon runs. Several studies have supported a procedure called carbohydrate loading.

There are various methods, but most experts recommend a procedure of eating a high carbohydrate diet and resting for one or two days before an event, such as a marathon run. This regime will not make a person run faster, but he or she may be able to run longer at a given speed.

Carbohydrate loading is most suitable for those in events that exceed one hour and involve high energy expenditure, such as running, swimming, cycling, cross-country skiing, and tournament play in soccer, tennis, or handball. Carbohydrate loading may be harmful to those with diabetes, hypertriglyceridemia, muscle enzyme deficiencies, or kidney disorders.

The timing may be more important than the makeup of the pre-event meal.

It is probably best to eat about three hours before competition or heavy exercise to allow time for digestion. Generally, the athlete can make his or her food selection on the basis of past experience. Tension, anxiety, and excitement are more apt to cause gastric distress than is food selection. It is generally accepted that fat intake should be minimal because it digests more slowly; "gas formers" should probably be avoided; and proteins and high cellulose foods should be kept to a moderate amount prior to prolonged events to avoid urinary and bowel excretion. Two or three cups of liquid should be taken to ensure adequate hydration.

As previously mentioned, carbohydrates should not be ingested within an hour or two of an event because they may cause an insulin response that results in weakness and fatigue. Sometimes they cause stomach distress, cramps, or nausea.

It should be noted that the excitement associated with competition is probably the main reason for having a special diet before participation. Because many people who exercise regularly usually are not competing, there is little reason to alter normal diet before regular exercise. Likewise, there is no need to delay exercise for long periods after the meal if exercise is moderate and noncompetitive.

"Health foods," tonics, and supplements will not contribute to health, fitness, weight control, or athletic performance.

The Food and Drug Administration labels the health food racket as the most widespread quackery in the United States. Whether athletic or sedentary, the individual on a well-balanced diet does *not* benefit from special organic foods, phosphate, alkaline salts, additional vitamins, choline, lecithin, wheat germ, honey, gelatin, aspartates, brewer's yeast, gelatin, royal jelly, or any other supplement, unless specifically prescribed for a medical purpose by a physician (also see Concept 19 regarding drugs).

Vitamins are not drugs and do not contain energy. Most people who take supplemental vitamins do not need them. There is no chemical difference between natural and synthetic vitamins, but the vitamins in food contain other associated nutrients, especially minerals. Megadoses of vitamins may even be harmful. Athletes most often abuse B complex, C, and E, as well as minerals. If you have a balanced diet, none of these will increase performance. (B_{15} [pangamic acid] is **not** a vitamin; it is a fraud and may be harmful.)

It is *not* true that emotional stress increases the need for vitamin B or C nor that taking a "stress formula" will reduce the effects of psychological stress.

Fad diets are not a satisfactory means to long-term weight reduction and may adversely affect the health.

There are hundreds of fad diets and diet books, but nutritionists warn that there is no scientific basis for drastic juggling of food constituents. Such diets are usually unbalanced and may result in serious illness or even death, especially for the obese person who is already apt to be suffering from a number of health disorders. Fad diets cannot be maintained for long periods of time; therefore, the individual usually regains any lost weight. Less than 5 percent of those who lose weight maintain the loss for more than a year. Constant losing and gaining, known as the "yo-yo syndrome" may be more harmful than the original obese condition.

Total fasting is dangerous as are crash (fast) diets. Crash diets that bring about weight loss by **dehydration** of only 5 percent in forty-eight hours have been shown to reduce the individual's working capacity by as much as 40 percent. The practice of **making weight** in athletics, whether by dehydration, induced vomiting, or starvation diets, is dangerous to health and should be condemned (see Concept 13 on weight control and Concept 19 on dehydration). Much of the weight lost on such fad diets is valuable lean muscle mass.

Pill popping, hormone injections, powder and liquid diets have little value in long-term weight control programs and present many health hazards. When in doubt, avoid diets that:

1. Promise fast, easy solutions.
2. Promise to help you achieve ideal weight without mental inspiration and perspiration.
3. Favor one food as the answer to weight problems.
4. Promise that your fat will melt away.

Exercise goes hand in hand with nutrition in health maintenance.

"Eat right and get plenty of exercise" is a common prescription (see table 14.2). The benefits of exercise specifically include the following: it can reduce blood lipids, burn excess calories to reduce weight, help prevent or improve cardiac heart disease, increase high-density lipoproteins that may protect against heart disease, train the heart muscle, reduce high blood pressure, have an insulin effect for the diabetic, reduce blood glucose, and reduce psychic stress and tension.

The only good diet is one balanced with the four food groups in amounts that provide the RDA of essential nutrients.

REFERENCES

American Alliance of Health, Physical Education, Recreation and Dance. *Nutrition for Athletes*. Washington, DC: AAHPERD, 1980.

Barrett, Stephen. *The Health Robbers*. Philadelphia: George F. Stickley Co., 1981.

Blackburn, G. L., and K. Pavlou. "Fad Reducing Diets: Separating Fads from Facts." *Contemporary Nutrition* 8:7(July 1983).

Clark, N. "Nutrition Update." *Sports Medicine Digest* 5:1(January 1983):3.

Clark, R., and G. Blackburn. "Danger Ahead? Fad Diets for Weight Control." *The Professional Nutritionist* (Summer 1982).

"Common Sense Approach to Athletic Training." *Sports Medicine Digest* 5(1983).

Consumer Reports Books, eds. *Health Quackery*. Mount Vernon, N.Y.: Consumers Union, 1980.

"Diet and Heart Disease." *Consumer Reports* (May 1981):256.

"Dieting, the Losing Game." *Time* (20 January 1986):54.

"Fear of Fat: The Medical Evidence." *Consumer Reports* (August 1985):455.

Haskell, W., J. Scala, and J. Whittam. *Nutrition and Athletic Performance*. Palo Alto, Calif.: Bull Publishing Co., 1982.

*Herbert, V. *Nutrition Cultism—Facts and Fiction*. Philadelphia: George F. Stickley Co., 1980.

Herbert, V. "Will Questionable Nutrition Overwhelm Nutrition Science." *The American Journal of Clinical Nutrition.* 34(December 1981):2848.

*Herbert, Victor, and Stephen Barrett. *Vitamins and Health Food Robbers: The Great American Hustle.* Philadelphia: George F. Stickley Co., 1981.

Kenny, J. J. "Is Your Nutritionist a Quack?" *Aerobics & Fitness.* (March–April 1985):22.

Milner, J. A. "Dietary Antioxidants and Cancer." *Contemporary Nutrition* 10:10(October 1985).

Moore, M. "Carbohydrate Loading: Eating Through the Wall." *Physician and Sportsmedicine* 9(1981):97.

Munnings, F. C. "Physicians Can Help Stop Nutrition Fraud." *Physician and Sportsmedicine* 14:6(June 1986):51.

Munnings, F. C. "College Athletes Are Losing to Food Quacks." *Physician and Sportsmedicine* 14:8(August 1986):38.

National Cancer Institute. *Diet, Nutrition, and Cancer Prevention: A Guide to Food Choices* (NIH Publication No. 85–2711). Washington, DC: U.S. Department of Health and Human Services, 1984.

"Nutrition Misinformation." *Dairy Council Digest* 52:4 (July–August 1981):19.

Nutrition References and Book Reviews. Rev. ed. Chicago: Chicago Nutrition Assoc., 1981, $8.00.

"Nutrition Update." *Sports Medicine Digest* 5(1983).

O'Connor, T. P. "Dietary Fat, Calories, and Cancer." *Contemporary Nutrition* 10:7(July 1985).

*"The Prudent Diet Has Been Endorsed by Experts." *Consumer Reports* (July 1985):423.

Serfas, R. C. "Nutrition for the Athlete Update." *Contemporary Nutrition* 7(1982):1.

Sherman, G., et al. "Effects of Exercise Diet Manipulation on Muscle Glycogen and Its Subsequent Utilization during Performance." *International Journal of Sports Medicine* 2(1981):114.

"Stress Formulas Theragran Vitamins." *Food For Thought.* (Orange County Nutrition Council) 12:3(May 1986).

U.S. Department of Agriculture and U.S. Department of Health and Human Services. *Dietary Guidelines for Americans.* Washington, DC: U.S. Government Printing Office, 1985.

"The Vitamin Pushers." *Consumer Reports* (March 1986):170.

Voy, R. O. "Water Soluble Vitamins Not Safe in Megadoses." *Physician and Sportsmedicine* 14:3(March 1986):52.

*Williams, M. H. *Nutrition for Fitness and Sport.* Dubuque, Iowa: Wm. C. Brown Publishers, 1983.

Willis, J. "Diet Books Sell Well But." *FDA Consumer* (March 1982).

*Wink, Dorothy. *Nutrition.* 2d ed. Reston, Va.: Reston Publishing Co., 1983.

▶ LAB RESOURCE MATERIALS (FOR USE WITH LABS 14A AND 14B, PAGES 251–254)

CHART 14A.1 Dietary Habits Questionnaire

Yes	No	
☐	☐	1. Do you eat regular meals?
☐	☐	2. Do you eat a good breakfast daily?
☐	☐	3. Do you eat lunch regularly?
☐	☐	4. Does your diet contain about 55 percent–60 percent carbohydrates with a high concentration of fiber?
☐	☐	5. Are less than ¼ of the carbohydrates you eat simple carbohydrates?
☐	☐	6. Does your diet contain 10–15% protein?
☐	☐	7. Does your diet contain less than 30% fat?
☐	☐	8. Do you limit the amount of saturated fat in your diet?
☐	☐	9. Do you limit salt intake to acceptable amounts?
☐	☐	10. Do you get adequate amounts of vitamins in your diet without a supplement?
☐	☐	11. Do you eat regularly from all food groups?
☐	☐	12. Do you drink adequate amounts of water?
☐	☐	13. Do you get adequate minerals in your diet without a supplement?
☐	☐	14. Do you limit your caffeine consumption to acceptable levels?
☐	☐	15. Is your average calorie consumption for the three day period reasonable for your body size and for the amount of calories you normally expend?

CHART 14A.2 Dietary Habits *Rating Scale*

Score	Rating
14–15	Very Good
12–13	Good
10–11	Marginal
9 or less	Poor

CHART 14A.3 Diet Record

Day _____

Breakfast Food	Amount	Calories	Basic Food Servings	Food Content
			Dairy group ☐ ☐ Meat/Fish/Eggs ☐ ☐ Vegetables/Fruits ☐ ☐ ☐ ☐ Breads/Cereals ☐ ☐ ☐ ☐	% Protein ————— % Fat ————— % Complex Carbohydrate ————— % Simple Carbohydrate —————

Lunch Food	Amount	Calories	Basic Food Servings	Food Content
			Dairy group ☐ ☐ Meat/Fish/Eggs ☐ ☐ Vegetables/Fruits ☐ ☐ ☐ ☐ Breads/Cereals ☐ ☐ ☐ ☐	% Protein ————— % Fat ————— % Complex Carbohydrate ————— % Simple Carbohydrate —————

Dinner Food	Amount	Calories	Basic Food Servings	Food Content
			Dairy group ☐ ☐ Meat/Fish/Eggs ☐ ☐ Vegetables/Fruits ☐ ☐ ☐ ☐ Breads/Cereals ☐ ☐ ☐ ☐	% Protein ————— % Fat ————— % Complex Carbohydrate ————— % Simple Carbohydrate —————

Snack Food	Amount	Calories	Basic Food Servings	Food Content
			Dairy group ☐ ☐ Meat/Fish/Eggs ☐ ☐ Vegetables/Fruits ☐ ☐ ☐ ☐ Breads/Cereals ☐ ☐ ☐ ☐	% Protein ————— % Fat ————— % Complex Carbohydrate ————— % Simple Carbohydrate —————

| **Total Calories for Day** | | | | |

15

SKILL-RELATED PHYSICAL FITNESS

CONCEPT 15

Skill-related fitness is essential
to performance in games
and sports as well as
to working efficiency.

INTRODUCTION

Skill-related fitness consists of six different components: balance, agility, coordination, speed, power, and reaction time (see Concept 2 for definitions). Although these aspects of physical fitness do not necessarily make you healthier, possessing these fitness characteristics makes you better at games and sports as well as improves your work efficiency. In a society that is becoming increasingly interested in leisure and recreation, skill-related physical fitness can be important to living a meaningful and enjoyable life.

TERMS

Motor Fitness—Another term commonly used for skill-related physical fitness.
Sports Fitness—A term commonly used for skill-related physical fitness.

THE FACTS

Good skill-related fitness may help you achieve good health-related fitness.

Individuals who achieve good skill-related fitness have the potential to succeed in sports and games. Regular participation in these activities can lead to improved health-related fitness throughout life. In addition, people who make an effort to learn activities involving skill-related fitness are more likely to be active in sports and games for a lifetime.

Skill-related fitness may improve your ability to work efficiently.

In manual labor, skillful performance improves efficiency. For example, a ditchdigger with great ditch-digging skills uses less energy than one who has not mastered the skill. Seemingly simple skills are often quite complex and may require some proficiency in each of the skill-related fitness components.

Skill-related fitness may improve your ability to meet emergency situations.

Good agility would enable you to dodge an oncoming car; good balance would lessen the likelihood of a fall; and good reaction time would decrease the chances of being hit by a flying object. Each aspect of skill-related fitness contributes in its own way to your ability to avoid injury and meet emergencies.

Good skill-related fitness is beneficial to carrying out the normal daily routine and enjoying your leisure time.

Walking, sitting, climbing, pushing, pulling, and other such tasks require varying degrees of skill-related fitness. Accordingly, improved fitness resulting from regular practice may improve efficiency in performing daily activities and in enjoying leisure or recreational time.

The potential for possessing outstanding skill-related fitness is based on hereditary predispositions, but all aspects of skill-related fitness can be improved through regular practice.

In order for a skill to be improved, it must be repeated. Some skill-related fitness components, such as power, agility, balance, and coordination, can be enhanced greatly with practice. Others, such as speed and reaction time, can be improved somewhat but are determined to a greater extent by heredity.

Exceptional athletes tend to be outstanding in more than one component of skill-related fitness.

Though people possess skill-related fitness in varying degrees, great athletes are likely to be above average in most, if not all, aspects. Indeed, exceptional athletes must be exceptional in many areas of skill-related fitness. Different sports require different skills, each of which requires varying degrees of the six components of skill-related fitness.

Excellence in one skill-related fitness component may compensate for lack in another.

Each individual possesses a specific level of each skill-related fitness aspect. The performer should learn his or her other strengths and weaknesses in order to produce optimal performances. For example, a tennis player may use coordination to compensate for lack of speed.

Excellence in skill-related fitness may compensate for lack of health-related fitness when playing sports and games.

As you grow older, health-related fitness potential declines. You may use superior skill-related fitness to compensate. For example, a baseball pitcher who lacks the strength and the power to dominate hitters may rely on a pitch such as a knuckleball, which is more dependent on coordination, than on power.

Skills are specific in nature.

An individual might possess ability in one area and not in another. For this reason, "general motor ability" probably does not really exist. Individuals do not have one general capacity for performing skills. Rather, the ability to play games or sports is determined by combined abilities in each of the separate motor skill components of agility, coordination, balance, reaction time, speed, and power. It is, however, possible and even likely that some performers will have above average skill in many areas.

Skill-related fitness can be improved by performing activities that require the use of specific skill-related fitness components.

Skill-related fitness components are prerequisite to the successful performance of many different sports skills. At the same time, the performance of sports skills, which require the use of different skill-related fitness components, will contribute to improvement in those fitness aspects. Table 15.1 shows the activities that require each different component of skill-related fitness. The table also gives you an idea about which activities tend to promote development of various skill-related fitness components. Though it is true that skill-related fitness is based on hereditary predispositions, all people can improve their skill-related fitness with participation in the appropriate activities.

TABLE 15.1 Skill-Related Benefits of Sports and Other Activities

Activity	Balance	Coordination	Reaction Time	Agility	Power	Speed
Archery	Good	Excellent	Poor	Poor	Poor	Poor
Backpacking	Fair	Fair	Poor	Fair	Fair	Poor
Badminton	Fair	Excellent	Good	Good	Fair	Good
Baseball	Good	Excellent	Excellent	Good	Excellent	Good
Basketball	Good	Excellent	Excellent	Excellent	Excellent	Good
Bicycling	Excellent	Fair	Fair	Poor	Poor	Fair
Bowling	Good	Excellent	Poor	Fair	Fair	Fair
Canoeing	Good	Good	Fair	Poor	Good	Poor
Circuit Training	Fair	Fair	Poor	Fair	Good	Fair
Dance, Aerobic	Fair	Good	Fair	Good	Poor	Poor
Dance, Ballet	Excellent	Excellent	Fair	Excellent	Good	Poor
Dance, Disco	Fair	Good	Fair	Excellent	Poor	Fair
Dance, Modern	Excellent	Excellent	Fair	Excellent	Good	Poor
Dance, Social	Fair	Good	Fair	Good	Poor	Fair
Fencing	Good	Excellent	Excellent	Good	Good	Excellent
Fitness Calisthenics	Fair	Fair	Poor	Good	Fair	Poor
Football	Good	Good	Excellent	Excellent	Excellent	Excellent
Golf (walking)	Fair	Excellent	Poor	Fair	Good	Poor
Gymnastics	Excellent	Excellent	Good	Excellent	Excellent	Fair
Handball	Fair	Excellent	Good	Excellent	Good	Good
Hiking	Fair	Fair	Poor	Fair	Fair	Poor
Horseback Riding	Good	Good	Fair	Good	Poor	Poor
Interval Training	Fair	Fair	Poor	Poor	Poor	Fair
Jogging	Fair	Fair	Poor	Poor	Poor	Poor
Judo	Good	Excellent	Excellent	Excellent	Excellent	Excellent
Karate	Good	Excellent	Excellent	Excellent	Excellent	Excellent
Mountain Climbing	Excellent	Excellent	Fair	Good	Good	Poor
Pool; Billiards	Fair	Good	Poor	Fair	Fair	Poor
Racquetball; Paddleball	Fair	Excellent	Good	Excellent	Fair	Good
Rope Jumping	Fair	Good	Fair	Good	Fair	Poor
Rowing, Crew	Fair	Excellent	Poor	Good	Excellent	Fair
Sailing	Good	Good	Good	Good	Fair	Poor
Skating, Ice	Excellent	Good	Fair	Good	Fair	Good
Skating, Roller	Excellent	Good	Poor	Good	Fair	Good
Skiing, Cross-Country	Fair	Excellent	Poor	Good	Excellent	Fair
Skiing, Downhill	Excellent	Excellent	Good	Excellent	Good	Poor
Soccer	Fair	Excellent	Good	Excellent	Good	Good
Softball (fast)	Fair	Excellent	Excellent	Good	Good	Good
Softball (slow)	Fair	Excellent	Good	Fair	Good	Good
Surfing	Excellent	Excellent	Good	Excellent	Good	Poor
Swimming (laps)	Fair	Good	Poor	Good	Fair	Poor
Table Tennis	Fair	Good	Good	Fair	Fair	Fair
Tennis	Fair	Excellent	Good	Good	Good	Good
Volleyball	Fair	Excellent	Good	Good	Fair	Fair
Walking	Fair	Fair	Poor	Poor	Poor	Poor
Waterskiing	Good	Good	Poor	Good	Fair	Poor
Weight Training	Fair	Fair	Poor	Poor	Fair	Poor

From C. B. Corbin, and R. Lindsey. *Fitness for Life,* 2d ed. (Glenview, IL: Scott, Foresman and Co. 1985) p. 127. Used by permission.

Important Note: Because skill-related physical fitness does not relate directly to good health, the rating charts used in this section differ from those used in earlier concepts. The rating charts that follow can be used to compare your scores to those of other people. You DO NOT have to have exceptional scores on skill-related fitness to be able to enjoy sports and other types of physical activity. After the age of thirty, you should adjust ratings by 1 percent per year.

Evaluating Skill-Related Physical Fitness

Evaluating agility: The Illinois agility run[1]

An agility course using four chairs, ten feet apart, and a thirty-foot running area will be set up as depicted in this illustration.

The test is performed as follows:

1. Lie prone with your hands by your shoulders and your head at the starting line. On the signal to begin, run the course as fast as possible.
2. Your score is the time required to complete the course.

CHART 15.1 Agility *Rating Scale*

Classification	Men	Women
Excellent	15.8 or faster	17.4 or faster
Very good	16.7–15.9	18.6–17.5
Fair	18.6–16.8	22.3–18.7
Poor	18.8–18.7	23.4–22.4
Very poor	18.9 or slower	23.5 or slower

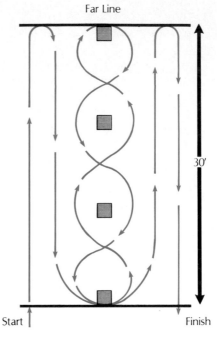

Agility Run

Evaluating balance: The Bass test of dynamic balance[2]

Eleven circles (9½-inch) are drawn on the floor as shown in the illustration. The test is performed as follows:

1. Stand on the right foot in circle X. *Leap* forward to circle one, then circles two through ten, alternating feet with each leap.
2. The feet must leave the floor on each leap and the heel may not touch. Only the ball of the foot may land on the floor.
3. Remain in each circle for five seconds before leaping to the next circle. (A count of five will be made for you, aloud.)
4. Practice trials are allowed.

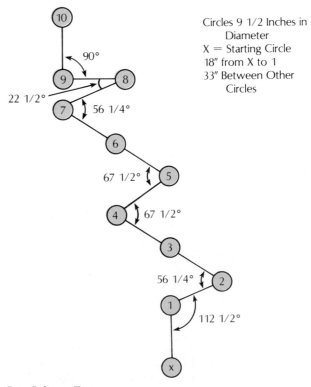

Circles 9 1/2 Inches in Diameter
X = Starting Circle
18″ from X to 1
33″ Between Other Circles

Bass Balance Test

[1]Adams et al., *Foundations of Physical Activity* (Champaign, IL: Stipes and Co., 1965), 111.

[2]From C. H. McCloy. *Tests and Measurements in Health and Physical Education* (New York: Appleton-Century-Crofts, 1954), 106.

5. The score is fifty, plus the number of seconds taken to complete the test, minus the number of errors.

6. For every error, deduct three points each. Errors include touching the heel, moving the supporting foot, touching outside a circle, or touching any body part to the floor other than the supporting foot.

7. Scores should be plotted on the appropriate rating scales.

Evaluating coordination: The stick test of coordination

The stick test of coordination requires you to juggle three wooden wands. The wands are used to perform a one-half flip and a full flip as shown in the illustrations.

1. *One-Half Flip*—Hold two twenty-four-inch (one-half inch in diameter) dowel rods, one in each hand. Support a third rod of the same size across the other two. Toss the supported rod in the air so that it makes a half turn. Catch the thrown rod with the two held rods.

2. *Full Flip*—Perform the preceding task, letting the supported rod turn a full flip.

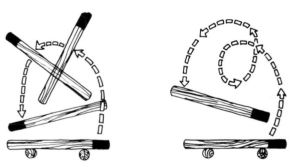

One-Half Flip   Full Flip

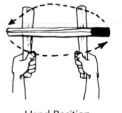

Hand Position

The test is performed as follows:

1. Practice the half-flip and the full flip several times before taking the test.

2. When you are ready, attempt a half-flip five times. Score one point for each successful attempt.

3. When you are ready, attempt the full flip five times. Score two points for each successful attempt.

CHART 15.2 Bass Test *Rating Scale*

Rating	Score
Excellent	90–100
Very good	80–89
Fair	60–79
Poor	30–59
Very poor	0–29

CHART 15.3 Coordination *Rating Scale*

Classification	Men	Women
Excellent	14–15	13–15
Very good	11–13	10–12
Fair	5–10	4–9
Poor	3–4	2–3
Very poor	0–2	0–1

Evaluating power: The vertical jump test

The test is performed as follows:

1. Hold a piece of chalk so its end is even with your fingertips.

2. Stand with both feet on the floor and your side to the wall and reach and mark as high as possible.

3. Jump upward with both feet as high as possible. Swing arms upward and make a chalk mark on a 5′×1′ wall chart marked off in half-inch horizontal lines placed six feet from the floor.

4. Measure the distance between the reaching height and the jumping height.

5. Your score is the best of three jumps.

CHART 15.4 Power *Rating Scale*

Classification	Men	Women
Excellent	25½″ or more	23½″ or more
Very good	21″–25″	19″–23″
Fair	16½″–20½″	14½″–18½″
Poor	12½″–16″	10½″–14″
Very poor	12″ or less	10″ or less

Evaluating reaction time: The stick drop test

To perform the stick drop test of reaction time, you will need a yardstick, a table, a chair, and a partner to help with the test. To perform the test, follow these procedures:

1. Sit in the chair next to the table so that your elbow and lower arm rest on the table comfortably. The heel of your hand should rest on the table so that only your fingers and thumb extend beyond the edge of the table.

2. Your partner holds a yardstick at the very top, allowing it to dangle between your thumb and fingers.
3. The yardstick should be held so that the twenty-four-inch mark is even with your thumb and index finger. No part of your hand should touch the yardstick.
4. Without warning, your partner will drop the stick and you will catch it with your thumb and index finger.
5. Your score is the number of inches read on the yardstick just above the thumb and index finger after you catch the yardstick.
6. Try the test three times. Your partner should be careful not to drop the stick at predictable time intervals so that you cannot guess when it will be dropped. It is important that you react to the dropping of the stick only.
7. Use the middle of your three scores (example: if your scores are 21, 18, and 19, your middle score is 19). The higher your score, the faster your reaction time.

Evaluating speed: Running test of speed
To perform the running test of speed, it will be necessary to have a specially marked running course, a stopwatch, a whistle, and a partner to help you with the test. To perform the test, follow this procedure:

1. Mark a running course on a hard surface so that there is a starting line and a series of nine additional lines, each two yards apart, the first marked at a distance ten yards from the starting line.
2. From a distance one or two yards behind the starting line, begin to run as fast as you can. As you cross the starting line, your partner starts a stopwatch.
3. Run as fast as you can until you hear the whistle that your partner will blow exactly three seconds after the stopwatch was started. Your partner marks your location at the time when the whistle was blown.
4. Your score is the distance you were able to cover in three seconds. You may practice the test and take more than one trial if time allows. Use the better of your distances on the last two trials as your score.

CHART 15.5 Reaction Time *Rating Scale*

Classification	Score in Inches
Excellent	More than 21
Very good	19–21
Fair	16–18¾
Poor	13–15¾
Very poor	Below 13

CHART 15.6 Speed *Rating Scale*

Classification	Men	Women
Excellent	24–26 yards	22–26 yards
Very good	22–23 yards	20–21 yards
Fair	18–21 yards	16–19 yards
Poor	16–17 yards	14–15 yards
Very poor	Less than 16 yards	Less than 14 yards

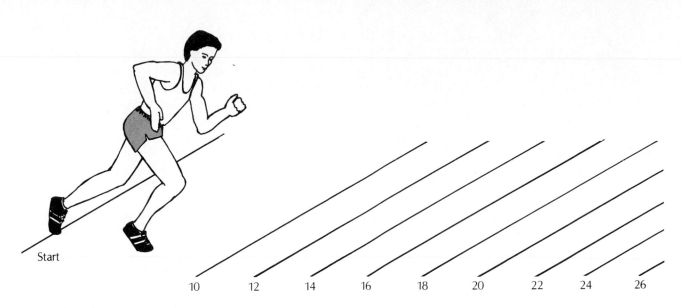

Start

| | | | | | | | | |
|10|12|14|16|18|20|22|24|26|

Running Speed

REFERENCES

*Corbin, C. B., ed. *A Textbook of Motor Development.* 2d ed. Dubuque, Iowa: Wm. C. Brown Publishers, 1980.

Corbin, C. B., and R. Lindsey. *The Ultimate Fitness Book.* New York: Leisure Press, 1984.

Csikszentmihalyi, M. *Beyond Boredom and Anxiety.* San Francisco: Jossey-Bass, 1977.

Fitness Canada. *Canada Fitness Survey—Highlights.* Ottawa, Ontario, Canada: Government of Canada, 1983.

Harris, L., and Associates. *The Perrier Study: Fitness in America.* New York: Great Waters of France, 1979.

Research and Forecasts, Inc. *The Miller Lite Report on American Attitudes toward Sports.* Milwaukee: Miller Brewing Co., 1983.

Snyder, E. E., and E. Spreitzer. "Adult Perceptions of Physical Education in the Schools and Community Sports Programs for Youth." *The Physical Educator* 40(1983):88.

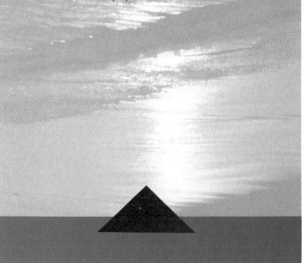

16

SPORTS AND PREPLANNED EXERCISE PROGRAMS

CONCEPT 16

Everyone, regardless of physical abilities,
can find a sport or physical activity
to enjoy for a lifetime.

INTRODUCTION

There are many kinds of exercise and physical activity programs. Some of these, including aerobic and anaerobic exercise, strength and endurance training, and stretching, have been discussed in previous concepts (7, 10, and 12). Other popular and effective types of physical activity including sports and preplanned exercise programs, are discussed in this concept.

TERMS

Lifetime Sport—A sport suitable for people of all ages; a sport that can be performed "from the cradle to the grave" (for a lifetime).

Preplanned Exercise Programs—Preplanned exercise programs are exercise regimes planned by someone other than the person doing the exercise. Often they are designed for a large group of people rather than for one individual.

Sport—An activity that involves competition between teams or individuals in which the goal is to beat the opponent or win the game. Except in the case of ties, there is a winner and a loser. Activities such as swimming, cycling, jogging/running are classified as sports by some writers; however, in this text, they are defined as aerobic activities rather than as sports because most adults do not perform these activities competitively.

THE FACTS ABOUT SPORTS

*Those **sports** in which youth are active are often not the activities performed by adults for a lifetime.*

Team sports are the most popular among school-age children, but the leading **lifetime sports** are bowling and tennis. However, many of the most popular lifetime activities are not even sports. Bowling is the only sport in the top five activities performed regularly by adults. The other four activities are walking, swimming, calisthenics, and bicycling. Only three of the top ten lifetime activities are sports. The top ten sports in which adults regularly participate (excluding swimming, cycling, and jogging/running) are listed in table 16.1.

More and more adults favor their children's involvement in aerobic activities and lifetime sports.

Though it is true that baseball, football, and basketball are still activities in which parents encourage children's participation, especially boys, many now prefer their children to become involved in lifetime sports or aerobic activities. Among the activities most preferred

TABLE 16.1 Achieving Fitness through Sports

Sport	Participants (in millions)	Cardiovascular	Muscular Endurance	Strength	Flexibility	Fat Control
Bowling	20.2	−	−	−	−	−
Tennis	14.0	**	**	*	*	*
Basketball	10.9	***	**	*	−	**
Softball	10.9	−	−	−	−	−
Baseball	9.3	−	−	−	−	−
Golf (walking)	7.8	*	*	−	*	*
Volleyball	7.8	*	**	*	*	*
Football	6.2	*	*	**	−	*
Frisbee	6.2	*	*	−	*	*
Table Tennis	6.2	−	−	−	*	−

***Very Good   **Good   *Minimum   −Low

for boys are tennis, swimming, bicycling, jogging/running, and camping. Among those preferred for girls are tennis, bowling, softball, swimming, bicycling, walking, and dance aerobics.

Participation in sports can contribute to good health-related physical fitness.

The ten most popular sports performed on a regular basis by adults are presented in table 16.1. Each has been assigned a value for building each of the health-related aspects of physical fitness.

Participation in a lifetime sport does not ensure good health-related physical fitness.

As seen in table 16.1, many popular lifetime sports lack sufficient frequency, intensity, or time to improve health-related physical fitness. For example, bowling, softball, and baseball are fun for many people but do very little to improve fitness.

The way a person plays a sport affects the amount of fitness he or she derives from it.

The way you play a sport will determine the fitness benefits you derive from the activity. If you play basketball, you may just shoot baskets or play on half the court, or you may play a vigorous full-court competitive game. In tennis, you may just hit the ball back and forth, play a recreational game, or play a vigorous competitive game. The benefits illustrated in table 16.1 are based on moderate recreational play. If you play less intensely or more vigorously, the benefits will vary accordingly.

Participation in lifetime sports can be a means of achieving physical fitness, but can also provide other valuable benefits as well.

One real benefit of regular participation in lifetime physical activities is improved health through improved cardiovascular fitness, muscular endurance,

strength, and flexibility. However, the participants may also derive personal satisfaction and meaning from the participation, and benefit from social interactions and release of emotional tensions.

In many cases, a person needs to exercise to get fit for sports rather than play sports to get fit.

Many sports require a considerable amount of fitness, especially those involving vigorous competition, yet the sport may do relatively little to develop fitness. For example, you need considerable strength, muscular endurance, and flexibility to play football. However, football is not a particularly good activity for developing these aspects of fitness.

Though recreational sports skills are learned by most people early in life, lifetime sports skills can be learned at any age.

Research evidence suggests that most skills are learned early in life. In fact, one study indicates that as many as 85 percent of all recreational skills are learned by the age of twelve. This does not mean that "old dogs cannot learn new tricks," but it does suggest a need to teach skills to children at an early age.

THE FACTS ABOUT PREPLANNED EXERCISE PROGRAMS

Preplanned exercise programs are a popular form of exercise.

The results of nationwide surveys in the United States and in Canada confirm that home calisthenics are among the most popular forms of exercise among adults. Preplanned programs are especially popular because someone else directs your performance.

There can be some problems in performing pre-planned exercise programs.

Because preplanned exercise programs are planned by one person (or group) for individuals of many different levels of fitness, they may not be equally effective for all people who use them.

When selecting a preplanned exercise program, the following suggestions may be useful.

1. Find out who wrote the program. Is the person(s) an expert? What makes the person an expert? Look for a program written by someone with a good educational background in physical education, exercise physiology, or sports medicine. Programs written by movie stars and television celebrities are rarely sound.
2. Choose a program with more than one level of exercise. A good program will have exercises for beginning, intermediate, and advanced levels of fitness. This allows you to select a program appropriate to your needs. Be skeptical of programs that include one set of exercises for all people.
3. Make certain that all exercises are "good" exercises. In Concept 18, some contraindicated or "bad" exercises are outlined. Avoid programs that include these exercises.
4. Choose a program that meets your needs. Because physical fitness has many components, you need a program that includes exercises and activities for the fitness areas in which you need improvement.
5. Choose a program that you enjoy enough to continue on a regular basis. No matter how good a program is, if you don't do it, it won't work.
6. Choose a program that can be adapted to your needs as your fitness improves.

Preplanned programs that are not well designed but provide motivation to exercise can be adapted to make them safe and effective programs.

Some preplanned exercise programs, especially those prepared by famous people with little exercise expertise, can be modified to improve them. Exercise programs on videotape and television can provide motivation to do regular exercise. Well-informed people can adapt these programs to make them safe and effective. You may want to use table 16.2 as a guide to making the necessary modifications.

There are many different kinds of preplanned exercise programs.

Popular preplanned programs include those developed by governmental agencies, such as the Adult Fitness Program (developed by the President's Council on Physical Fitness and Sport) and the Royal Canadian XBX and 5BX exercises. Some are developed commercially, such as videotapes of home exercises, programs published in books and magazines, and those already discussed in Concept 7 (dance aerobics routines and aqua dynamics). The benefits of preplanned programs are described in table 16.3.

One preplanned program that has been widely used over the last thirty years is the Royal Canadian program. Because it is a good example of one of the better preplanned programs, more details concerning it are presented here.

TABLE 16.2 Guidelines for Adapting Preplanned Exercise Programs

1. If the program contains contraindicted or "bad" exercises, don't do them or substitute safe exercises.
2. Determine if the program gets you to exercise in the target zone for all parts of fitness. If not, supplement it with appropriate exercises. Many programs emphasize one component of fitness while neglecting others.
3. If the program is too difficult, don't continue. Modify with easier exercises that are more suited to your needs. For cardiovascular exercises, you may slow the speed of the exercise or eliminate arm movements to make them easier. Don't feel that you need to keep up with the instructor.
4. If you experience pain, stop exercising or reduce the intensity of the exercise. The "no pain, no gain" idea is an incorrect idea!
5. If the program is too easy, supplement it with additional exercises.
6. Rotate programs regularly to keep your interest level high.

TABLE 16.3 Achieving Fitness through Preplanned Exercise Programs

Program Type	Cardiovascular Fitness	Strength and Muscular Endurance	Flexibility	Body and Fat Control	Skill-Related Fitness	Enjoyment or Fun[1]
Aquadynamics	**	**	**	**	*	**
Dance Exercise[2]	***	**	***	***	*	**
XBX-5BX	*	***	**	*	—	*

***Very Good   **Good   *Minimum   —Low

[1]Enjoyment and fun are relative, and for this reason, it is impossible to classify activities accurately. However, for the average person, some activities seem to be more enjoyable than others. The above listed classifications reflect the opinions of the typical person. *Any of the activities listed above can be fun and enjoyable for a given person in the right circumstances.*
[2]All dance exercise classes are not "equal." If taught well by a professional, these rankings would be accurate.

Royal Canadian XBX and 5BX Programs

The Royal Canadian XBX and 5BX programs are progressive exercise plans designed to build total physical fitness. These plans, originally developed for use by the Royal Canadian Air Force, require eleven to twelve minutes a day. They were, like the Aerobics Program, originally designed to develop and maintain the physical fitness of military personnel. However, the programs have been widely received by the public.

The Canadian Air Force program consists of two separate parts: 5BX for men and XBX for women, though either set of exercises is appropriate for either sex. These graduated programs are arranged so that a specific number of exercises and repetitions are performed, depending upon your initial fitness. The more fit people select exercises from a chart listing more difficult exercises, while the less fit people select exercises from a chart illustrating less difficult exercises.

The XBX plan contains four charts of ten exercises, each chart more difficult than the preceding one. The 5BX includes six charts of five exercises each; each chart is divided into twelve fitness "levels." Intensity of exercise increases progressively as you move from level to level and from chart to chart.

A sample from the Royal Canadian program is shown here. It is one of the many included in the program, and is of moderate intensity. Some exercises have been modified to improve them.

THE CANADIAN XBX AND 5BX EXERCISES (SAMPLE PROGRAM)*

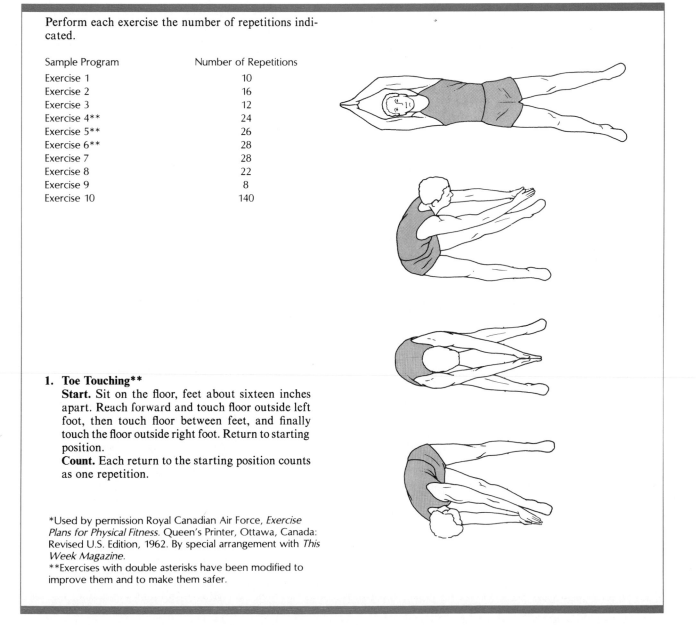

Perform each exercise the number of repetitions indicated.

Sample Program	Number of Repetitions
Exercise 1	10
Exercise 2	16
Exercise 3	12
Exercise 4**	24
Exercise 5**	26
Exercise 6**	28
Exercise 7	28
Exercise 8	22
Exercise 9	8
Exercise 10	140

1. **Toe Touching****
   Start. Sit on the floor, feet about sixteen inches apart. Reach forward and touch floor outside left foot, then touch floor between feet, and finally touch the floor outside right foot. Return to starting position.
   Count. Each return to the starting position counts as one repetition.

*Used by permission Royal Canadian Air Force, *Exercise Plans for Physical Fitness*. Queen's Printer, Ottawa, Canada: Revised U.S. Edition, 1962. By special arrangement with *This Week Magazine*.
**Exercises with double asterisks have been modified to improve them and to make them safer.

2. Knee Raising**
Start. Stand erect, feet together, arms at sides. Raise left knee as high as possible, grasping behind the upper leg with hands. Pull leg against body. Keep straight throughout. Lower foot to floor. Repeat with right leg. Continue by alternating legs.
Count. Left knee raise plus right knee raise counts as one repetition.

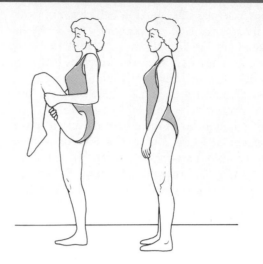

3. Lateral Bending
Start. Stand erect, feet twelve inches apart, right arm extended over head, bent at elbow. Bend sideward from waist to left. Slide left hand down leg as far as possible, and at the same time press to left with right arm. Return to starting position and change arm positions. Repeat to right. Continue by alternating to left, then right.
Count. Bend to left plus bend to right counts as one repetition.

4. Arm Circling**
Start. Stand erect, feet twelve inches apart, arms at sides. Make large circles with arms in a windmill action—one arm following the other and both moving at the same time. Make backward circles only. Keep palms up.
Count. Each full circle by both arms counts as one repetition.

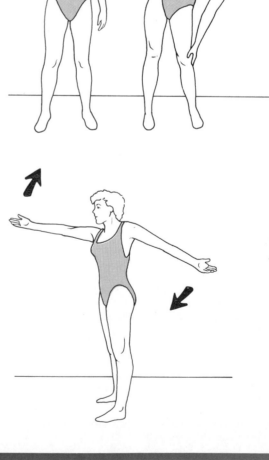

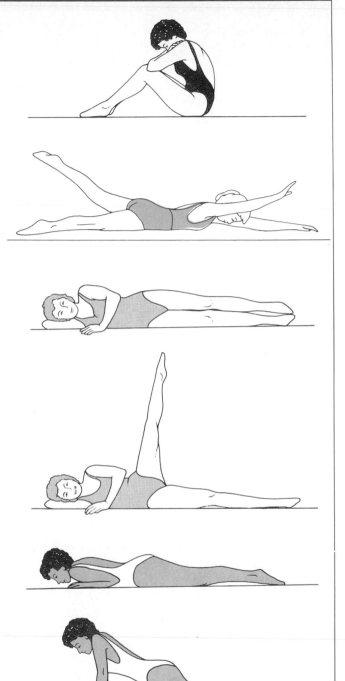

5. **Sit-ups****

   Start. Lie on back, knees bent and together, arms across chest. Roll shoulders and trunk forward to a sitting position. Return to starting position.

   Count. Each return to the starting position counts as one repetition.

6. **Arm and Leg-lift****

   Start. Lie face down, legs straight and together; arms straight, together, and forward. First lift the left leg and the right arm. Return to starting position. Next lift the right leg and the left arm. Return to starting position. Keep the chin on the floor.

   Count. Each return to the starting position counts as one repetition.

7. **Side Leg Raising**

   Start. Lie on side with the legs straight along floor, top arm used for balance. Raise upper leg until it is perpendicular to floor. Lower to starting position.

   Count. Each leg raise counts as one. Do half the number of repetitions raising the left leg. Roll to other side and do half with the right leg.

8. **Modified Push-up**

   Start. Lie face down, hands directly under shoulders, knees on the floor. Raise body from floor by straightening it from head to knees. In the "up" position, the body should be in a straight line with palms of hands and knees in contact with floor. Lower to starting position. Keep head up throughout.

   Count. Each return to the starting position counts as one repetition.

9. Leg-overs—Tuck

Start. Lie on back, legs straight and together, arms stretched sidewards at shoulder level, palms down. Raise both legs from floor, bending at hips and knees until in a tuck position. Lower legs to left, keeping knees together and both shoulders on floor.

Twist hips and lower legs to floor on right side. Twist hips to tuck position and return to starting position. Keep knees close to abdomen throughout.
Count. Each return to the starting position counts as one repetition.

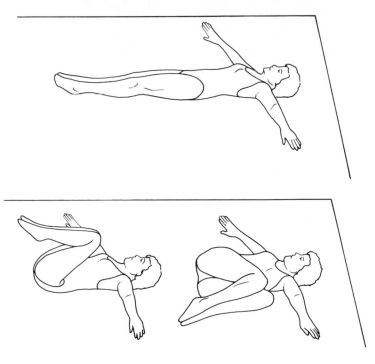

10. Run and Half Knee Bends

Start. Stand erect, feet together, arms at sides. Starting with left leg, run in place raising feet at least six inches from floor.
Count. Each time the left foot touches the floor counts as one repetition. After each fifty counts do ten half knee bends.

Half Knee Bends. Start with hands on hips, feet together, body erect. Bend at knees and hips, lowering body until thigh and calf form an angle of about 90 degrees. Do not bend knees past a right angle. Keep back straight. Return to starting position.

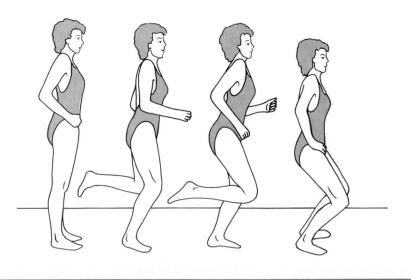

REFERENCES

*Cooper, K. H. *The Aerobics Program for Total Well-Being.* New York: M. Evans, 1982. (Contains information on aerobic dance and various sports.)

*Corbin, C. B., and R. Lindsey. *Fitness for Life.* 2d ed. Glenview, Ill.: Scott, Foresman and Co., 1985.

Corbin, C. B., and R. Lindsey. *The Ultimate Fitness Book.* New York: Leisure Press, 1984.

Fitness Canada. *Canada Fitness Survey—Highlights.* Ottawa, Ontario, Canada: Government of Canada, 1983.

Harris, L., and Associates. *The Perrier Study: Fitness in America.* New York: Great Waters of France, 1979.

President's Council on Physical Fitness and Sports. *Adult Physical Fitness* (Publication No. 017–000–00172–1). Washington, D.C.: U.S. Government Printing Office. Copies available from Superintendent of Documents.

Research and Forecasts, Inc. *The Miller Lite Report on American Attitudes toward Sports.* Milwaukee: Miller Brewing Co., 1983.

*Royal Canadian Air Force. *Exercise Plans for Physical Fitness.* Ottawa, Ontario, Canada: Queen's Printer. Rev. U.S. ed. published by Simon and Schuster, Inc., by special arrangement with *This Week Magazine.* Copies available from *This Week Magazine,* P.O. Box 77–E, Mt. Vernon, NY.

Snyder, E. E., and E. Spreitzer. "Adult Perceptions of Physical Education in the Schools and Community Sports Programs for Youth." *The Physical Educator* 40(1983):88.

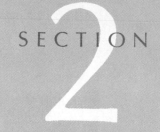

SECTION

2

IMPORTANT FITNESS FACTORS

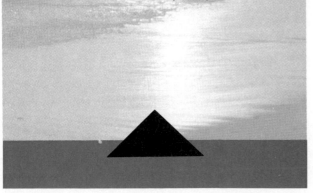

17

BODY MECHANICS

CONCEPT 17

Because the human body is a system of
weights and levers, its efficiency and
effectiveness at rest or in motion
can be improved by the application
of sound mechanical
and anatomical principles.

INTRODUCTION

"Body mechanics" is the application of physical laws
to the human body. The bones of the body act as levers
or simple machines, with the muscles supplying the
force to move them. Therefore, mechanical laws can be
applied to the body to aid in performing more and better
work with less energy while avoiding strain or injury.

This concept focuses on three aspects of body
mechanics. The first part of the concept discusses the
mechanics of body alignment while sitting or standing
(*static postures*). The second part of the concept emphasizes the *prevention of low back and neck pain*
through proper body mechanics. The third section of
the concept stresses *dynamic postures* for activities of
daily living.

TERMS

Center of Gravity—The center of the mass of an object.

Effectiveness—The degree to which the purpose is accomplished.

Efficiency—The relationship of the amount of energy
used to the amount of work accomplished.

Head Forward—The head is thrust forward in front of
the gravity line; also called "poke neck."

Herniated Disc—The soft nucleus of the spinal disc
protrudes through a small tear in the surrounding
tissue; also called prolapse.

Hyperextended Knees—The knees are thrust backward in a locked position.

Kyphosis—Increased curvature (flexion) in the upper
back; also called "hump back."

Linear Motion—Movement in a straight line.

Lumbar Lordosis—Increased curvature (hyperextension) in the lower back (lumbar region), with a forward pelvic tilt; commonly known as "swayback."

Myofascial Trigger Points—See Concept 11 terms.

Posture—The relationship of body parts, whether
standing, lying, sitting, or moving. "Good posture"
is the relationship of body parts that allows you to
function most effectively, with the least expenditure
of energy and with a minimum amount of strain on
muscles, tendons, ligaments, and joints.

Referred Pain—Pain that appears to be located in one
area, while in reality it originates in another area.

Round Shoulders—The tips of the shoulders are drawn
forward in front of the line of gravity.

Ruptured Disc—Spinal disc crushed from a severe blow
or jolt.

Sciatica—Pain radiating down the sciatic nerve in the
back of the hip and leg.

Scoliosis—A lateral curvature with some rotation of
the spine; the most serious and deforming of all postural deviations.

THE FACTS ABOUT STATIC POSTURES

*Good **posture** has aesthetic benefits.*

The first impression one person makes on another is usually a visual one. Good posture can help convey an impression of alertness, confidence, and attractiveness.

There is probably no one best posture for all individuals, because body build affects the balance of body parts. In general, certain relationships are desirable however.

In the standing position, the head should be centered over the trunk, the shoulders should be down and back, but relaxed, with the chest high and the abdomen flat. The spine should have gentle curves when viewed from the side, but should be straight as seen from the back. When the pelvis is tilted properly, the pubis falls directly underneath the lower tip of the sternum. The knees should be relaxed, with the kneecaps pointed straight ahead. The feet should point straight ahead and the weight should be borne over the heel, on the outside border of the sole, and across the ball of the foot and toes.

Clinical evidence cited by physicians and opinions of educators indicate that poor posture can cause a number of health problems.

For example:

1. Protruding abdomen and **lumbar lordosis** may contribute to painful menstruation, back injury, and backache.
2. A forward position of the head can result in headache, dizziness, and neck, shoulder, and arm pain.
3. **Rounded shoulders** may impair respiratory capacity.
4. **Hyperextended knees** may predispose a person to knee injury.
5. Unbalanced postural lines can cause excessive tension in muscle groups, produce joint strain, stretch ligaments, damage joint cartilage, and become a factor in arthritic changes.
6. Poor posture creates mechanical stresses that perpetuate **myofascial trigger points.**

If one part of the body is out of line, other parts must move out of line to balance it, thus increasing the strain on muscles, ligaments, and joints.

The body is made in segments that are held balanced in a vertical column by muscles and ligaments. If gravity or a short muscle pulls one segment out of line, other portions of the body will move out of alignment

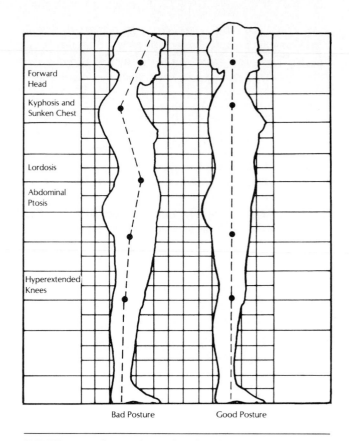

FIGURE 17.1 Comparison of Bad and Good Posture

to compensate, producing worse posture, more stress and strain, and possible deformity of the musculoskeletal system (figure 17.1).

There are many causes of poor posture, including hereditary, congenital, and disease conditions, as well as certain environmental factors.

Some factors that may contribute to poor posture include ill-fitting clothing, chronic fatigue, improperly fitting furniture (including poor beds and mattresses), emotional and personality problems, poor work habits, lack of physical fitness due to inactivity, and lack of knowledge relating to good posture. Some posture problems, especially **scoliosis,** are congenital, but can often be corrected with exercise, bracing, and/or other medical procedures. Early detection is critical in treating these problems.

Approximately 80 percent of the adult population suffers from acquired foot defects.

Most foot defects are acquired and are preventable. They are most often caused by improperly fitting shoes and socks; excessive hard use (such as in athletics); long standing or walking on hard surfaces; obesity or rapid weight gain (as in pregnancy); and improper bearing of weight through poor foot and leg alignment.

Exercises for the correction of postural deviations are generally based on this assumption: if the problem is a functional deformity, regardless of the factors causing it, muscular imbalance will be present.

If the muscles on one side of a joint are stronger than the muscles on the opposite side of that joint, the body part is pulled in the direction of the stronger muscles. Corrective exercises are usually designed to strengthen the long, weak muscles and to stretch the short, strong ones in order to have equal pull in both directions. For example, persons with lumbar lordosis may need to strengthen the abdominals and stretch the lower back muscles.

THE FACTS ABOUT BACK AND NECK ACHES

Poor posture, especially lordosis, can cause back strain and pain and make the back more susceptible to injury.

The forward tilt of the pelvis may cause the sacral bone or one of the lumbar vertebrae to press on nerve roots with consequent low back pain and **sciatica.** To be on the safe side, some authorities advise those who have lordosis and weak abdominals to eliminate all exercises that hyperextend the spine. Incidence of lordosis is about the same for men as it is for women, except that women experience an added back strain during pregnancy, and high heels may also contribute to spinal strain.

The neck is probably strained more frequently than the lower back.

The neck is constructed with the same curve and has the same mechanical problems as the lower back. The postural fault of **head forward** places a chronic strain on the posterior neck muscles. Tension in these muscles can lead to myofascial trigger points, causing headache or **referred pain** in the face, scalp, shoulder, arm, and chest.

The overwhelming majority of back and neck aches are avoidable. A common cause of backache is muscular strain, frequently precipitated by poor body mechanics in daily activities or during exercise.

When lifting improperly, there is great pressure on the lumbar discs and severe stress on the lumbar muscles and ligaments. Many popular exercises place great strain on the back (see Concept 19). Sleeping flat on the back or abdomen on a soft mattress can also cause lower back strain.

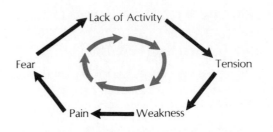

FIGURE 17.2 The Viscious Cycle of Back Pain

Muscular fatigue and weak muscles are frequent causes of backache.

Backache has been referred to as a "hypokinetic disease," meaning that it is caused by insufficient exercise. Lack of exercise results in weak muscles that are easily strained and fatigued. Sedentary workers are particularly susceptible to spinal strain, and weak abdominal and back muscles are especially to blame. If the abdominals are weak, the pelvis is apt to tilt forward, causing lordosis.

Most people agree excessive muscle tension is a contributing factor in painful spines.

Backaches may be precipitated by a minor injury or strain that sets off a muscle spasm; this causes pain, worry, excitement, fear, and stimulation of already hypersensitive muscular areas, referred to as "trigger points." These tender, painful spots occur frequently in the neck, shoulders, back, and hip as a result of constant tension, strain, or muscle spasm. When these tense muscles shorten, lose elasticity, and are weakened by lack of exercise, the "low back syndrome" occurs. With a weak back, the mildest movement can trigger back pain.

Back pains may result from referred pain caused by muscle tension in other areas. In some cases, the pain is "referred" from the back of the legs if the hamstring muscles have been overstretched or injured.

There is no such thing as a slipped disc.

Disc problems are frequently misunderstood. Vertebral discs may **herniate** or **rupture,** but they do not slip. Disc material pressure on nerves causes pain, and a protective reflex (muscle spasm) occurs to protect it. This causes more pain, beginning a vicious cycle (figure 17.2). The discs in the lumbar area are subjected to greater pressure, partly because they are at the bottom of the spine. Therefore, they are more apt to be damaged by severe jolts or strains.

Most backaches can be prevented or alleviated by good sense, proper exercise, and relaxation.

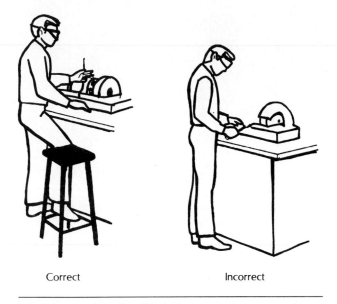

Correct   Incorrect

FIGURE 17.3 Standing Work Postures

Several "good sense" suggestions for taking care of the back are listed here:

1. Avoid the swayback position at all times by taking such precautions as the following:
   a. To relieve back strain during prolonged standing, try to keep the lower back flat by propping one foot on a stool, bar, or rail; alternate feet occasionally (see figure 17.3). (Dentists, beauticians, barbers, and store clerks are particularly susceptible to back problems because they must stand to work.)
   b. When sitting, use a hard chair with a straight back, placing the spine against it; keep one or both knees higher than the hips by crossing the legs (alternate sides) or by using a foot rest and keeping the knees bent.
   c. When driving a car, place a hard seat-and-backrest combination over the seat of the automobile; pull the seat forward so the legs are bent when operating the pedals.
   d. When lying, keep the knees and hips bent; avoid lying on the abdomen. When lying on the back, a pillow or lift should be placed under the knees.
   e. Avoid lifting and carrying improperly. Especially avoid bending over or straightening up while twisting the trunk.
2. To prevent neck strain, avoid the head forward position. The forward thrust is apt to occur in such activities as card playing, sewing, studying, and watching television. Sleeping on a high pillow may also cause back or neck strain.
3. Do corrective exercises to strengthen the abdominal muscles and stretch the lower back muscles.

Avoid exercises that strain or arch the lower back (see Concepts 18 and 19).

4. General exercises, involving the entire body, are important in preventing weak muscles and lack of flexibility.
5. Warm up before engaging in strenuous activity.
6. Get adequate rest and sleep. Avoid pushing yourself mentally or physically to the point of exhaustion.
7. Vary the working position by changing from one task to another before feeling fatigued. When working at a desk, get up and stretch occasionally to relieve tension.
8. Sleep on a firm mattress or place a three-fourths-inch-thick plywood board under the mattress.
9. Avoid sudden, jerky back movements.
10. The smaller the waistline, the lesser the strain on the lower back. Avoid being overweight.

THE FACTS ABOUT DYNAMIC POSTURE: LIFTING AND CARRYING

The best method for lifting or carrying a given object depends upon its size, weight, shape, and position in space. However, there are some general principles that are applicable in all situations.

1. *Stand close to the object and assume a wide base.* Stand in a forward-backward stride position with the object at the side of the body, or assume a side-stride position with the object between the knees. The purpose of lifting from this position is to allow you to lift straight upward from a stable position, utilizing the most efficient leverage.
2. *Keep the back straight and bend at the hips and knees. Squat, do not bend, regardless of how light the object may be.* The back was never meant to be used as a lever for lifting. Orthopedists constantly caution against leaning forward to pick up objects without bending the knees because of the strain placed on the muscles and joints of the spine. This kind of back strain can occur when improperly making a bed or when lifting a child out of a crib. When bending from the waist, the body's **center of gravity** is higher than when squatting, thus the bending posture is less stable as well as more injurious than the squatting position.
3. *Lower your body only as far as necessary, directly downward, keeping the hips tucked.* Squatting lower than is necessary is a waste of energy, but more importantly perhaps, deep knee bends can damage the structures of the knee joints. The deeper the flexion, the greater the twist on the joint and the greater the tension in the leg muscles.

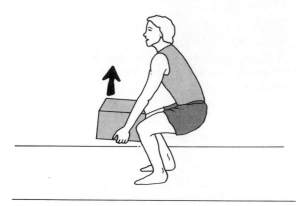

FIGURE 17.4 Lifting an Object

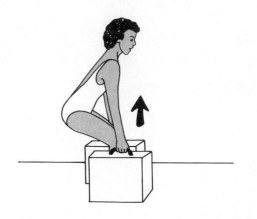

FIGURE 17.5 Dividing the Load

4. *Grasp the object and lift with your leg muscles, keeping the object close to the center of the body's gravity.* (See figure 17.4.) The leg muscles are the strongest in the body. If the back is kept erect, use of the legs for lifting allows a maximal force to be applied to the load without wasting energy.

5. *Carry the object close to the body's center of gravity and no higher than waist level (except when carrying on the shoulder, head, or back).* When objects are carried in front of the body above the level of the waist, you must lean backward to balance the load, producing an undesirable arch in the lower back. Carrying loads at the midline of the body, such as in a knapsack or on the head or shoulders, is **effective** in reducing the stress on the skeletal system.

6. *Push or pull heavy objects, if this can be done efficiently, rather than lifting them.* Theoretically, it takes about thirty-four times more force to lift than to slide an object across the floor. The size, shape, and friction of the object determine whether or not it is feasible to push or pull it.

7. *Divide the load if possible, carrying half in each arm. If the load cannot be divided, alternate it from one side of the body to the other.* (See figure 17.5.) When walking with the weight carried on one side of the body, the force on the opposite hip is much greater than when the load is distributed on both sides. This is true even when the bilateral load is twice as great as the unilateral load. If the weight must be carried on only one side, the opposite arm should be raised to counterbalance the load and to help keep the center of gravity over the base.

8. *Avoid arching the back when lifting and lowering an object from overhead. Any lift above waist level is inefficient.* Occasionally, you must reach overhead to lift an object from a high shelf. To avoid back strain, climb a ladder or stand on a stool so you don't have to raise your arms overhead. If this is not practical, reach for the object with your weight on the forward foot, and then step backward on the rear foot as the object is lowered.

9. *Do not try to lift or carry burdens too heavy for you.* The most economical load for either a man or a woman is about thirty-five percent of his or her body weight. Obviously, with strength training, you can safely lift a greater load.

THE FACTS ABOUT DYNAMIC POSTURES: PUSHING AND PULLING

The choice to push or to pull depends upon the nature of the task.

When deciding whether to push or pull, you must consider such factors as desired direction, type of movement, distance to be moved, and friction. If a downward force is desired, pushing would be best. If an upward force is desirable, pulling is probably better. Pushing tends to increase friction because of the downward force, but may offer better control because the object is closer to the person.

Pushing and pulling are forms of lifting; therefore, the same mechanical principles may be applied.

When pushing or pulling, the back should be kept as straight as possible, a wide stance should be used, and the leg muscles should do the work rather than the back or arms. You may alternate the working muscles by changing positions occasionally; that is, face forward, then backward, then sideward.

Force should be applied as nearly as possible in the desired line of direction.

If **linear motion** is desired, you should apply force at the center of the object's gravity and push or pull in the desired direction by leaning from the hips in that direction. To move an object horizontally, the upward and downward components of the push or pull should be reduced to a minimum. When pulling, increasing the length of the handle reduces the vertical component.

If there is a great deal of friction, the force should be applied below the object's center of gravity. Sufficient force should be applied continuously to keep the load moving, because it takes more force to start an object moving (overcoming inertia) than to keep it going.

When rotary motion is desired, apply force away from the center of gravity of the object.

Objects that are too heavy or too awkward to be moved as a whole, such as a refrigerator or couch, can be moved by applying force alternately at one end and then the other, so that a pivoting or "walking" action is employed to rotate the object.

THE FACTS ABOUT DYNAMIC POSTURES: SAVING ENERGY DURING WORK

When working with the arms in front of the body, a pulling motion is easier than a pushing motion.

The pulling motion uses the stronger flexor muscles, while a pushing motion employs the seldom used extensors that are usually weaker. Thus, counterclockwise circular movements are easier for the right hand, and clockwise circular movements easier for the left hand.

Organize work to avoid stooping or unnatural positions.

1. Sideward flexion of the trunk is more strenuous than forward trunk flexion.
2. Avoid constant arm extension, whether forward or sideward.
3. Whenever possible, sit while working but stand occasionally.
4. The arms should move either together or in opposite directions. When the conditions allow, use both hands in opposite and symmetrical motions while working.
5. Tools most often used should be the closest to reach.
6. When working with the hands, the workbench or kitchen cabinet should be about 5 to 10 centimeters (2 to 4 inches) below the waist. The office desk should be about 74 to 78 centimeters (29 to 30 inches) high for the average man and about 70 to 74 centimeters (27 to 29 inches) high for the average woman.

Some types of arm movements are more accurate than others.

Horizontal movements are more precise than vertical ones. Circular movements are better than zigzag ones. Movements toward the body are easier to control than those away from the body. Rhythmic movements are more accurate and less tiring than abrupt movements.

REFERENCES

Allman, F. L. "Rehabilitation Following Athletic Injuries." In O'Donoghue, D. H., *Treatment of Athletic Injuries.* 4th ed. Philadelphia: W. B. Saunders Company, 1984, 677.

Basmajian, J. V., ed. *Manipulation, Traction, and Massage.* Baltimore: Williams and Wilkins, 1985.

Belkin, S. C., and H. H. Banks. *Backaches.* Tufts-New England Medical Center, Inc. Wellesly: Arandel Publishing Co., 1978.

*Calliet, R. *Neck and Arm Pain.* 2d ed. Philadelphia: F. A. Davis Co., 1981.

*Calliet, R. *Low Back Pain Syndrome.* 3d ed. Philadelphia: F. A. Davis Co., 1981.

Calliet, R. *Soft Tissue Pain and Disability.* Philadelphia: F. A. Davis Co., 1977.

Daniels, L., and C. Worthingham. *Therapeutic Exercise.* 2d ed. Philadelphia: W. B. Saunders Co., 1977.

Edgar, M. "Pathologies Associated with Lifting." *Physiotherapy* 65(1979):245.

Fisk, J. W. *The Painful Neck and Back.* Springfield, Ill.: C. C. Thomas, 1977.

Forsell, M. Z. "The Swedish Back School." *Physiotherapy* 66(1980):4.

Hall, H. "The Canadian Back School." *Physiotherapy* 66(1980):4.

Keim, H. A., and W. H. Kirkaldy-Willis. "Low Back Pain." *Clinical Symposia* 32(1980):6.

Kennedy, J. B. "An Australian Programme for Management of Back Problems." *Physiotherapy* 66(1980):4.

Kornfield, J. "Getting Aggressive about Conservative Therapy for Back Pain." *Medical World News* (5 July 1982).

Kottke, F. J., G. K. Stillwell, and J. F. Lehmann. *Krusen's Handbook of Physical Medicine.* 3d ed. Philadelphia: W. B. Saunders Co., 1982.

Kraus, H. "Ecology and Backaches." *Journal of Physical Education* 69(1972):111.

Kreighbaum, E., and K. M. Barthels. *Biomechanics.* Minneapolis: Burgess Publishing Co., 1985.

Lehmkuhl, L. D., and L. K. Smith. *Brunnstrom's Clinical Kinesiology.* Philadelphia: F. A. Davis Co., 1983.

Lindsey, R., B. Jones, and A. V. Whitley. *Fitness for Health, Figure/Physique, Posture.* 5th ed. Dubuque, Iowa: Wm. C. Brown Publishers, 1983.

Luttgens, K., and K. F. Wells. *Kinesiology.* 7th ed. Philadelphia: Saunders College Publishing, 1982.

Mattmiller, A. W. "The California Backschool." *Physiotherapy* 66(1980):4.

McKenzie, R. *The Lumbar Spine.* Waikanae, New Spinal Publishers, 1981.

Rovere, G. D. "Low Back Pain among Athletes." *Physician and Sportsmedicine* 15(1987):105.

Sherrill, C. *Adapted Physical Education and Recreation.* Dubuque, Iowa: Wm. C. Brown Publishers, 1981.

Soderberg, G. L. *Kinesiology: Application to Pathological Motion.* Baltimore: Williams and Wilkins, 1986.

Stamford, B. "Posture Perfect Performance." *Physician and Sportsmedicine* 14(June 1986):197.

Stanitski, C. L. "Low Back Pain in Young Athletes." *Physician and Sportsmedicine* 10(1982):77.

Travell, J. G., and D. G. Simons. *Myofascial Pain and Dysfunction.* Baltimore: Williams and Wilkins, 1983.

*Williams, P. C. *Low Back and Neck Pain: Causes and Conservative Treatment.* Springfield, Ill.: C. C. Thomas, 1974.

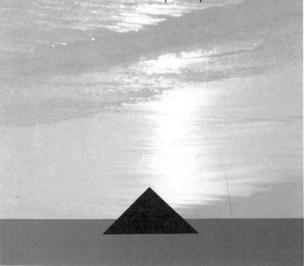

18

EXERCISES FOR CARE OF THE BACK AND GOOD POSTURE

CONCEPT 18

Exercise plays an important role in the prevention and correction of backaches and poor posture.

INTRODUCTION

The mechanics of back care and both static and dynamic postures are discussed in Concept 17. However, the vast majority of the population should do exercises similar to the samples included in this concept because backache and poor posture are so prevalent. Eighty percent of all Americans will see a physician about a backache during their lifetime. An estimated 75 million Americans have recurring back problems, and two million can't hold jobs as a result. Low back pain causes 93 million days of lost work per year and $10 billion in workers' compensation.

Incorrect postures, when standing, sitting, lying, or working, are responsible for many back problems. Compounding this are weak muscles that result from lack of exercise. Much can be done to prevent poor postures using proper education and proper exercise.

Treatment for painful spines ranges from surgical removal of a disc or fusion, to more conservative measures, such as injections, electrical stimulation, muscle relaxants, anti-inflammatory drugs, vapocoolant spray, bracing, traction, bed rest, heat, ice massage, and therapeutic exercise.

The exercises that follow are designed to strengthen or stretch certain muscles that are most often involved in back problems and most common in postural problems. (See figure 18.1.) If you have had surgery or an injury, you should wait until your physician advises you to start exercising. If you have been inactive for a period of time, it would be wise to perform these exercises below your threshold level initially so as to avoid muscle soreness.

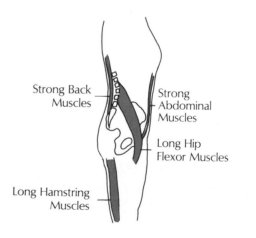

FIGURE 18.1 Muscles for Care of the Back and Good Posture

The exercises suggested here should be performed as described until you are able to increase repetitions. Muscles depicted in color are those primarily involved in the exercises.

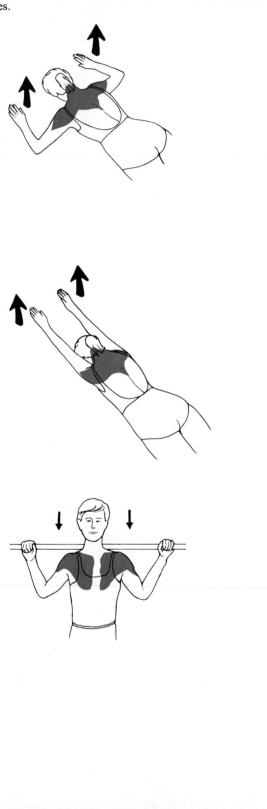

1. Bent-Arm Lift

Purpose

To help prevent or correct round shoulders and kyphosis by strengthening adductors.

Position

Lie prone, arms in reverse T; forehead resting on floor.

Movement

Lift the arms vertically by contracting the muscles between the shoulder blades (adductors). Maintain the 90° angle at the elbow and the shoulder. Hold; relax and repeat. If the arms are pressed into the floor before being lifted, this is a PNF exercise, and range of motion may be greater.

2. Straight-Arm Lift

Purpose

To help prevent and correct round shoulders and kyphosis by strengthening adductors.

Position

Lie prone, arms extended overhead and held close to ears; forehead resting on floor.

Movement

Raise both arms as high as possible without lifting head. Hold; relax; repeat. Pressing downward on the floor before lifting may allow you to lift the arms higher.

3. Wand Exercise

Purpose

To help prevent and correct round shoulders and kyphosis by stretching the muscles on the anterior side of the shoulder joint.

Position

Sit with wand grasped at ends. Raise wand overhead. Be certain that the head does not slide forward into a "poke neck" position. Keep the chin tucked and neck straight.

Movement

Bring wand down behind shoulder blades. Keep spine erect. Hold. Hands may be moved closer together to increase stretch on chest muscles.

Note

If this is an easy exercise for you, try straightening the elbows and bringing the wand to waist level in back of you.

4. Lateral Trunk Exercise

Purpose

To help prevent and correct backaches by maintaining flexibility in the spine.

Position

Stand with feet shoulder width apart.

Movement

Stretch left arm overhead to right. Bend to right at waist reaching as far to right as possible with left arm; reach as far as possible to the left with right arm; hold. Do not let trunk rotate. Repeat on opposite side.

Note

This exercise is made more effective if a weight is held in the hand opposite the side being stretched. More stretch occurs also if the hip on the stretched side is dropped and most of the weight is borne by the opposite foot.

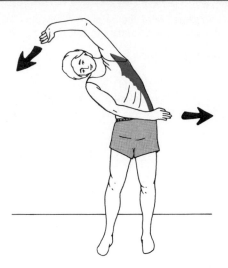

5. Lateral Neck Flexion

Purpose

To prevent or correct forward head and cervical lordosis, as well as upper back and cervical trigger points.

Position

Sit erect.

Movement

Apply resistance to left side of head as you try to bend the head and neck sideward in that direction. This is an isometric strengthening exercise for the lateral flexors of the neck. Hold the contraction six seconds. Repeat to threshold, and then exercise the right side of the neck using the right hand as resistance. For neck exercises, it is probably best to use less than a maximal contraction. This is particularly true in the presence of arthritis, degenerated discs, and injury.

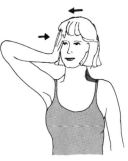

6. Neck Flexion Exercise

Purpose

To prevent or correct forward head or cervical lordosis, as well as upper back and cervical trigger points.

Position

Place hands on forehead.

Movement

Resist forward flexion. Keep the chin tucked to avoid the forward head position. This isometric exercise strengthens the neck and head flexors.

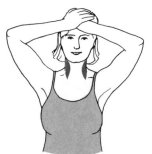

7. Neck Extension Exercise

Purpose

To prevent and correct forward head or cervical lordosis, as well as upper back and cervical trigger points.

Position

Place hands on back of head.

Movement

Apply resistance on back of head and isometrically push the head backward, keeping the neck straight. This strengthens the head and neck extensor muscles.

8. Neck Rotation Exercise

Purpose

This PNF exercise strengthens and stretches the neck rotators. It should always be done with the head and neck in axial extension (good alignment). It is particularly useful for relieving trigger point pain and stiffness.

Position

Place palm of left hand against left cheek; point fingers toward ear and point elbow forward.

Movement

Try to turn head and neck left while resisting with left hand. Hold several seconds. Relax and turn head to right as far as possible; hold. Repeat.

9. Bent-Leg Stretcher

Purpose

To help prevent or correct backache caused in part by short hamstrings.

Position

Sit on the floor with the feet against the wall or an immovable object. Bend left knee and bring foot close to buttocks. Clasp hands behind back.

Movement

Bend forward from hips, keeping lower back as straight as possible. Let bent knee rotate outward so trunk can move forward. Use static or gentle ballistic stretch to lengthen hamstring and calf muscles.

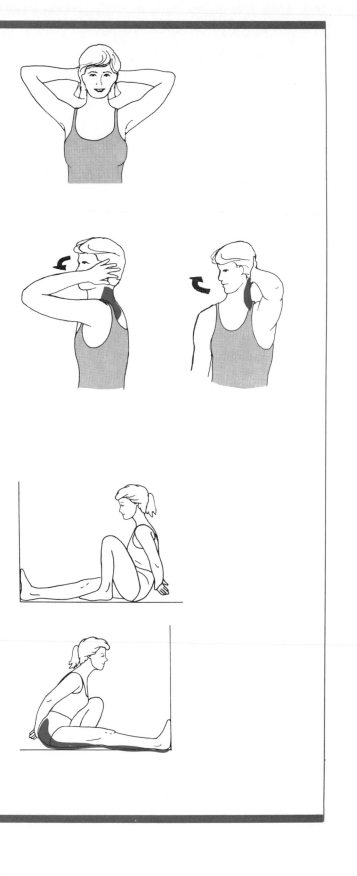

10. Iliopsoas Muscle Stretcher

Purpose

To help prevent or correct forward pelvic tilt and lumbar lordosis or backache.

Position

Place knee directly above right ankle and stretch left leg backward so knee touches floor. If necessary, place hands on floor for balance.

Movement

Press pelvis forward and downward; hold. Repeat on opposite side. *Caution:* Do not bend front knee more than 90°.

Note

This exercise uses the weight of the body to stretch the flexor muscles on the front of the hip joint, particularly the iliopsoas group.

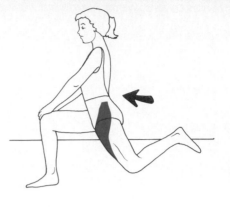

11. Low Back Stretcher

Purpose

To help prevent or correct lumbar lordosis and backache.

Position

Supine position.

Movement

Draw one knee up to the chest and pull it down tightly with the hands, then slowly return to the original position. Repeat with the other knee. Do not grasp knee; grasp thigh. If a partner or a weight stabilizes the extended leg, the iliopsoas muscle on that leg will also be stretched.

Note

This same exercise may be done on a table with one leg hanging over the edge approximately one-third of the length of the thigh. If a partner, weight, or strap stabilizes the leg, the iliopsoas muscle will be stretched more effectively.

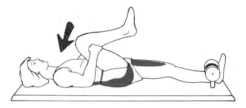

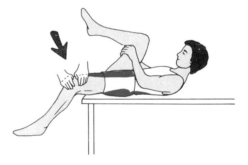

12. Knee-to-Chest Exercise

Purpose

To prevent or correct lordosis and backache; the fetal stretch.

Position

Bring both knees to chest and grasp thighs.

Movement

Pull knees to chest and curl both pelvis and upper body off of floor. Hold for 30–60 seconds. Stretches lumbar muscles and gluteals (hip extensors).

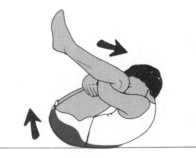

13. Single Knee-to-Chest Back Flattener

Purpose

To help prevent or correct lordosis and backache.

Position

Supine with knees bent.

Movement

Draw one knee to the chest, then extend the knee and point the foot toward the ceiling; hold. Return to the starting position by drawing the knee back to the chest before sliding the foot to the floor. Repeat with other leg (stretches lumbar muscles).

14. Double Knee-to-Chest Back Flattener

Purpose

To help prevent or correct lordosis and backache (advanced exercise).

Position

Supine with knees bent.

Movement

Draw both knees to the chest, then extend both legs toward the ceiling, keeping the lower back flat. Return to the starting position by drawing the knees to the chest before placing the feet on the floor (stretches lumbar muscles).

Note

This is a more strenuous exercise and the weak person should not attempt it until the other exercises have been performed for three or four weeks.

15. Pelvic Tilt

Purpose

Help prevent or correct lumbar lordosis, abdominal ptosis, and backache.

Position

Supine with knees bent.

Movement

Tighten the abdominal muscles and try to flatten the lower back against the floor. At the same time, tighten the hip and thigh muscles. Hold, then relax. Breathe normally during the contraction, do not hold the breath (strengthens abdominals).

16. Trunk Curl ("Crunch")

Purpose

To help prevent or correct lumbar lordosis, abdominal ptosis, or backache.

Position

Supine with the knees bent.

Movement

Roll the head and neck forward, then the shoulders. Roll as far forward as possible without lifting the lower back off the floor. Hold. Return to start and repeat (strengthens abdominals).

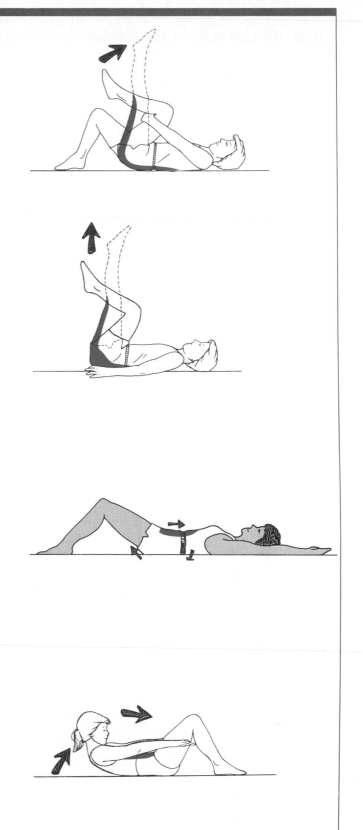

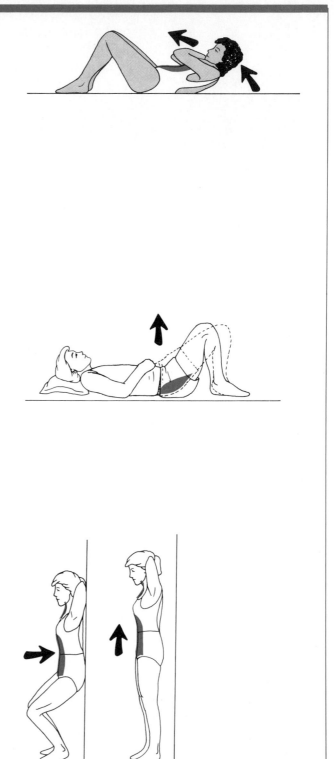

17. Sit-Up

Purpose

To help prevent or correct lumbar lordosis, abdominal ptosis, or backache.

Position

Assume a hook-lying position with arms crossed and hands on shoulders.

Movement

Roll up, making elbows touch knees, then roll down to the starting position. Repeat. For more overload, place hands on top of head or place index fingers by ears (do not put hands behind neck and do not anchor feet).

Note

If you are weak, start in the sitting position and gradually curl down. Stop and hold and return to sit, gradually getting lower until full sit-up can be done.

18. Bridging

Purpose

To help prevent and correct lordosis and forward pelvic tilt.

Position

Supine with knees bent and feet close to buttocks.

Movement

Contract gluteals, lifting buttocks off the floor as high as possible without raising the back off the floor above the waistline. Hold; relax; repeat. Strengthens hip extensor muscles, particularly the gluteus maximus. Do not allow the lower back to arch.

19. Wall Slide

Purpose

To help prevent or correct poor spinal alignment by teaching the feel of flattening the neck and back and tilting the pelvis.

Position

Stand with heels 4–6 inches from wall, arms at sides.

Movement

Flatten neck and lumbar region to wall by flexing knees and sliding down wall until spine can be forced against it. Slide up wall, maintaining flat spine. Walk away from wall, keeping curves flat. Return to wall and check alignment. Repeat with hands behind neck and elbows touching wall. Repeat with arms at sides and sandbag on head. Repeated flexion and extension of the knees can develop strength in the quadriceps muscles on the front of the thigh.

Testing for Back Weakness and Muscular Imbalance

Test 1—Back to wall

Stand with your back against a wall, with head, heels, shoulders, and calves of legs touching the wall as shown in the diagram. Try to flatten your neck and the hollow of your back by pressing your buttocks down against the wall. Your partner should just be able to place a hand in the space between the wall and the small of your back. If this space is greater than the thickness of his/her hand, you probably have lordosis with shortened lumbar and hip flexor muscles.

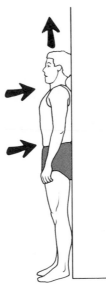

Test 2—Supine leg-lift

Lie on your back with hands behind your neck. The partner on your right should stabilize your right leg by placing his/her left hand on the knee. With the right hand, your partner should grasp your left ankle and raise your left leg as near to a right angle if possible. In this position (as shown in the diagram), your lower back should be in contact with the floor. Your right leg should remain straight and on the floor throughout the test. If your left leg bends at the knee, short hamstring muscles are indicated. If your back arches and/or your right leg does not remain flat on the floor, short lumbar muscles or hip flexor muscles (or both) are indicated. Repeat the test on the opposite side.

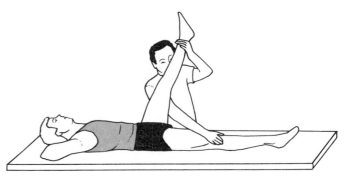

Test 3—Knee to chest

Lie on your back on a table or bench with your left leg extended beyond the edge of the table (approximately one-third of the thigh off the table). Bring your right knee to your chest and pull the thigh down tightly with your hands. Your lower back should remain flat against the table as shown in the diagram. Your left thigh should remain on the table. If your left thigh lifts off the table while your right knee is hugged to chest, a tight hip flexor (iliopsoas) on that side is indicated. Repeat on the opposite side.

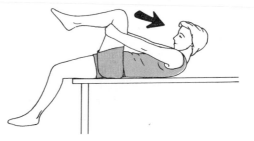

CHART 18A.1 Back "Health" *Rating Scale*

Rating	Number of Tests Passed
Good Fitness Zone	3
Marginal Zone	2
Low Zone	0–1

CHART 18B.1 Posture Evaluation

Side View	Points	Back View	Points
Head forward	_____	Tilted head	_____
Sunken chest	_____	Protruding scapulae	_____
Round shoulders	_____	Symptoms of scoliosis:	
		Shoulders uneven	_____
Kyphosis	_____	Hips uneven	_____
Lordosis	_____	Lateral curvature of spine (Adams position)	_____
Abdominal ptosis	_____	One side of back high (Adams position)	_____
Hyperextended knees	_____		
Body lean	_____		

Total score _____

CHART 18B.2 Posture *Rating Scale*

Classification	Total Score
Excellent	0–2
Very good	3–4
Fair	5–7
Poor	8–11
Very poor	12 or more

19

EXERCISE CAUTIONS

CONCEPT 19

Some exercises should be

used with caution or

not used at all because they are

"high risk" exercises or because

they may cause

more harm than good.

INTRODUCTION

There are literally thousands of exercises to choose from—some good, some bad, and some of little consequence. In some exercises, there are certain inherent hazards that can and should be minimized with proper technique, knowledgeable instructors, proper equipment, appropriate apparel, and careful adherence to the principles mentioned in the first four concepts. As a general rule, when in doubt, don't do it. There is always a safe and effective alternative exercise for any specific muscle group.

TERMS

Dehydration—Excessive loss of water from the body, usually through perspiration, urination, or evaporation.

Hyperflexion—Bending (flexing) a joint more than normal; excessive bending.

Hyperextension—Straightening (extending) a joint past its normal position.

Hyperventilation—"Overbreathing;" forced, rapid, or deep breathing.

Epiglottis—The lidlike structure that closes the entrance to the windpipe.

Pyriformis Syndrome—Muscle spasm and nerve entrapment in the pyriformis muscle of the buttocks region causing pain similar to sciatica.

Valsalva Maneuver—Exerting force with the epiglottis closed, thus increasing pressure in the thorax and raising arterial pressure. When released, arterial pressure drops rapidly, blood vessels expand and are then filled, causing a lag in blood flow to the left ventricle. Peripheral arterial blood pressure then drops and dizziness or fainting occurs.

THE FACTS

*As a general rule, exercises that cause **hyperextension** of the lower back should be avoided.*

Objections to hyperextension of the lower back are: (1) the abdominal muscles, which are too long and weak in most people, should not be over stretched; (2) the possibility of a vertebrae impinging on a nerve, or causing compression and even herniation of the disc, and producing myofascial trigger points. Examples of exercises in which lower back hyperextension can occur include back bends, straight leg-lifts, straight leg situps, prone or all-four leg-lifts, prone swans, and backward trunk circling.

Back arching, abdominal stretches (figures 19.1 and 19.2) are not recommended except for special circumstances.

One of the back hyperextension exercises commonly seen is the back arching, abdominal stretch. When prescribed, as in the McKenzie program, for certain patients with low back pain or when done occasionally as a static stretch following vigorous abdominal strengthening exercises, it will probably not be harmful. If used, do *not* hyperextend the neck as shown and *do* stretch slowly and gently. Stop if it hurts.

The same is true of the exercise shown in figure 19.2. This exercise can stretch the hip flexors, quadriceps, and shoulder flexors (such as the pectorals), as well as the abdominals, but it has the additional problem of possibly **hyperflexing** the knee joint, which can be precipitated by the arm pull (see later discussion of the knee). If used for hip flexors and quadriceps, try substituting the "hip and thigh stretcher" (exercise 8, p. 111). If used for the shoulders, substitute the "pectoral stretch" (exercise 5, p. 110) or test 2 (p. 106).

The "kneeling donkey kick" (figure 19.3) is not recommended if the spine hyperextends.

The donkey kick exercise is performed for the purpose of developing strength and/or endurance of the buttocks muscles (hip extensors; gluteus maximus). It may involve touching the nose with the knee followed by a ballistic backward kick, a lifting of the head (neck hyperextension), and hyperextension of the lower back. As discussed earlier, hyperextension of the back is generally undesirable in an exercise. The same is true for the neck (see discussion of the neck later in the concept).

This exercise should be modified as shown in the "knee-to-nose touch" (exercise 15, p. 83), so the leg does not lift higher than the hips and the neck and lower back are not allowed to hyperextend. Another exercise that might be substituted is the "lower trunk lift" (exercise 16, p. 83).

The double leg-lift exercise (figure 19.4) may hyperextend the lower back and is not recommended for most people.

The double leg lift is usually used with the intent of strengthening the lower abdominals, when in fact it is primarily a hip-flexor (iliopsoas) strengthening exercise. That muscle attaches to the lower back and tilts the pelvis forward, arching the back. Most people have overdeveloped the hip flexors and do not need to strengthen those muscles further. Even if the abdominals are strong enough to contract isometrically and prevent hyperextension of the lower back, the exercise produces excess compression on the discs. Examples of

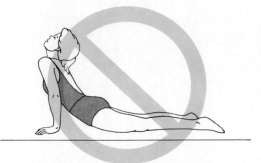

FIGURE 19.1 Back Arching, Abdominal Stretch

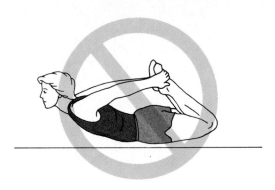
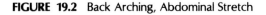

FIGURE 19.2 Back Arching, Abdominal Stretch

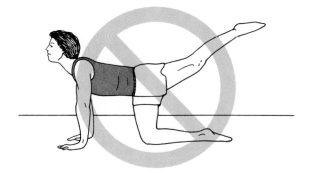

FIGURE 19.3 Back Arching, Neck Arching (Donkey Kick)

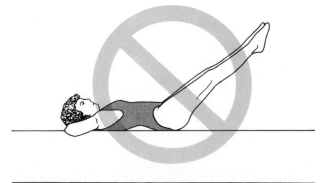

FIGURE 19.4 Double Leg Lift

safer and better exercises to strengthen the lower abdominals are the "reverse sit-up" (exercise 6, p. 81) and "sitting tucks" (exercise 13, p. 82).

The bench press (figure 19.5) is a good exercise for developing strength or endurance in the arms and the chest (pectorals), but back hyperextension should be prevented.

To prevent hyperextension and possible strain on the lower back when performing the bench press or similar exercises on a bench, bend the knees and place the feet on the bench in a hook-lying position as shown in exercise 6, page 89.

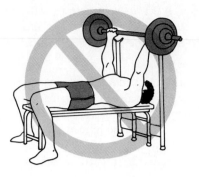

FIGURE 19.5 Back Arching (Bench Press)

As a general rule, exercises that hyperextend the neck should be avoided.

Tipping the head backward during any exercise, such as is done in neck circling (figure 19.6), can pinch arteries and nerves in the neck and at the base of the skull, grind down the discs, and result in dizziness or myofascial trigger points. It also aggravates arthritis and degenerated discs. Exercises 1, 2, and 3 in this concept also show improper neck positions. If the purpose of the exercise is relaxation of the neck, substitute the "neck stretch" (exercise 1, p. 180). If your purpose in doing the exercise is strengthening, try some of the isometric or PNF exercises (exercises 5, 6, 7, 8, pp. 160 and 161) or perform the "wall slide" (exercise 19, p. 164).

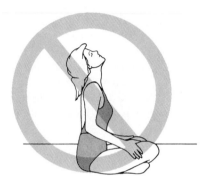

FIGURE 19.6 Neck Hypertension

As a general rule, exercises that force the neck and upper back into hyperflexion should not be used.

It has been estimated that 80 percent of the population has forward head and kyphosis (hump back) with accompanying weak muscles. Hyperflexion of the neck can be as harmful as hyperextension by causing excessive stretch on the ligaments and nerves, especially. It can aggravate already thin discs and arthritic conditions.

Exercises that tend to promote these conditions by further stretching already elongated muscles and ligaments should be avoided. Examples of such exercises are vertical bicycling (figure 19.7) and Yoga positions called the "plough" and the "plough shear."

If the purpose for these exercises is to reduce gravitational effects on the circulatory system or internal organs, try lying on a tilt board with the feet elevated, or assume a kneeling position similar to the "leg extension exercise" (exercise 8, p. 81).

If the purpose is to warm up the muscles in the legs, try the "stationary leg change" (exercise 14, p. 83); or, if the purpose for doing the exercise is to stretch the lower back, try the "low back stretcher," "knee-to-chest," or "single knee-to-chest" exercises (exercises 11, 12, 13, pp. 162 and 163).

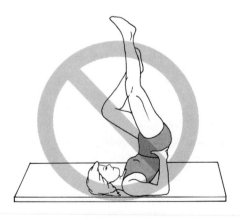

FIGURE 19.7 Shoulder Stand Bicycle

Pulling on the neck with hands during sit-ups (figure 19.8) and curl-ups ("crunches") produces hyperflexion of the head and neck and should be avoided.

Placing the hands behind the neck or head during the sit-up and "crunch" exercises allows the arms to pull the head and neck into hyperflexion, stretching the posterior ligaments, as described in the preceding section. If the hands are not placed at the sides or across the chest, then the hands should be placed so the palms cover the ears (see "crunch," exercise 16, p. 163) or the index fingers are in the ears to prevent stretching the neck.

Standing ballistic toe touches (figure 19.9) are not the best way to stretch the back and the hamstrings.

Like the neck and lower back, *the knee joint should not be hyperextended.* This action stretches the ligaments and joint capsule of the knee. Bending the back while the legs are straight may cause back strain (see Concept 17), particularly if the movement is done ballistically. Safer stretches of the lower back, which are just as effective, are found on page 162 and include "low back stretcher" (exercise 11), "knee to chest" (exercise 12), "single knee to chest" (exercise 13) and "double knee to chest" (exercise 14). To stretch the hamstrings, substitute a sitting or lying stretch such as "hamstring stretcher" (exercise 13, p. 113) or the "back saver toe touch" (exercise 2, p. 32).

Leg stretches on a bar (figure 19.10) may be potentially harmful.

Some experts have found that stretches on a bar in which the extended leg is raised 90 degrees or more and the trunk is bent over the leg may lead to sciatica and **pyriformis syndrome,** especially in the person who has limited flexibility. Substitute some of the back and hamstring stretching exercises suggested in Concept 18.

Quadriceps stretching exercises (figure 19.11) should avoid hyperflexion of the knee joint.

When the knee is hyperflexed 120 degrees or more, the ligaments and joint capsule are apt to be stretched and the cartilage may be damaged. Among the many exercises that place this type of stress on the knee joint are certain quadriceps stretching exercises. Figure 19.11 depicts this position and also shows the shin muscle being stretched. It is usually not necessary to stretch the shin muscles, because they tend to be weak and elongated; however if you need to stretch them to relieve muscle soreness, try the "shin stretcher" (exercise 11, p. 112). To avoid injuring the knee when stretching the quadriceps, substitute the "hip and thigh stretcher" (exercise 8, p. 111).

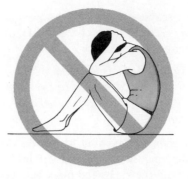

FIGURE 19.8 Hands-Behind-the-Head Sit-Up

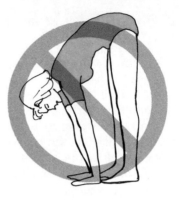
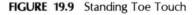

FIGURE 19.9 Standing Toe Touch

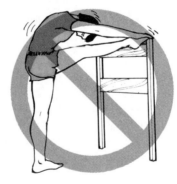

FIGURE 19.10 Ballistic Bar Stretch

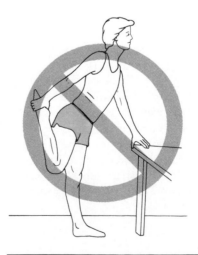

FIGURE 19.11 Shin and Quadriceps Stretch

Deep squatting (knee bend) exercises (figure 19.12) have been found to damage the knee joint.

Deep squatting exercises, with or without weights, place the knee joint in hyperflexion and tend to "wedge it open," stretching the ligaments, irritating the synovial membrane, and possibly damaging the cartilage. There is even greater stress on the joint when the lower leg and foot are not in straight alignment with the knee. If you are performing squats to strengthen the quadriceps and gluteal muscles, then substitute the "forward lunge" (exercise 12, p. 82), "stationary leg change" (exercise 14, p. 83), "half squat" (exercise 3, p. 85), "leg extension" (exercise 5, p. 92), and "knee extension" (exercise 14, p. 95 or exercise 8, p. 89).

The "hero" stretch (figure 19.13) and the "hurdler's" stretch produce too much torque on the knee joint.

The hero places the knee in a rotated position with lateral forces on the flexed knee, which are apt to stretch the ligaments and capsule and damage the cartilage. It may also strain the groin muscles and lower back. If the exercise is used to stretch the quadriceps, read the section in this concept regarding quadriceps stretching. The hurdler's stretch is a sitting toe-touch exercise with one leg turned out as shown in the hero. It produces the same kind of stress on the knee joint. Hamstring stretches have been discussed previously, but if you have been using this exercise you may wish to substitute the safer bent-leg stretcher (exercise 9, p. 161).

Hugging the knee and pulling it to the body (figure 19.14) with the arms or hands places undue stress on the knee joint.

The knee pull-down exercise is one of many exercises in which the knee is pulled to the body. (This hyperflexed position of the knee is depicted in exercises 11, 12, and 13 in this concept.) In this case, the exercise is intended to stretch the lower back. The hand position should be changed to hug the thigh rather than the shin to make this a good exercise. See low back stretches (exercises 11, 12, and 13, pp. 162 and 163) and the "leg hug" (exercise 4, p. 110) for examples.

Repeatedly rising on the toes and heels may weaken the long arches of the feet.

Tiptoeing exercises will develop the calf muscles, but at the same time, they will stretch the muscles and ligaments that help support the long arch of the foot. "Heel walking" may have the same effect; that is, it may develop strong shin muscles while further weakening the arch. The potential harm is lessened if these exercises are performed with the toes turned in slightly.

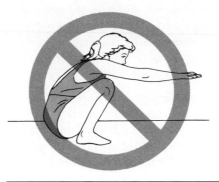

FIGURE 19.12 Deep Knee Bends

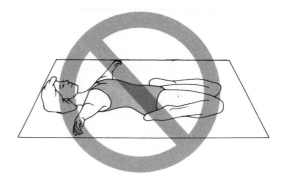

FIGURE 19.13 The Hero

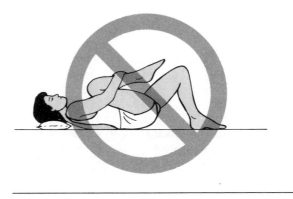

FIGURE 19.14 Knee Pull-Down

Isometric exercises may be harmful to some people.

Isometric exercises have advantages (see Concept 8) but they may be more dangerous to heart patients than isotonic exercises, because they cause a marked rise in blood pressure and may produce irregular heartbeats. Those with high blood pressure or heart trouble should not perform isometrics. Isometric exercise (as well as heavy weight training) for adolescents is also questionable because the bones of adolescents have not matured and growth may be stunted.

Jogging and aerobic dance exercises are excellent exercise for cardiovascular conditioning, weight control, and improvement of a variety of conditions; however, reasonable caution should be observed.

Jogging has been used successfully in rehabilitating cardiac patients and those with pulmonary emphysema; in weight reduction of diabetics; in relaxing insomniacs, the emotionally disturbed, and migraine patients; and in reducing the discomfort accompanying arthritis in the legs and back. Like many other exercises, jogging should not be done without a physician's approval for those with arthritis, osteoporosis, and heart and circulatory diseases. It is *not* harmful to women, although some women may need to wear a special bra as a comfort measure. Jogging can cause shin splints, blisters, and foot, ankle, knee, and hip problems. Using the proper footwear and learning how to jog correctly will minimize these hazards. If you have poor leg or foot alignment, you would be wise to jog only three or four days per week because studies show that the risk of injury is greatest for those who jog every day. The same fitness levels will result with less risk of injury.

Aerobic dance exercise has some of the same hazards as jogging; these include the overstress syndromes from too many hours of high impact landings on the floor. The most common problems are shin splints, Achilles tendon injuries, arch strains, and pain under the knee cap. Most of these problems can be prevented by warming up and stretching properly before exercising, by using low impact movements, and by avoiding hazardous exercises such as those described in this concept. A qualified physical education teacher will be more apt to teach/lead safe classes than a person with no qualifications other than being a good dancer and looking good in a leotard.

Some exercise equipment is potentially harmful.

Most exercise equipment is safe when used properly, but there is still the potential for abuse. One piece in particular is very difficult to use safely—the "slimming wheel." This wheel, with a handle passing through its axis, is used in a push-up type exercise and is advertised as a back and abdomen strengthener. Unfortunately, the wheel is difficult to control and may roll too rapidly, causing the users to fall flat on their faces. When this occurs, the abdominals may be overstretched and hemorrhaging of that muscle may develop or back strain may occur.

Another piece of equipment that can be hazardous for some people is the "gravity inversion boot" and similar devices designed to allow a person to hang upside down. They are supposed to be effective for the treatment of backache. However, studies have shown that during hanging (inactively or while oscillating) significant increases occur in systemic blood pressure; intraocular and retinal arterial pressure (in the eye) doubles; and pulse and other heart irregularities occur. Therefore, this type of equipment is potentially dangerous to the elderly and medically compromised; and to persons with high blood pressure, glaucoma, diabetes, and heart abnormalities.

Dehydration, a hazard in certain sports and exercise situations, is a serious medical problem.

Dehydration can impair performance and lead to illness, heat stroke, and even death. Weight losing gimmicks that cause dehydration, such as high protein/low carbohydrate diets, steam baths, or plastic sweat suits, are dangerous, especially for athletes (e.g., wrestlers trying to "make weight"). Exercisers subjected to heat stress should weigh themselves before and after exercises and replace the water-weight loss. Water should not be restricted during exercise. The person who regularly exercises under heat stress conditions may benefit from drinking a quart of milk and two eight-ounce glasses of orange juice per day. It is *not* necessary to take salt tablets because evidence suggests that many people already consume ten to sixty times the daily salt requirement. Sweating releases more water than it does salt from the body, thus increasing, rather than decreasing, the body's salt concentration.

You are more susceptible to heat stroke if you are obese, older, have had previous heat strokes, or are dehydrated, poorly conditioned, or not adjusted to a warmer climate.

When exercising out-of-doors in cold weather, certain precautions should be taken.

During cold weather exercising, stay warm, but don't wear bulky clothes that interfere with movement. Wear a thin absorbent layer next to the skin and two removable layers on top of that, such as a sweat suit and windbreaker. This outfit enables you to peel off layers as you become warm from the exercise. Do wear a cap and mittens (they are warmer than gloves) and wool socks. Change clothes immediately after coming indoors.

Breathing cold air will not freeze the lungs, but it does slow the heart. Those with heart disease should be wary of exercising in extreme cold.

Some people can be allergic to exercise.

It is rare, but there is a shocklike syndrome associated with vigorous exercise known as "exercise-induced anaphylaxis." This syndrome can occur in anyone, whether a beginner or a well-conditioned athlete. The syndrome's symptoms include itching, swelling of the throat, and generalized swelling. Treatment is the same as for allergic reactions to insect bites—an injection of epinephrine. Because this syndrome is rare, an emergency kit is probably not necessary equipment, but it is a good idea always to exercise with a partner. If you experience the symptoms, seek emergency care immediately.

There are times when you should not exercise, but pregnancy is not one of them.

Regular exercise is important, but you should not exercise when your body temperature is above 100° F. Certain diseases or injuries are also aggravated by exercise. Extreme temperatures and humidity should discourage most people, and smog alerts certainly should be heeded.

Pregnant women, contrary to some beliefs, can exercise and even jog safely, but they should first consult their physician, as should anyone with disease or injury or who is taking medication regularly.

Exercise can alter the effect of drugs on the body, as well as the effect of certain disorders.

The effect of drugs used to treat thyroid disease may be altered by exercise. Likewise, patients taking certain medicine for asthma and collagen diseases may not be able to perform exercises that require moderate or heavy exertion in a normal fashion. Exercise alters the effect of nonsteroidal analgesics and anti-inflammatory drugs (like aspirin). During exercise, these drugs can cause increased oxygen consumption and increased carbon dioxide production, as well as promote sweating and dehydration. Muscle relaxants may cause depression and hinder coordination.

There is some evidence that anabolic androgenic steroids enhance performance when taken in massive doses. There *is,* however, clear-cut evidence that these steroids have serious side effects, including hepatitis, carcinoma, and myeloid leukemia. It is best to consult your physician about any drugs you are taking before beginning an exercise program.

Too much exercise can result in "overtraining" or "burnout."

Overworking—doing too much too soon—so that there is not enough time for recovery between workouts will lead to weight loss, depression, insomnia, increased resting heart rate, decreased work capacity, poorer performance, and lack of enjoyment and motivation. When these symptoms occur, cut back on the intensity, frequency, or duration of your training.

The valsalva maneuver should be avoided when exerting great force in weight lifting, calisthenics, or isometrics.

Dizziness, blackouts, and inguinal hernias may result from the valsalva maneuver. This can be prevented in weight lifting by avoiding **hyperventilation,** squatting as briefly as possible, and raising the weight as rapidly as possible to a position where it can be supported while breathing normally. In all activities, breathe normally! Do *not* hold your breath during exercise.

Commercial establishments, such as health clubs, reducing salons, and aerobic dance centers, may not employ personnel qualified to prescribe exercise programs.

Studies indicate that many commercial enterprises do not employ properly trained instructors. Those who are qualified to advise you about exercise have college degrees and four to eight years of study in such courses as anatomy, physiology, kinesiology, preventive and therapeutic exercise, and physiology of exercise. These qualified individuals are physical educators, corrective therapists, and physical therapists. On-the-job training, a good physique or figure, and good dancing ability are not sufficient qualifications for teaching or advising about exercise.

Hazardous exercises can be avoided by following these general rules.

1. Do not hyperflex the knee or neck.
2. Do not hyperextend the knee, neck, or lower back.
3. Do not apply a twisting or lateral force to the knee.
4. Avoid holding your breath during exercise.
5. Avoid stretching already long/weak muscles and avoid shortening already short/strong muscles.
    a. Most people should especially avoid aggravation of head forward, kyphosis, abdominal ptosis, medial rotation of the thigh, and pronation of the foot.
    b. Most people need to stretch the chest, hip flexor, calf, hamstring, lower back, and medial thigh rotator muscles.
    c. Most people need to strengthen the abdominals, the muscles between the shoulder blades, the upper back muscles, the lateral hip rotators, and the shin muscles.
6. Avoid overstretching any joint so that ligaments and joint capsules are stretched.
7. Avoid passive stretches by another person, especially ballistic passive stretches.
8. Avoid movements that place acute compressional forces on spinal discs, such as extending and rotating the spine simultaneously, trunk and neck circling, and double leg-lifts.
9. Avoid movements that cause joint impingements or cartilage damage, such as arm circles in palm-down position.

REFERENCES

Allman, F. L. "Rehabilitation Following Athletic Injuries." In O'Donoghue, D. H., *Treatment of Injuries to Athletes*, 14th ed. Philadelphia: W. B. Saunders Co., 1984, 677.

Alsop, K. "Potential Hazards of Abdominal Exercises." *JOHPERD*. 42(January 1971):89.

American College of Sports Medicine. "Position Stand on the Use of Anabolic-Androgenic Steroids in Sports." *Sports Medicine Bulletin* (1984):1.

American College of Sports Medicine. "Weight Loss in Wrestlers: Position Stand of American College of Sports Medicine." In *P.E. Conditioning and Physical Fitness*, edited by P. E. Allsen, Dubuque, Iowa: Wm. C. Brown Publishers, 1978.

Anderson, S. D. "Drugs Affecting the Respiratory System with Particular Reference to Asthma." *Medicine and Science in Sports and Exercise* 13(1981):259.

"Back Specialists Hit 'Inversion' Fad," *Medical World News* (28 March 1983).

Basmajian, J. V. *Therapeutic Exercise*. 3d ed. Baltimore: Williams and Wilkins, 1984.

Beaulieu, J. E. "Developing a Stretching Program." *Physician and Sportsmedicine* 9(1981):59.

Blackburn, S. E., and I. G. Portney. "Electromyographic Activity of Back Musculature during Williams' Flexion Exercises." *Physical Therapy* 61(1981):878.

Cailliet, R. *Neck and Arm Pain*. Philadelphia: F. A. Davis Co., 1981.

Corbin, C. B., and R. Lindsey. *The Ultimate Fitness Book*. New York: Leisure Press, 1984.

Day, R. O. "Effects of Exercise Performance on Drugs in Musculoskeletal Disorders." *Medicine and Science in Sports and Exercise* 13(1981):272.

*Dominguez, R. H., and R. S. Gajda. *Total Body Conditioning*. New York: Charles Scribners Sons, 1982.

Flint, M. "Selecting Exercises." *JOHPERD* 35 (February 1964): 1984.

Flint, M., and J. Gudgell. "Electromyographic Study of Abdominal Muscular Activity during Exercise." *Research Quarterly* 36(March 1965):1.

Forman, J. "Focus: DeAnza College Older Adult Education." *American Corrective Therapy Journal* 36:2(March–April 1982):44.

Getchell, B., and P. Cleary. "The Caloric Cost of Rope Skipping and Running. *Physician and Sportsmedicine* 8:2(February 1980):56.

Goldman, R. M. "Dr. Goldman Replies." *Physician and Sportsmedicine* 13:7 (July 1985):15.

Hage, P. "Exercise and Pregnancy Compatible, M. D. Says." *Physician and Sportsmedicine* 9(1981):23.

"Hanging a Health Hazard?" *Medical World News* (22 August 1983).

Kaufman, W. C. "Cold Weather Clothing for Comfort or Heat Conversion." *Physician and Sportsmedicine* 10(1982):71.

Kavanaugh, T. "Postcoronary Joggers Need Precise Guidelines." *Physician and Sportsmedicine* 4(1976):63.

*Kelly, D. L. "Exercise Prescription and the Kinesiological Imperative." *Journal of Health, Physical Education, Recreation and Dance* 53(1982):18.

Kendall, F. P., and E. K. McCreary. *Muscles: Testing and Function*. 3d ed. Baltimore: Williams and Wilkins, 1983.

Kisner, C. and L. A. Colby, *Therapeutic Exercise: Foundations and Techniques*. Philadelphia: F. A. Davis Co., 1985.

Klatz, R. M., et al. "Effects of Gravity Inversion on Hypertensive Subjects." *Physician and Sportsmedicine* 13:3(March 1985):85.

Klein, K. K. "The Deep Squat as Utilized in Weight Training for Athletics and Its Effect on the Ligaments of the Knee." *Journal of Physical and Mental Rehabilitation* 15:6(January–February 1961):10.

Koszuta, L. E. "Low Impact Aerobics: Better Than Traditional Aerobic Dance?" *Physician and Sportsmedicine* 14(July 1986):156.

Kuntzleman, C. "Dangerous Exercises. Which, When, and Why." *Fitness For Living* (January–February 1974):5.

Kuntzleman, C. "Winter Fitness Guide." *Family Weekly* (23 January 1983):15.

Kuntzleman, C., and the Editors of *Consumer Guide*. *Rating the Exercises*. New York: William Morrow and Co., 1978.

Kusinitz, I., M. Fine, and the Editors of *Consumer Reports*. *Physical Fitness for Practically Everybody: The Consumers Union Report on Exercise*. Mount Vernon, NY: Consumers Union, 1983. Lamb, L. *Health Newsletter* 1:10(1973).

Levy, R. L., et al. "Lateral Medullary Syndrome After Neck Injury." *Neurology* 30(July 1980):788.

*Lindsey, R., B. Jones, and A. V. Whitley. *Fitness for Health, Figure/Physique, Posture*. 5th ed. Dubuque, Iowa: Wm. C. Brown Publishers, 1983.

Lowman, C., and C. Young. *Postural Fitness, Significance and Variance*. Philadelphia: Lea and Febiger. 1960.

Luttgens, K., and K. Wells. *Kinesiology: Scientific Basis of Human Movement*. Philadelphia: Saunders College Publishing, 1982.

Maitland, G. D. *Vertebral Manipulation*. Boston: Butterworth. 1984.

McGlynn, G. H. "A Reevaluation of Isometric Strength Training." *Journal of Sports Medicine and Physical Fitness* 12(1972):258.

Mirkin, G. "Overtraining of Athletes: A Round Table." *Physician and Sportsmedicine* 11(1983):93.

Morehouse, C. A. "Evaluation of Knee Abduction and Adduction. The Effects of Selected Exercise Programs on Knee Stability and Its Relationship to Knee Injuries in College Football" (Grant No. RD2815M). Washington, DC: Department of Health, Education, and Welfare, Division of Research and Demonstration.

Nirschl, R. P. "Health Clubs are A Great Source of Business for Orthopedists." Quoted in "Scanning Sports." *Physician and Sportsmedicine* 14(March 1986):54.

Norkin, C., and P. Levangie. *Joint Structure and Function: A Comprehensive Analysis*. Philadelphia: F. A. Davis Co., 1983.

Powles, A. C. P. "The Effect of Drugs on the Cardiovascular Response to Exercise." *Medicine and Science in Sports and Exercise* 13(1981):252.

Rasch, P., and F. Allman. "Controversial Exercises." *American Corrective Therapy Journal* 26:4(July–August 1972):95.

Rasch, P. J. *Weight Training*, 4th ed. Dubuque, Iowa: Wm. C. Brown Publishers, 1982.

Ricci, B., M. Marchetti, and F. Figura. "Biomechanics of Sit-Up Exercises" *Medicine and Science in Sports and Exercise* 13(1981):54.

Robertson, L. D. "Article Not Conclusive." *Physician and Sportsmedicine* 13:7(July 1985):15.

Ryan, A. J. "Hazardous Exercises." *Fitness for Living*. (September–October 1970):5.

Shefer, A. quoted in "Exercise Can Provoke Allergic Reaction." *Atlanta Journal* (February 1980).

Shyne, K. "Richard H. Dominguez, M.D.: To Stretch or Not to Stretch." *Physician and Sportsmedicine* 10(September 1982):137.

Skinner, J. "The Misinformation Crisis." *ACSM Newsletter* (1976).

Soderburg, G. *Kinesiology: Application to Pathological Motion.* Baltimore: Williams and Wilkins, 1986.

Soderberg, Gary L. "Exercises for the Abdominal Muscles." *JOHPER,* 37:2(September 1966):67.

Stevenson, E. "Recycled Exercise." *CAHPERD Journal Times* 44:2 (November 1981):13.

Stevenson, E. "Double Leg Raising." *CAHPERD Journal Times* 44(1982):18.

Stevenson, E. "The Mad Cat." *CAHPERD Journal Times* 44(1982):23.

Stevenson, E. "The Sit-Up." *CAHPERD Journal Times* 44(1982):17.

Stevenson, E. "Specificity of Exercise." *CAHPERD Journal Times* 45(1982):6.

Stevenson, E. "Head Circling." *CAHPERD Journal Times* 45(1983):6.

Stevenson, E. "The Shoulder Stand." *CAHPERD Journal Times* 45(1983):19.

Stevenson, E. "The Bench Press." *CAHPERD Journal Times* 45(May 1983):14.

Stevenson, E. "Trunk Circling." *CAHPERD Journal Times* 46:2(November 1983):20.

Stevenson, E. "Hurdle Stretch." *CAHPERD Journal Times* 46(January 1984):16.

Stevenson, E. "Hamstring Stretcher." *CAHPERD Journal Times* 46:6(March 1984):10.

Stevenson, E. "The New Fitness Test." *CAHPERD Journal Times* 48 (November 1985):16.

Stevenson, E. "Hamstring Stretches." *CAHPERD Journal Times* 48:6 (March 1986):6.

Stevenson, E. "Stretches (calf)." *CAHPERD Journal Times* 48:8(May 1986):14.

Stevenson, E. "Hip Flexor Stretches." *CAHPERD Journal Times* 46(May 1986):17.

Sutton, J. R. "Drugs Used in Metabolic Disorders." *Medicine and Science in Sports and Exercise* 13(1981):266.

Sutton, J. R. "The Effects of Drugs on Exercise Performance." *Medicine and Science in Sports and Exercise* 13(1981):246.

Sweeney, G. D. "Drugs—Some Basic Concepts." *Medicine in Sports and Exercise* 13(1981):247.

Travell, J. G., and D. G. Simons. *Myofascial Pain and Dysfunction: The Trigger Point Manual.* Baltimore: Williams and Wilkins, 1983.

Weltman, A., and G. Stamford. "Exercising Safely in The Winter." *Physician and Sportsmedicine* 10(1982):130.

Williams, P. *Low Back and Neck Pain.* Springfield, Ill.: C. C. Thomas. 1974.

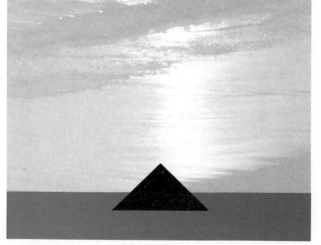

20

STRESS, TENSION, AND RELAXATION

CONCEPT 20

Mental and physical health are affected by
an individual's ability to avoid
or adapt to stress,
emotional factors, and tension.

INTRODUCTION

Stress can trigger an emotional response that, in turn, evokes the autonomic nervous system to a "fight or flight" response. This adaptive and protective device stimulates the ductless glands to hypo- or hyperactivity in preparation for what is perceived as a threat or assault on the whole organism. In some instances, this alarm reaction (the body's warning signal that a stressor is present) of the body may be essential to survival, but when evoked inappropriately or excessively, it may be more harmful than the effects of the original stressor. For example, a fight or flight response may cause a coronary spasm that could lead to a heart attack.

TERMS

Adaptation—The body's efforts to restore normalcy.

Alarm Reaction—The body's warning signal that a stressor is present.

Anxiety—A state of apprehension with a compulsion to do something; excessive anxiety is a tension disorder with physiological characteristics.

Chronic Fatigue—Constant state of entire body fatigue.

Distress—Negative stress or stress that contributes to health problems.

Eustress—Positive stress or stress that is mentally or physically stimulating.

Hypostress—Lack of stress.

Neuromuscular Hypertension—Unnecessary or exaggerated muscle contractions; excess tension beyond that needed to perform a given task; also called hypertonus.

Physiological Fatigue—A deterioration in the capacity of the neuromuscular system as the result of physical overwork and strain; also referred to as "true fatigue."

Psychological Fatigue—A feeling of fatigue usually caused by such things as lack of exercise, boredom, or mental stress that results in a lack of energy and depression; also referred to as "subjective" or "false" fatigue.

Relaxation—The release or reduction of tension in the neuromuscular system.

Stress—The nonspecific response (generalized adaptation) of the body to any demand made upon it in order to maintain physiological equilibrium.

Stressor—Anything that produces stress or increases the rate of wear and tear on the body.

THE FACTS

All living creatures are in a continual state of stress (some more; some less).

There are many kinds of stressors. Environmental stressors include heat, noise, overcrowding, climate, and terrain. Physiological stressors may be such things as drugs, caffeine, tobacco, injury, infection, or disease. Mental and physical effort as well as emotions can be stressors.

Psychosocial stimuli are probably the most common stressors affecting humans. These include "life-change events," such as a change in work hours or line of work, family illnesses, problems with superiors, deaths of relatives or friends, and increased responsibilities. In school, the pressures of grades, term papers, and oral presentations may induce **stress.**

Too little stress (hypostress) is undesirable and distressful.

Stress is not always harmful. In fact, too little stress, sometimes called "rust out," is not best for optimal health. Moderate stress may enhance behavioral adaptation and is necessary for maturation and health. It stimulates psychological growth. It has been said that "freedom from stress is death" and "stress is the spice of life."

Excessive stress reduces the effectiveness of our immune system.

Between 50 and 70 percent of all illnesses are linked to stress response. Too much stress—**distress**—can result in various health disorders. Some mental and physical conditions that can be psychosomatic (or stress caused) include high blood pressure and heart disease; psychiatric disorders, such as depression and schizophrenia; indigestion; colitis; ulcers; headaches; insomnia; diarrhea; constipation; increased blood clotting time; increased cholesterol concentration; diuresis; edema; and low back pain. Even serious diseases, such as cancer, can be influenced by a person's state of mind.

In some cases, there is considerable time between a major **stressor** and the onset of a disease, so we do not always associate the two. With too much stress, rather than "rust out" we "burnout."

Individuals react and adapt differently to different stressors.

What one person finds stressful may not be for others, and stress affects people differently. It mobilizes some to greater efficiency, while it confuses and disorganizes others. For example, skydiving or riding a roller coaster would be fun for some people, but for others it would be very stressful.

An individual's response to stress depends upon the intensity of the threat, the type of situation in which

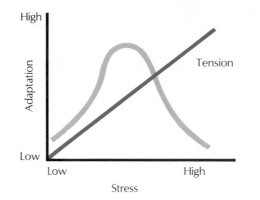

FIGURE 20.1 Stress and Adaptive Responses

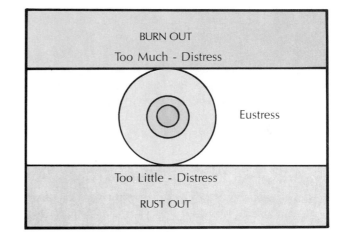

FIGURE 20.2 Stress Target Zone

it occurs, and such personal variables as cultural background, tolerance levels, past experience, and personality. You can't make a racehorse out of a turtle and vice versa. Some people react by biting their nails; others eat too much, chain smoke, or drink excessively.

An individual's capacity to adapt is not a static function, but fluctuates with energy, drive, and courage. The better your fitness, the better you can withstand the rigors of tension without becoming susceptible to illness or other disorders.

Individuals tend to adapt best to moderate stress.

You would expect mild stress to produce mild adaptations, and strong stress to produce strong adaptive responses, but this is not so. High levels of threat tend to evoke ineffective, disorganized behavior. Figure 20.1 shows this relationship between stress and adaptive responses.

The amount of stress that you can adapt to comfortably is what Selye (1978) calls **eustress** (see figure 20.2) and would, in a sense, be our target zone for stress.

Stress can be self-induced and pleasurable or un-pleasurable.

Some people may deliberately place themselves in stressful situations; for example, athletes place themselves under maximum strain; lawyers and surgeons are challenged by difficulties; pregnancy imposes psychological and physiological stress on a woman. Self-induced stress may also be an unpleasant but necessary interlude that cannot be avoided. For example, there is a risk of falling that is necessary in learning to ride a bicycle.

Occupations are common sources of stress and some are more stressful than others.

One study showed that the twelve most stressful jobs were laborer, secretary, inspector, clinical lab technician, office manager, foreman, manager/administrator, waiter/waitress, machine operator, farm owner, miner, and painter. Air traffic controller is currently considered a most stressful job. Business and industry often hire psychologists to counsel employees about occupational stress to help reduce absenteeism, boredom, and the number of accidents and resignations.

Neuromuscular hypertension may be both a cause and an effect of stress.

Tension is a primary index of stress. **Anxiety** is an emotional response caused by stressors and is manifested in muscular tension. Muscular tension may also be physical in origin, resulting from overuse of a muscle group. This tension can cause muscle spasms and pain that, in turn, become additional stressors. Trigger points and the myofascial pain syndrome that lead to backache and headache are good examples of muscular tension.

Some tension is normally present in muscles and contributes to the adjustment of the individual to the environment.

Some tension is needed to remain awake, alert, and ready to respond. In fact, a certain degree of tension aids some types of mental activity. It appears that each individual has an optimum level of tension to facilitate the thought process. However, too much tension can inhibit some types of mental activity and physical skills (such as those requiring accuracy and steadiness in held postures).

Fatigue and neuromuscular hypertension are closely related.

High levels of tension are a source of fatigue. Fatigue from lack of rest or sleep, emotional strain, pain, disease, and muscular work may produce too much muscle tension. **Fatigue** may be either **psychological** or **physiological** in origin, but both can result in a state of exhaustion or **chronic fatigue** with muscle tenseness.

One cardiologist says: "Rule 1 is don't sweat the small stuff; and rule 2 is its all small stuff and if you can't fight it and you can't flee—go with the flow" (American Heart Association, 1984).

Excessive tension can be avoided or relieved by proper "coping strategies."

Psychologists say stressful situations must be recognized and people trained to withdraw psychologically to a state of reflection, meditation, or **relaxation.** "Moderation in all things" may still be a helpful maxim. Work must be balanced with rest. Provision should be made for recreational activities and diversions. Diversions may be even more important than rest, because stress on one system helps to relax another. This may range from a temporary change from one task to another (e.g., from studying to lawn mowing), or a change of scenery, a change in job, a vacation, or even retirement. The approach to life may even need to be altered.

These strategies are beyond the scope of this book, but there are some helpful books on stress reduction such as those listed in the references. Courses and workshops are offered in most communities for the person who needs additional help.

Some methods of relieving tension are less desirable or are not recommended.

There is no magic cure for stress or tension, but there are a variety of therapeutic approaches. Some treatments are less desirable than others because they act only as "crutches" or "fire extinguishers" and do not get at the root of the problem. Hypnosis may lead to fantasy and dependency. Alcoholic beverages, tranquilizers, and painkillers may give temporary relief and may be prescribed by a physician as part of the treatment, but they do not resolve the problem and may even mask symptoms or cause further problems. Drugs do not provide a long-term solution to chronic tension. Contrary to vitamin and mineral advertisements, there are no proven benefits to supplementing the diet with such products as vitamin C or special "stress" formulations.

Primal scream, EST, transactional analysis, psychoanalysis, transcendental meditation (TM), and other popular methods may provide temporary reduction of physical tension but may be hazardous to your mental well-being.

Exercise is one of the best ways to relieve stress and aid muscle tension release.

Exercise is especially useful to relieve white-collar job stress. Hans Selye (1977) believes physical fitness serves as a sort of "inoculation against stress."

If you feel tense, take a run or a stretch instead of a tranquilizer!

Stretching exercises and rhythmical exercises especially aid in relaxation. Some good relaxation exercises are illustrated in the box on page 180.

Those who work long hours at a desk can release tension by getting up frequently and stretching, by taking a brisk walk down the hall, or by performing "office exercises" [See Austin (1984), MacLennon (1980), and Murphy (1984)].

Massage, heat, and deep breathing aid relaxation of tense muscles.

Gentle effleurage, a type of massage; heat in the form of a hot bath (or shower or sauna); and deep breathing with prolonged exhalation, when combined with conscious relaxation techniques described in this concept, are effective for most people.

There are several satisfactory methods of releasing tension through techniques of conscious relaxation.

In some way not fully understood, certain involuntary bodily functions can be controlled by an act of will (voluntarily). Relaxation of the muscles is a skill that can be learned through practice just as other muscle skills are learned, and it works! It is no gimmick.

Conscious relaxation techniques usually employ the "three Rs" of relaxation: (1) reduce mental activity, (2) recognize tension, and (3) reduce respiration.

Some examples of these systems are described here:

1. *Jacobson's Progressive Relaxation Method*—You must recognize how a tense muscle feels before you can voluntarily release the tension. In this technique, contract the muscles strongly then relax. Each of the large muscles is relaxed first, later the small ones. The contractions are gradually reduced in intensity until no movement is visible. Always, the emphasis is placed on detecting the feeling of tension as the first step in "letting go," or "going negative." Jacobson (1961, 1978), a pioneer in muscle relaxation research, emphasizes the importance of relaxing eye and speech muscles, because he believes these muscles trigger reactions of the total organism more than other muscles. A sample contract-relax exercise routine for relaxation is presented on page 181.

2. *Autogenic (self-generated) Relaxation Training*—Several times daily, the individual lies down in a quiet room and, with eyes closed, passively concentrates on preselected phrases. This technique has been used to focus on heaviness of limbs, warmth of limbs, heart regulation, breathing regulation, and coolness in the forehead. It evokes changes opposite to those produced by stress. Research has shown that those who are skilled in this technique can decrease oxygen consumption, change the electrical activity of the brain, slow the metabolism, decrease blood lactate, lower body temperature, and slow the heart rate.

   Transcendental meditation (TM), as used by the Eastern religions, falls into this category. The individual sits quietly and attempts to block out distracting thoughts by mentally repeating a personal, secret word or phrase.

3. *Biofeedback-Autogenic Relaxation Training*—Biofeedback training utilizes machines that monitor certain physiological processes of the body and provide visual or auditory evidence of what is happening to normally unconscious bodily functions. When combined with autogenic phrases, subjects have learned to relax and reduce the electrical activity in their muscles, lower blood pressure by increasing the temperature of their hands, decrease heart rate, change their brain waves, and decrease headaches, asthma attacks, and some psychosomatic disorders.

4. *Imagery*—Thinking autogenic phrases, you can visualize such feelings as "sinking into a mattress or pillow," or you can think of being a "limp, loose-jointed puppet with no one to hold the strings." You can imagine being a "half-filled sack of flour resting on an uneven surface" or pretend to be "a sack of granulated salt left out in the rain, melting away." Some people seem to respond better to the concept of "floating" than to feeling "heavy," but whatever the image you wish to conjure, imagery is a form of self-hypnosis that helps to take your mind off anxieties and distractions, and at the same time, releases unwanted tension in the muscles using "mind over matter."

RELAXATION EXERCISES

1. **Neck Stretch**—Roll the head slowly in a half circle, first right then left. Close your eyes and feel the stretch. Do *not* make a full circle by tipping the head back. Repeat several times.

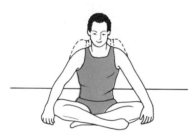

2. **Shoulder Lift**—Hunch the shoulders as high as possible and then let them drop. Repeat several times. Inhale on the lift; exhale on the drop.

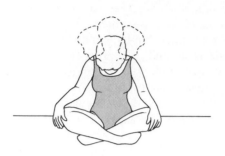

3. **Trunk Stretch and Drop**—Stand and reach as high as possible; tiptoe and stretch every muscle, then collapse completely, letting knees flex and trunk, head, and arms dangle (see trunk swing illustration). Repeat two or three times.

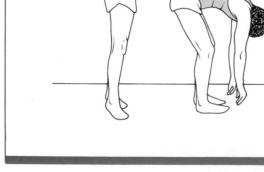

4. **Trunk Swings**—Following the trunk drop (preceding illustration), bounce gently with a minimum of muscular effort. Set the trunk swinging from side to side by shifting the weight from one foot to the other, letting the heels come off the floor alternately. Then with a slight springing movement of the lower back, gently bob up and down, keeping the entire body (especially the neck) limp.

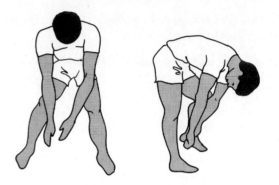

5. **Tension Contrast**—With arms extended overhead, lie on your side. Tense the body as "stiff as a board," then "let go," and relax, letting the body fall either forward or backward in whatever direction it loses balance. Continue "letting go" for a few seconds after falling and allow yourself to feel like you are still "sinking." Repeat on the other side.

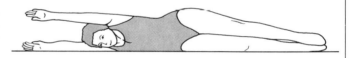

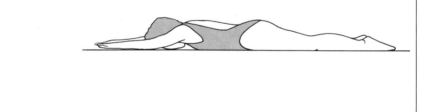

CONTRACT-RELAX EXERCISE ROUTINE FOR RELAXATION*

1. Hand and forearm—Contract your hand, making a fist; relax.

2. Biceps—Flex the elbow and contract your biceps; relax.

3. Forehead—Raise your eyebrows and wrinkle your forehead; relax.

4. Cheeks and nose—Make a face; wrinkle your nose and squint; relax.

5. Jaws—Clench your teeth; relax.

6. Lips and tongue—With teeth apart, press lips together and press tongue to roof of mouth; relax.

7. Neck and throat—Push head backward while tucking chin, pushing against floor or pillow if lying; if sitting, push against high chair back; relax.

8. Shoulders and upper back—Hunch shoulders to ears; relax.

9. Abdomen—Suck in abdomen; relax.

10. Thighs and buttocks—Squeeze your buttocks together and push your heels into the floor (if lying) or against a chair rung (if sitting); relax.

11. Calves—Pull instep and toes toward shin; relax.

12. Toes—Curl toes; relax.

*Note: Eventually, you should progress to a combination of muscle groups and gradually eliminate the "contract" phase of the program. Refer to Jacobson's relaxation method page 179 for more instructions.

► LAB RESOURCE MATERIALS (FOR USE WITH LABS 20A, PAGE 267 AND 20C, PAGE 271)

TABLE 20A.1 Stressful Life Events for College Students*

	Event	Score		Event	Score
_____	Death of a close family member	100	_____	Problems with your boss or professor	25
_____	Jail term	80	_____	Outstanding personal achievement	25
_____	Final year or first year in college	63	_____	Failure in some course	25
_____	Pregnancy (to you or caused by you)	60	_____	Final exams	20
_____	Severe personal illness or injury	53	_____	Increased or decreased dating	20
_____	Marriage	50	_____	Change in working conditions	20
_____	Any interpersonal problems	45	_____	Change in your major	20
_____	Financial difficulties	40	_____	Change in your sleeping habits	18
_____	Death of a close friend	40	_____	Several-day vacation	15
_____	Arguments with your roommate (more than every other day)	40	_____	Change in eating habits	15
_____	Major disagreements with your family	40	_____	Family reunion	15
_____	Major change in personal habits	30	_____	Change in recreational activities	15
_____	Change in living environment	30	_____	Minor illness or injury	15
_____	Beginning or ending a job	30	_____	Minor violations of the law	11

*Adapted from the Social Readjustment Scale devised by Thomas Holmes and Richard Rahe. Used by permission.

TABLE 20A.2 Stressful Life Events*

Event	Score	Event	Score
Death of spouse	100	Son/daughter leaves home	29
Divorce	73	Trouble with in-laws	29
Marital separation	65	Outstanding achievement	28
Jail term	63	Spouse begins work	26
Death of close family member	63	Start or finish school	26
Personal injury/illness	53	Change in living conditions	25
Marriage	50	Revision of personal habits	24
Fired from work	47	Trouble with boss	23
Marital reconciliation	45	Change in work hours, conditions	20
Retirement	45	Change in residence	20
Change in family member's health	44	Change in schools	20
Pregnancy	40	Change in recreational habits	19
Sex difficulties	39	Change in church activities	19
Addition to family	39	Change in social activities	18
Business readjustment	39	Mortgage/loan under $50,000	18
Change in financial status	38	Change in sleeping habits	16
Death of close friend	37	Change in number of family gatherings	15
Change in number of marital arguments	35	Change in eating habits	15
Mortgage/loan over $50,000	31	Vacation	13
Foreclosure of mortgage/loan	30	Christmas season	12
Change in work responsibilities	29	Minor violation of law	11

Adapted from the Social Readjustment Scale devised by Thomas Holmes and Richard Rahe. Used by permission.

CHART 20A.1 Stressful Life Events *Rating Scale*

Rating	Score	Implication for Illness
Low stress	150 or less	35% chance of getting a stress-related disease in the next two years
Moderate stress	151–300	51% chance of getting a stress illness in the next two years
High stress	301 or higher	80% chance of getting a stress illness in the next two years

Evaluating Muscular Tension

A trained person can diagnose neuromuscular hypertension by observation and by manual testing. While there is insufficient time in this course to master either the technique of relaxing or the techniques of evaluation, it is possible to learn the procedures for both.

1. Following the procedure outlined in Lab 20C, page 271, look for visual signs of tension outlined in section A of chart 20C.1. Place a check mark in the appropriate column.

2. Quietly and gently, the tester should grasp the subject's right wrist with his or her fingers, and slowly raise it about three inches from the floor, letting it hinge at the elbow; then let the hand drop. Observe the signs of tension outlined in section B of chart 20C.1. Record results.
3. After all visual and manual symptoms have been recorded on the chart, determine the total number of symptoms checked yes.
4. Find your total score on chart 20C.2 to determine your rating.

CHART 20C.1 Signs of Tension Observed by Tester

	No	Yes
A. Visual Symptoms		
Frowning	☐	☐
Twitching	☐	☐
Eyelids fluttering	☐	☐
Breathing	☐	☐
shallow	☐	☐
rapid	☐	☐
irregular	☐	☐
Mouth tight	☐	☐
Swallowing	☐	☐
B. Manual Symptoms		
Assistance (subject helps lift arm)	☐	☐
Resistance (subject resists movement)	☐	☐
Posturing (subject holds arm in raised position)	☐	☐
Perseveration (subject continues upward movement)	☐	☐

CHART 20C.2 Tension-Relaxation *Rating Scale*

Classification	Total Score
Excellent (relaxed)	0
Very good (mild tension)	1–3
Fair (moderate tension)	4–6
Poor (tense)	7–9
Very poor (marked tension)	10–12

REFERENCES

American Lung Association of California. *Breathe Easy Relaxation Exercises.* Adapted from Davis, McKay, and Eshelman. *The Relaxation and Stress Workbook.* Oakland, Calif.: New Harbinger Publications, 1980.

Austin, D. *Tone Up at the Terminals.* Verbatim Corp., 1984, 323 Soquel Way, Sunnyvale, CA 94086.

Benson, H. *Beyond the Relaxation Response.* New York: Berkley Publishers, 1985.

Benson, Herbert. *The Relaxation Response.* New York: Avon, 1975.

Brown, B. B. *Between Health and Illness: New Notions on Stress and the Nature of Well Being.* New York: Bantam, 1985.

*"Focus: Stress Management Overview." *Fitness Leader.* 1:1 (September 1982):1–10.

*Freudenberg, H. *Burnout: The High Cost of High Achievement.* New York: Anchor Press, Doubleday, 1980.

Gunderson, E., and R. Rahe, eds. *Life Stress and Illness.* Springfield, Ill.: C. C. Thomas, 1979.

Hollis, M. *Practical Exercise Therapy,* 2d ed. Boston: Blackwell Scientific Publications, 1981.

"How to Deal with Stress on the Job." *U.S. News and World Report* (13 March 1978):80.

Jacobson E. *Anxiety and Tension Control.* Philadelphia: J. B. Lippincott Co., 1964.

*Jacobson, E. *You Must Relax.* New York: McGraw-Hill, 1978.

Kipp, D. "Stress and Nutrition." *Contemporary Nutrition.* 9:7 (July 1984).

Leatz, C. A. *Unwinding.* Englewood Cliffs, N.J.: Prentice-Hall, 1981.

Lindsey, R., B. Jones, and A. V. Whitley. *Fitness for Health, Figure/Physique, Posture.* 5th ed. Dubuque, Iowa: Wm. C. Brown Publishers, 1983.

MacLennan, D. *How to Keep Fit at Your Desk the Deskercize Way.* Fitness Institute, Totem Books, 1980, 255 Yorkland Blvd., Willowdale, Ontario, Canada M2J.1S3.

Mason, J. *Guide to Stress Reduction.* Culver City, Calif.: Peace Press, 1980.

Menninger, R. W. "Coping with Life's Strains." *U.S. News and World Report* (1 May 1978):80.

Murphy, P. "Office Stress: Is a Solution Shaping Up?" *Physician and Sportsmedicine.* 12:12(December 1984):114.

Pelletier, K. *Mind as Healer, Mind as Slayer.* New York: Dell Publishers. 1977.

Perry, P. "You Can Relax on the Job." *American Health* (May 1986):42.

Pollock, M., et al. *Exercise in Health and Disease: Evaluation and Rehabilitation.* Philadelphia: W. B. Saunders Co., 1984.

Pollock, M., J. Willmore, and S. M. Fox. *Health and Fitness through Physical Activity.* New York: John Wiley, 1978.

Rosen, Gerald. *The Relaxation Book.* Englewood Cliffs, NJ: Prentice-Hall, 1977.

*Selye, H. *Stress without Distress.* Philadelphia: J. B. Lippincott Co., 1974.

Selye, H. "Secret of Coping with Stress." *U.S. News and World Report* (21 March 1977):51.

*Selye, H. *The Stress of Life.* New York: McGraw-Hill, 1978.

American Heart Association, Greater Long Beach Chapter. "Stress—Bona Fide A.H.A. Risk Factor." *Heart Lines* 41:1 (February 1984).

Taylor, L. P. *Electromyometric Biofeedback Therapy.* Los Angeles: Biofeedback and Advanced Therapy Institute, 1981.

Travell, J. G., and D. G. Simons. *Myofascial Pain and Dysfunction.* Baltimore: Williams and Wilkins, 1983.

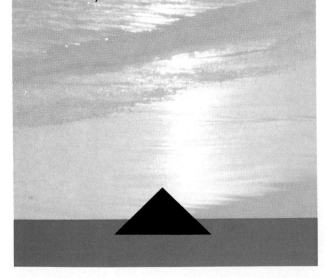

21

HYPOKINETIC DISEASE RISK FACTORS

CONCEPT 21

There are many factors that contribute

to increased risk of hypokinetic disease.

Many of these are controllable.

INTRODUCTION

As the name indicates, hypokinetic diseases and conditions are caused or compounded by a lack of regular exercise. Such hypokinetic conditions as heart disease and back pain, however, are caused by many factors other than lack of exercise. These factors associated with hypokinetic conditions are called risk factors. It cannot be proven that all risk factors cause hypokinetic disease, but the link between them is strong. Some risk factors such as sex and age cannot be altered. They are predetermined by heredity and the passing of time. Other factors can be controlled by modifying your life-style. You can do something about these.

TERMS

Blood Lipids—Fats in the bloodstream, including cholesterol and triglicerides.
Diastolic Blood Pressure—Commonly referred to as resting blood pressure; it is the lower of the two blood pressure readings.
Hypertension—Another word for high blood pressure.
Hypokinetic Disease or Condition—A disease or condition associated with physical inactivity.
Risk Factor—A factor or circumstance that relates to the increased risk of acquiring a disease or medical condition; in this case, increased risk of hypokinetic conditions such as heart disease and back pain.
Systolic Blood Pressure—Commonly referred to as working blood pressure, systolic blood pressure is the higher of the two blood pressure readings. It is the pressure necessary to force movement of the blood through the artery and is measured (usually at the brachial artery on the inside of the upper arm) just after the heart beats, forcing a surge of blood through the artery.

THE FACTS

There are many risk factors associated with hypokinetic diseases and conditions.

Some major risk factors associated with hypokinetic disease, especially heart disease and back pain, are presented in the box on page 185.

Certain risk factors cannot be altered by changes in life-style.

There is nothing you can do about some risk factors, such as age, heredity, and sex. For example, an older male with a family history of heart disease has a higher risk of heart disease than a young female without a history of heart disease. If you possess risk factors you cannot control, it is especially important that you do what you can to alter those you can control.

Some risk factors can be altered by changing your lifestyle.

Risk of hypokinetic conditions can be reduced by controlling body fatness; altering diet to include good basic foods low in fat and salt; following your doctor's advice to control existing medical conditions (including taking medicine as prescribed); exercising regularly; eliminating smoking; avoiding excessively stressful situations; and learning how to cope effectively with stress. The person at risk must make lifestyle changes in order to reduce the incidence of hypokinetic disease effectively.

Altering risk factors can help reduce the risk of more than one adverse condition at the same time.

By altering the risk factors that are controllable, you can reduce the risk of several hypokinetic conditions. For example, controlling body fatness reduces the risk of diabetes, **hypertension,** and back problems. Altering your diet can reduce the chances of developing high levels of **blood lipids,** and thus reduce the risk of atherosclerosis.

HYPOKINETIC DISEASE RISK FACTORS

Factors That Cannot Be Altered

1. *Age*—As you grow older, your risk of hypokinetic diseases increases. For example, the risk of heart disease is approximately three times as great after sixty than before. The risk of back pain and ulcer disease is considerably greater after forty.

2. *Heredity*—Those people who have a family history of hypokinetic disease are more likely to develop a hypokinetic condition. Heart disease, hypertension, ulcers, back problems, obesity, high blood lipid levels, and other problems have been shown to be more prevalent among those who have a family history of these conditions than among those with no family history. Black Americans are 45 percent more likely to have high blood pressure than whites, therefore, they suffer strokes at an earlier age and sustain more severe results than whites.

3. *Gender*—Men have a higher incidence of many hypokinetic conditions than women. Although the number of women with heart disease is increasing, women still have only about half the incidence of the disease as men have; however, the incidence increases sharply in women after menopause.

Factors That Can Be Altered

4. *Body Fatness*—Having too much body fat is considered by many to be a hypokinetic condition because it may limit your ability to function efficiently and effectively. Even those who do not classify overfatness as a hypokinetic condition agree that it does increase the risk of other hypokinetic conditions. For example, loss of fat can result in relief from symptoms of adult-onset diabetes; can reduce problems associated with certain types of back pain; and can reduce the risks of surgery.

5. *Diet*—There is a clear association between hypokinetic disease and certain types of diets. The excessive intake of saturated fats, such as animal fats, is linked to atherosclerosis and other forms of heart disease. Excessive salt in the diet is associated with high blood pressure.

6. *Diseases*—People who have one hypokinetic disease are more likely to develop a second, or even a third, condition. For example, if you have diabetes, atherosclerosis, or high blood pressure, your risk of having a heart attack or stroke increases dramatically. People with poor posture have a high risk of experiencing back pain and those with too much body fat have a greater than normal risk of diabetes. Although you may not be entirely able to alter the extent to which you develop certain diseases and conditions, reducing your risk and following your doctor's advice can improve your "odds" significantly.

7. *Regular Exercise*—As noted throughout this book and especially in Concept 3, regular exercise can help reduce the risk of hypokinetic disease.

8. *Smoking*—Smokers have a much higher risk of developing and dying from heart disease than nonsmokers. The risk of heart attack is twice as great among young smokers as among young nonsmokers. (Most striking is the difference in risk between older women smokers and nonsmokers.) Smokers have five times the risk of heart attack. Smoking is also associated with increased risk of high blood pressure, cancer, and several other medical conditions. Apparently the more you smoke, the greater the risk. To stop smoking, even after years, can significantly reduce the hypokinetic disease risk.

9. *Stress*—There is evidence that people who are subject to excessive stress are predisposed to various hypokinetic diseases including heart disease and back pain. Statistics indicate that hypokinetic conditions are common among those in certain high-stress jobs and those having "type A" personality profiles.

10. *High Blood Pressure* (Hypertension)—Though high blood pressure is a disease mentioned in item 6 above, it deserves special mention. Hypertension is considered to be a primary risk factor as one of the factors especially likely to increase risk of heart disease.

Certain heart disease risk factors are considered to be primary.

Some risk factors are more likely to contribute to heart disease than others. These are considered to be primary risk factors. High blood pressure (hypertension), particularly high **systolic pressure,** high blood-fat levels (cholesterol and other fats), and smoking are considered to be primary risk factors. Others noted in the chart below, such as age, exercise, and stress, are considered as secondary risk factors.

Risk reduction does not guarantee freedom from disease.

Reducing risk alters the probability of disease, but does not assure disease immunity.

Some risk factors are present at a very early age.

It is never too early to begin controlling hypokinetic disease risk factors. Studies of very young children show that even these youngsters exhibit early stage symptoms of atherosclerosis, type A personality traits, obesity, and even high blood pressure. Establishing healthy lifestyles early in life can be effective in reducing the risk of hypokinetic disease.

It is never too late to begin altering risk factors.

More than one person has said, "It's too late for me," implying that eliminating a risk factor is of little value. This is just not true! For example, eliminating smoking can result in an almost immediate decrease in risk of heart disease and cancer. The same is true for other risk factor modifications.

▶ LAB RESOURCE MATERIALS (FOR USE WITH LAB 21, PAGE 275)

Heart Disease Risk Factor Questionnaire*

Circle the appropriate answer to each question.

	Risk Points				
	1	**2**	**3**	**4**	**Score**
Unalterable Factors					
1. How old are you?	30 or less	31–40	41–54	55+	_____
2. Do you have a history of heart disease in your family?	none	grandparent with heart disease	parent with heart disease	more than one with heart disease	_____
3. What is your gender?	female		male		_____
				Total Unalterable Risk Score	_____
Alterable Factors					
4. What is your percent of body fat?	F =20%↓ M=15%↓	25%↓ 20%↓	30%↓ 25%↓	35%↑ 30%↑	_____
5. Do you have a high-fat diet?	no	slightly high in fat	above normal in fat	eat a lot of meat, fried and fatty foods	_____
6. What is your blood pressure? (systolic or upper score)	120↓	121–135	136–155	155↑	_____
7. Do you have other hypokinetic diseases?	no	ulcer	diabetes	both	_____
8. Do you exercise regularly?	4–5 days a week	3 days a week	less than 3 days a week	no	_____
9. Do you smoke?	no	cigar or pipe	less than 1/2 pack a day	more than 1/2 pack a day	_____
10. Are you under much stress?	less than normal	normal	slightly above normal	quite high	_____

Total Alterable Risk Score _____

Grand Total Risk Score _____

Adapted from W. J. Stone, CAD Risk Factor Scoring Scale (Tempe: Arizona State University, 1984).

CHART 21.1 Heart Disease Risk *Rating Scale*

Rating	Unalterable Score	Alterable Score	Total Score
Very High	9 or More	21 or More	31 or More
High	7–8	15–20	26–30
Average	5–6	11–14	16–25
Low	4 or Less	10 or Less	15 or Less

REFERENCES

*American Heart Association. *1986 Heart Facts Reference Sheet.* Dallas: American Heart Association, 1986.

Anderson, K. M., W. P. Costelli, and D. Levy. Cholesterol and Mortality. *Journal of the American Medical Association* 257 (April 1987): 2,176.

Blair, S. N., et al. "Changes in Coronary Heart Disease Risk Factors Associated with Increased Treadmill Time in 753 Men." *American Journal of Epidemiology* 118(1983):352.

Blair, S. N., et al. "Physical Fitness and Incidence of Hypertension in Healthy Normotensive Men and Women." *Journal of the American Medical Association* 252(1984):487.

Brewer, V., et al. "Role of Exercise in Prevention of Involutional Bone Loss." *Medicine and Science in Sports and Exercise* 15(1983):445.

Corbin, C. B., and R. Lindsey. *The Ultimate Fitness Book.* New York: Leisure Press, 1984.

Gibbons, L. W., et al. "Association Between Coronary Heart Disease, Risk Factors, and Physical Fitness in Healthy Adult Women." *Circulation* 67(1983):977.

*Gilliam, T. B., et al. "Exercise Programs for Children: A Way to Prevent Heart Disease?" *Physician and Sportsmedicine* 10(1982):96.

Jennings, G., et al. "The Effects of Changes in Physical Activity on Major Cardiovascular Risk Factors, Hemodynamics, Sympathetic Function, and Glucose Utilization in Man: A Controlled Study of Four Levels of Physical Activity." *Circulation* 73(1986):30–40.

Monahan, T. "Exercise and Depression: Swapping Sweat for Serenity." *Physician and Sportsmedicine* 14(1986):192.

Nash, H. J. "Can Exercise Make Us Immune to Disease?" *Physician and Sportsmedicine* 14(1986):250.

Paffenbarger, R. S., et al. "Physical Activity, All-Cause Mortality, and Longevity of College Alumni." *New England Journal of Medicine* 314(1986):605.

*Pollock, M. L., et al. *Exercise in Health and Disease.* Philadelphia: W. B. Saunders Co., 1984.

Smith, E. L. "Exercise for Prevention of Osteoporosis: A Review." *Physician and Sportsmedicine* 10(1982):72.

Stillman, R. J. "Physical Activity and Bone Mineral Content in Women Aged 30 to 85 Years." *Medicine and Science in Sports and Exercise* 18(1986):576.

Stone, W. J. "Exercise and Long-Term CV Risk Reduction in Corporate Executives." *Health Education* 14(1983):26.

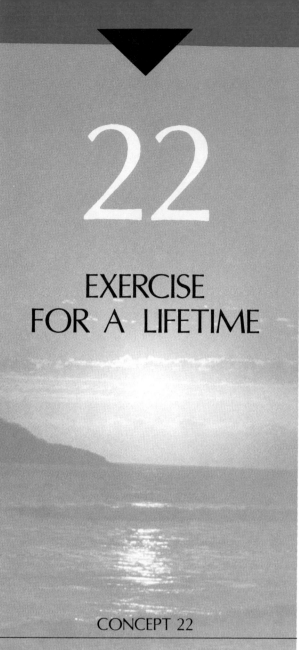

22

EXERCISE FOR A LIFETIME

CONCEPT 22

Exercise can contribute to physical fitness, good health, and an improved quality of life for people of all ages.

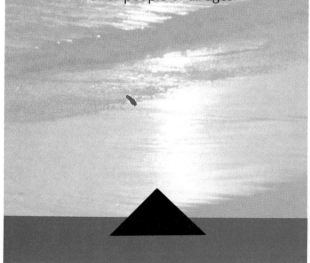

INTRODUCTION

In our culture, some think activity is only appropriate for children and youth. Yet research evidence indicates that *all people need* regular physical activity.

TERMS

Acquired Aging—The acquisition of characteristics commonly associated with aging but which are, in fact, caused by immobility or inactivity.

Time-Dependent Aging—The loss of function resulting from growing older.

THE FACTS: PHYSICAL ACTIVITY FOR CHILDREN

The risk factors associated with hypokinetic disease begin to develop very early in life.

The most recent research evidence indicates that the risk factors of such hypokinetic conditions as coronary heart disease and back pain begin to evidence themselves very early in life. Fat deposits on the walls of the arteries have been found in school-age children, and too many children are overfat. Tests of the fitness components that promote good posture and a healthy back show that a large percentage of children are physically unfit. This is, in part, due to the fact that children are not as active as you might expect. All children do *not* voluntarily engage in vigorous activity. Usually, the children most likely to need exercise are the ones most likely to avoid it.

Children, even very young children, are quite capable of vigorous physical activity. However, the optimal time for development of high levels of health-related fitness occurs after adolescence.

Children can exercise regularly. The typical child needs several hours of large muscle activity daily. For their body size, children can perform as well as young adults, but should not be expected to compete with adolescents and young adults (because of their smaller size and because they are not mature emotionally).

A healthy child cannot physiologically injure his or her heart with physical exercise.

Parents should not be concerned about the old wives' tale suggesting that exercise for children will result in heart damage. Research has dispelled this myth. At the same time, children are not miniature adults and programs of exercise for health-related fitness, including cardiovascular fitness, should be designed to meet both the physical and psychological needs and interests of children. Too much too soon may breed dislike for any type of physical activity.

Children should be exposed to a wide variety of physical activities in order to establish a basis for a lifetime of activity.

Recent research indicates that nearly all Americans have had some physical education during their school years. Nevertheless, less than 40 percent of all schoolchildren have physical education in the elementary school. Most skills are learned by age twelve or by the end of the sixth grade. For this reason, it is important that children *not* specialize in one activity too early, thus allowing more time to learn as many activities as possible during the school years. Just as a child learning to read must first learn the alphabet and grammar, the child should be exposed to many fundamental activities relating to physical fitness early in life so that he or she can take advantage of more than one lifetime activity in adulthood.

Certain types of activities, particularly weight training and weight lifting, are not recommended for preadolescents.

Although there is evidence that children can build muscle as a result of overload training, the best current information suggests that this type of training program should start after bone growth is relatively complete.

THE FACTS: PHYSICAL ACTIVITY FOR THE ADOLESCENT

Like children, adolescents are often physically unfit.

During the teen years, the potential for health-related fitness improvement is great. However, the results of physical fitness tests indicate that many teenagers never achieve optimal fitness levels. Regular exercise and sound nutrition is especially important during this age period.

Exercise contributes the most dramatic improvements in health-related physical fitness during adolescence.

During adolescence, hormonal changes occur that promote dramatic increases in cardiovascular fitness and strength with regular exercise. Fitness in both boys and girls can improve significantly at this age with regular exercise.

Adolescence is a time when the social aspects of sports competition and participation can provide great satisfaction for both the participant and the spectator.

Because adolescence is a social age, and because sports and sporting events are social experiences, sports can be a significant part of adolescent life. However, for a lifetime of exercise, the adolescent should be encouraged to become involved in sports as a participant, not only as a spectator.

Adolescence is a good time to refine lifetime sports skills.

Most skills are learned during childhood, but during adolescence lifetime sports skills are refined. Adolescents acquire the health-related, as well as the skill-related, fitness necessary to refine and become efficient in sports skills. They should be exposed to a variety of skills that can be used for a lifetime.

THE FACTS: PHYSICAL ACTIVITY FOR ADULTS (AGE 17 PLUS)

It is during young adulthood that the greatest potential for high level fitness and physical performance exists.

For many people, "their best level of fitness" will be achieved during the school years because they become less active after this time. However, with continued regular exercise, fitness and performance will reach peak levels in the young adult years.

The activity level of adults does more than contribute to personal fitness.

Parents who are active are more likely to have fit and active children than parents who are sedentary. The regular activity in which adults engage is important to personal fitness, but also appears to promote active lifestyles among children. Active-women role models are especially important for young girls.

Most limitations on adults concerning exercise are self-imposed.

Of those who do not exercise regularly, it is their own lack of fitness from years of inactivity that makes them feel unable to participate. While one of five American adults has been told by a physician to exercise, rarely does a physician suggest inactivity except for short periods of time for a specific ailment.

The "weekend" adult athlete may create, rather than solve, exercise problems.

A "weekend athlete" exercises, sometimes vigorously, only on the weekend. This person may avoid exercise during the "busy" weekdays and attempt to "make up" for a week of inactivity on Saturday or Sunday. To be effective, exercise must be regular (at least three times a week). Vigorous exercise done only one day a week can be dangerous because the weekly exercise is not sufficient to produce improvements in fitness. Thus, the unfit person may be exercising when the body is unprepared.

Being "too busy" is not a good excuse for inactivity.

The most common reason for inactivity among adults is, "I can't take the time." If business or other obligations make such weekday activities as golf or tennis impossible, then walking, jogging, or calisthenics are appropriate. These activities take relatively little time, and if planned properly, can provide important fitness and health benefits. After the inactive person has had a heart attack or some other hypokinetic disease, he or she will have more free time than is really wanted. Exercise may be as important as food and, like meals, should be scheduled on a regular basis.

THE FACTS: PHYSICAL ACTIVITY FOR OLDER ADULTS

Adults are never "too old" to begin exercising.

Physical fitness for old age should begin in the early years in order to enjoy maximum benefits. If this does not occur for one reason or another, a person is never too old to begin exercising. Studies conducted over a period of years indicate that properly planned exercise for older people is not only safe, but that older men and women are *not* significantly different from youth in their abilities to improve fitness through exercise.

Regular exercise can significantly delay the aging process.

Though exercise cannot stop aging, at least one researcher suggests that "exercise is the closest thing to an antiaging pill now available" (Butler 1975, p. 67). Another indicates that continued mental and physical activity is ". . . the only antidote for aging that I know" (Klump 1975, p. 93).

*There is a difference between **acquired aging** and **time-dependent aging**.*

Forced inactivity in young adults can cause losses in function (acquired aging) very much like those that are generally considered to occur with aging (time-dependent aging). Studies suggest that acquired aging is a product of a sedentary lifestyle. In Africa, Asia, and South America, where older adults (age sixty-five and older) maintain an active lifestyle, individuals do not "acquire" many of the characteristics commonly associated with aging.

In our culture, middle-aged and older people are encouraged (and sometimes compelled) to reduce their physical activity to the extent that they cannot continue to function on their own.

In our society, the attitude toward older people is often one of overprotection, placing the person in a dependent position. Physical fitness can enhance the quality of life for the elderly by increasing independence. The ability to go places and do things without being dependent on others is very important. It has been suggested that "we don't stop exercising because we get old, we get old because we stop exercising."

Participation in regular activity has benefits other than improved physical health and fitness.

A general feeling of well-being is frequently reported to be one real benefit of regular fitness for older people. Nervous tension, which detracts from the feeling of well-being, is a problem for many older adults. One recent study showed that exercise can be more effective than tranquilizers in the treatment of nervous tension in older people.

Participation in regular physical activity has many physical health benefits for the older adult.

In addition to the health benefits exercise promotes, which have already been presented in this book, older people can enjoy other benefits from regular physical activity.

1. "The syndrome of shaky hand and tottery gait is responsible in a large degree for much of the dependency of the aged. The treatment (for this condition) is physical exercise" (Swartz, 1975, p. 7). Merely fifteen minutes of exercise a day will not do it, rather there must be a shift from a sedentary to an active lifestyle.
2. Active older adults have fewer illnesses and fewer early deaths than do those who are inactive.
3. Reductions in physical working capacity, which is the most obvious result of aging, does not occur in older men who engage in regular exercise.
4. Regular exercise can help older adults in the "war with gravity." With time, if muscles are not kept fit, gravity can cause a "bay window" or protruding abdomen, sagging shoulders, poor posture, and joint immobility. These problems result from lack of strength, muscular endurance, and flexibility, but can be forestalled with regular activity.
5. Bones that are not used tend to decalcify. Regular exercise for older adults can delay bone decalcification.
6. Regular exercise can forestall the decline in circulatory function. In addition, increases in atherosclerosis, blood pressure, and EKG abnormalities that occur with age can be prevented with appropriate, regular exercise.
7. Decreased skeletal muscle, gain in body fat, decrease in oxygen-use capacity, and decreased respiratory function can be postponed with regular exercise.

Older adults can participate in a variety of sports and physical activity.

It has been shown that with appropriate, progressively maintained exercise, older adults can participate in most sports for a lifetime. For example, one eighty-five-year-old man regularly plays handball. The increased participation in masters (over fifty) classifications in track and field, swimming, and tennis are well documented. Golf is an activity well suited for older Americans and is good for promoting fitness if the participant walks. For those who do not wish to choose a sport, walking, jogging, bicycle riding, swimming, and calisthenics are forms of physical activity widely used by people of all ages.

REFERENCES

*American Academy of Pediatrics. "Weight Training and Weight Lifting: Information for the Pediatrician." *Physician and Sportsmedicine* 11(1983):157.

Bar-Or, O. *Pediatric Sports Medicine.* New York: Springer-Verlag, 1983.

Butler, R. N. "Psychological Importance of Physical Fitness." *Testimony on the Physical Fitness of Older People.* Washington, D.C.: National Association for Human Development, 1975.

*Corbin, C. B., ed. *A Textbook of Motor Development.* 2d ed. Dubuque, IA: Wm. C. Brown Publishers, 1980.

Corbin, D. E., and J. Metal-Corbin. *Reach for It! A Handbook of Exercise and Dance for Older Adults.* Dubuque, Iowa: Eddie Bowers and Co., 1983.

Gilliam, T. B., et al. "Physical Activity Patterns Determined by Heart Rate Monitoring in 6–7-Year-Old Children." *Medicine and Science in Sports and Exercise* 13(1981):65.

*Gilliam, T. B. "Exercise Programs for Children: A Way to Prevent Heart Disease?" *Physician and Sportsmedicine* 10(1982):96.

Gorman, D., and B. Brown. "Fitness and Aging: An Overview." JOPERD 57(1986):50.

Hazzard, W. "Preventative Gerontology: Strategies for Healthy Aging." *Postgraduate Medicine* 72(1983):279.

Hollozy, J. O. "Exercise, Health, and Aging: A Need for More Information." *Medicine and Science in Sports and Exercise* 15(1983):1.

Klump, F. "Physical Activities and Older Americans." *Testimony on the Physical Fitness of Older People.* Washington, D.C.: National Association for Human Development, 1975.

Londeree, B. R., and M. L. Moeschberger. "Effects of Age and Other Factors on Maximal Heart Rate." *Research Quarterly for Exercise and Sports* 53(1983):297.

Montoye, H. J., et al. "Bone Mineralization in Tennis Players." *Scandinavian Journal of Sport Science* 2(1980):26.

Ostrow, A. C. *Physical Activity and the Older Adult.* Princeton: Princeton Book Co., 1984.

Pangrazi, R. P., et al. "From Theory to Practice: A Summary." *Motor Development: Theory into Practice.* Monograph 3(1981):65.

Research and Forecasts, Inc. *The Miller Lite Report on American Attitudes toward Sports.* Milwaukee: Miller Brewing Co., 1983.

Sager, K. "Exercise to Activate Seniors." *Physician and Sportsmedicine* 12(1984):144.

Smith, E. L., and S. L. Zook. "The Aging Process: Benefits of Physical Activity." *Journal of Physical Education, Recreation and Dance* 57(1986):32.

Spirduso, W. W. "Exercise and the Aging Brain." *Research Quarterly for Exercise and Sports* 54(1983):208.

*Stovas, J. "Seniors Walk Away from Sedentary Life." *Physician and Sportsmedicine* 12(1984):22.

Swartz, F. C. "Statement on Physical Fitness and the Elderly." *Testimony on the Physical Fitness of Older People.* Washington, D.C.: National Association for Human Development, 1975.

PLANNING FOR FITNESS

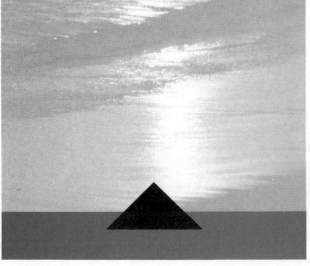

23

ENJOYING EXERCISE

CONCEPT 23

Exercise is for everyone.
No matter who you are, there is some
form of exercise that you can enjoy.

INTRODUCTION

Many adults are now participating in a variety of physical activities on a regular basis. However, roughly 64 million American adults over the age of eighteen do not exercise during their leisure time. Of those who are active, many spend only a few minutes a week participating in some activity. One reason is that many do not enjoy exercise; they feel that it is "just not for them."

All people, regardless of age, gender, or ability, can enjoy exercise if they carefully choose activities, carefully perform the activities, and follow some basic guidelines for making physical activities fun.

TERMS

Catharsis—The release or purifying of emotions; in this book, the release of stress and tension.
Mental Practice—Imagining the performance of a skill without physically performing it.
Overlearning—Practicing a skill over and over many times in an attempt to make the skill a "habit."
"Paralysis by Analysis"—Overanalysis of skill behavior. This occurs when more information is supplied than the performer can really use or when concentration on too many details of a skill results in interference with performance.
Skill Analysis—Breaking the performance of a skill into component parts and critically evaluating each phase of the performance.

THE FACTS

Those who are prepared for exercise are likely to enjoy it.

If you are sore, injured, or afraid of irritating a medical problem, exercise can become something to fear rather than something to enjoy. It is especially important to be well prepared for exercise. Review the information in Concept 4 to make sure you are well prepared before you begin regular exercise. Consider the following factors: be medically ready, start slowly, warm up before and cool down after exercise, and dress properly.

Having a "positive" attitude may enhance exercise enjoyment.

As noted in Concept 1, there are many reasons people do and do not exercise regularly. Earlier you assessed your own feelings concerning physical activity. You may want to reassess them at this time (Lab 23). If you can determine the reasons you especially enjoy activity, you can focus on them, and if you can determine those things you dislike about exercise, you may be able to change your attitudes so that active participation is more enjoyable. All people do not exercise for the same reasons. Consider your feelings about physical activity as you select activities as part of your exercise program.

Selecting "personalized" physical activities can help make exercise more enjoyable.

There is no such thing as a single best activity for all people. Everyone has different abilities and feelings about exercise. There are, however, some factors that are useful in selecting personalized activities *just* for you.

1. *Some people especially enjoy social activities.* If you are a social person, you may want to consider group activities. In fact, exercising in a group can sometimes help motivate you. Friends can encourage each other and make exercise something to enjoy.

2. *Competition may or may not make exercise fun.* Some people especially enjoy competition. Others, however, avoid competitive activities because they have not had success in competitive games. Whatever the benefits of regular physical activity, none should be exaggerated to the point of detracting from a fuller life. Overemphasis on sports can cause anxiety and even neurosis. In fact, people who create stress for themselves by being excessively competitive may increase their chances of getting stress-related diseases.

3. *Variety may enhance exercise enjoyment.* Some people enjoy doing the same basic activities day in and day out, year after year. Others like a change from time to time. You may want to consider a variety of activities to keep your exercise interesting.

4. *Self-criticism may reduce exercise enjoyment.* If an activity makes you angry with yourself, it may decrease your enjoyment of the activity. Improving your skills may reduce self-criticism. Selecting an activity that requires less skill may also reduce self-criticism. Jogging/running, walking, cycling, swimming, and home calisthenics are quite popular because they do not take a great amount of physical skill, and they do not produce as much self-criticism as other activities. Remember that most people are far more critical of their own abilities than they are of the abilities of others.

5. *What "feels good" to others may not "feel good" to you.* Choose an activity that feels good to YOU. Sometimes you find yourself doing those things others do, or others want you to do. You should, however, select activities that feel good to you, regardless of what others do.

A person does not have to be a "great" performer to enjoy sports and physical activity for a lifetime.

Many Americans discontinue participation in physical activity as they get older because they "are not very good at sports." There are many different types of sports and activities and each requires different abilities.

Failure in the past does not mean that you cannot find enjoyment in sports in the future. Some activities require coordination; some require agility and balance; while others may require health-related physical fitness, such as cardiovascular fitness, strength, and flexibility; and still others require daring or ability to use strategy.

Skill proficiency in a sport and selection of a partner of similar ability are both important for the enjoyment of the sporting experience.

Those who have some skill in an activity are more likely to participate in that activity than those with little or no skill. For this reason, it is advisable to practice and perhaps seek instruction to enhance enjoyment of a lifetime activity. People with greater skill are more likely to get involved because they are more likely to be successful. However, there is another way to increase satisfaction from sports participation. Research indicates that you must be 65 to 75 percent as good as your partner if either of you is to enjoy the activity. For this reason, it is not only advisable to improve your skills, but you should find a playing partner or group of similar ability.

There are certain guidelines that can be followed to help you learn and enjoy lifetime sports and physical activities.

1. *When learning a new activity, concentrate on the "general idea" of the skill first; worry about details later.* For example, a diver who concentrates on pointing the toes and keeping the legs straight at the end of a "flip" may land flat on his or her back. To make it "all the way over," he or she should concentrate on merely doing the flip. When the general idea is *mastered,* then concentrate on details.

2. *The beginner should be careful not to emphasize too many details at one time.* After the general idea of the skill is learned, the learner can begin to focus on the details, one or two at a time. Concentration on too many details at one time may result in **paralysis by analysis.** For example, a golfer who is told to keep the head down, the left arm straight, and the knees bent, cannot possibly concentrate on all of these details at once. As a result, neither the details nor the general idea of the golf swing are performed properly.

3. *In the early stages of learning a lifetime sport or physical activity, it is not wise to engage in competition.* Beginners who compete are likely to concentrate on "beating their opponent" rather than on learning a skill properly. For example, in bowling, the beginner may abandon the newly learned hook ball in favor of the "sure thing" straight ball. This may make the person more successful immediately, but is not likely to improve the person's bowling skills for the future.

4. *To be performed well, lifetime sports skills must be **overlearned**.* Oftentimes, when you learn a new activity, you begin to "play the game" immediately. The best way to learn a skill is to overlearn it, or practice it until it becomes "habit." Frequently, game situations do not allow you to overlearn skills. For example, it is not a good time to learn the tennis serve during a game because there may be only a few opportunities to serve. For the beginner, it would be much more productive to hit many services (overlearn) with a friend until the general idea of the serve is well learned at least. Further, the beginner *should not* sacrifice speed to concentrate on serving for accuracy. Accuracy will come with practice of a properly performed skill.

5. *Once the general idea of a **skill** is learned, an **analysis** of the performance may be helpful.* Be careful not to overanalyze; it may be helpful to have a knowledgeable person help you locate strengths and weaknesses. Movies and videotapes of performances have been shown to be of help to learners.

6. *When "unlearning" an old (incorrect) skill and learning a new (correct) skill, a person's performance may get worse before it gets better.* Frequently, a performer hopes to unlearn a "bad habit" so as to be able to "relearn" the new or correct skill. For example, a golfer with a "baseball swing" may want to learn the correct golf swing. It is important for the learner to understand that the score may worsen during the relearning stage. As the new skill is overlearned, skill will improve, as will the golf score.

7. ***Mental practice** may aid skill learning.* Mental practice may benefit performance of motor skills, especially if the performer has had previous experience in performing the skill. Mental practice might be used for golf, tennis, and other sports when the performer cannot participate regularly because of weather, business, or lack of time.

8. *For beginners, practicing in front of other people may be detrimental to learning a skill.* Research indicates that an audience may inhibit the beginner's learning of a new sports skill. This is especially true if the learner feels that his or her performance is being evaluated by someone in the audience.

Women can enjoy and benefit from the same activities as men.

In the past, many sports and physical activities were considered appropriate for men only. The benefits of regular exercise are similar for men and women, so there is no reason why both cannot choose to become involved in enjoyable activities.

To enjoy physical activities, give yourself a chance to succeed.

Some people avoid exercise because they see it as a source of failure. If done properly, anyone can succeed in exercise. As already noted, practice and becoming skilled in an activity can enhance your chances of success. Some other suggestions are listed here.

1. *Set realistic goals for yourself.* Set small and realistic goals at first. Gradually increase your expectations, but only after your performance increases. If you set your goals too high, you increase the chances of failure.

2. *Do not equate success with winning.* Sports psychologists agree that one problem experienced by many adults is that they cannot enjoy competitive activities unless they win. Though most people enjoy winning, it must be realized that only 50 percent of the participants in most activities can win. Playing well and enjoying the sport also makes you a "winner."

3. *Avoid comparing yourself and your accomplishments to those of other people.*

4. *Consider long-term improvement over time as a successful accomplishment.*

5. *Try using a handicap system when competing with those of unequal skill.* Such systems as those used in golf and bowling can be adapted for other activities to help "even up" the competition.

The "psychological benefits" of exercise can be a source of enjoyment to those who exercise.

Although some studies have indicated that participation in highly competitive athletics may not contribute to character development or good sportsmanship, there is evidence that those who are involved in regular exercise throughout life reap both social and emotional benefits. Some psychological benefits are presented in Concepts 2 and 3, others are listed here.

1. Participation in physical activity can provide a **catharsis,** or emotional release, from the pent-up tensions of regular, daily activity.

2. Physically fit individuals are more likely to try new leisure time activities, which can provide for a meaningful social life.

3. Those who exercise regularly are more likely to have good physical health, which in turn contributes to good mental health.

4. As noted in a previous concept, people who suffer from psychological depression can benefit from regular exercise. Regular exercise and fitness are associated with a sense of well-being. If you exercise regularly, you can develop what some call a "positive addiction" to exercise. A positive addiction is a need to do something for which the consequences are positive.

Movement has meaning.

Movement is a means to many ends. Through movement, you perform work, achieve health and physical fitness, and accomplish other useful objectives. However, movement can be an end in itself. Those who have performed a dance, played a game, or jogged a mile realize that the mere performance of any of these tasks is an accomplishment in itself. Movement and physical activity do not always have to be purposeful; you can derive satisfaction merely from your involvement in a movement experience.

▶ LAB RESOURCE MATERIALS (FOR USE WITH LAB 23, PAGE 279)

CHART 23.1 The Physical Activity Questionnaire

The term "physical activity" in the following statements refers to all kinds of activities, including sports, formal exercises, and informal activities, such as jogging and cycling. Check your answers first, and then read the directions for scoring at the end of the questionnaire.

	Strongly Agree	Agree	Undecided	Disagree	Strongly Disagree	Score
1. Doing regular physical activity can be as harmful to health as it is helpful.	☐	☐	☐	☐	☐	———
2. One of the main reasons I do regular physical activity is because it is fun.	☐	☐	☐	☐	☐	———
3. Participating in physical activities makes me tense and nervous.	☐	☐	☐	☐	☐	———
4. The challenge of physical training is one reason why I participate in physical activity.	☐	☐	☐	☐	☐	———
5. One of the things I like about physical activity is the participation with other people.	☐	☐	☐	☐	☐	———
6. Doing regular physical activity does little to make me more physically attractive.	☐	☐	☐	☐	☐	———
7. Competition is a good way to keep a game from being fun.	☐	☐	☐	☐	☐	———
8. I should exercise regularly for my own good health and physical fitness.	☐	☐	☐	☐	☐	———
9. Doing exercise and playing sports is boring.	☐	☐	☐	☐	☐	———
10. I enjoy taking part in physical activity because it helps me to relax and get away from the pressures of daily living.	☐	☐	☐	☐	☐	———
11. Most sports and physical activities are too difficult for me to enjoy.	☐	☐	☐	☐	☐	———
12. I do not enjoy physical activities that require the participation of other people.	☐	☐	☐	☐	☐	———
13. Regular exercise helps me to look my best.	☐	☐	☐	☐	☐	———
14. Competing against others in physical activities makes them enjoyable.	☐	☐	☐	☐	☐	———

Score the physical activity questionnaire as follows:

1. For items 1, 3, 6, 7, 9, 11, and 12 give one point for strongly agree, two for agree, three for undecided, four for disagree, and five for strongly disagree. Put the correct number in the blank to the right of these statements.
2. For items 2, 4, 5, 8, 10, 13, and 14 give five points for strongly agree, four for agree, three for undecided, two for disagree, and one for strongly disagree. Put the correct number in the blank to the right of each statement.
3. Determine each of the following seven scores by adding the numbers to the right of the items listed here (two numbers for each score).

Score

a. Health and fitness score   Item 1 _____ + Item 8 _____ = _____

b. Fun and enjoyment score   Item 2 _____ + Item 9 _____ = _____

c. Relaxation and tension release score   Item 3 _____ + Item 10 _____ = _____

d. Challenge and achievement score   Item 4 _____ + Item 11 _____ = _____

e. Social score   Item 5 _____ + Item 12 _____ = _____

f. Appearance score   Item 6 _____ + Item 13 _____ = _____

g. Competition score   Item 7 _____ + Item 14 _____ = _____

Total Score _____

4. Determine your total score by adding each of the previous seven scores. Write your total score in the bottom blank.
5. Use Chart 23.2 to determine your rating on each score.

CHART 23.2 Physical Activity Questionnaire *Rating Scale*

Classification	Each of Seven Scores	Total Score
Excellent	9–10	63–70
Good	7–8	50–62
Fair	6	42–49
Poor	4–5	30–41
Very Poor	3 or Less	29 or Less

REFERENCES

Appengeller, O. "What Makes Us Run?" Editorial, *New England Journal of Medicine* 305(1983):578.

Chalip, L., et al. "Variations of Experience in Formal and Informal Sport." *Research Quarterly for Exercise and Sport* 55(1984):109.

Corbin, C. B. "Self-Confidence of Women in Sports." In *Clinics in Sports Medicine: Women in Sports,* edited by W. M. Walsh. Philadelphia: W. B. Saunders Co., 1984.

*Corbin, C. B., and R. Lindsey. *The Ultimate Fitness Book.* New York: Leisure Press, 1984.

Csikszentmihaliyi, M. "The Value of Sports." In *Sports in Perspective,* edited by J. T. Parlington et al. Ottawa: Coaching Association of Canada, 1982.

Dishman, R. K. "Exercise Compliance: A New View for Public Health." In *Physicians and Sportsmedicine* 14(May 1986):127.

Eliot, R. S., and D. L. Breo. *Is It Worth Dying For?* New York: Bantam, 1984.

*Glasser, W. *Positive Addiction.* New York: Harper and Row, 1976.

Gruger, C. E., C. B. Corbin, and A. B. Nielsen, et al. "General Commitment to Physical Activity." In *Exercise Physiology.* New York: AMS Press, Inc., 1986.

Little, J. C. "The Athlete's Neurosis: A Deprivation Crisis." In *Psychology of Running,* edited by M. H. Sacks and M. L. Sacks. Champaign, Ill.: Human Kinetics, 1981.

Mehrabran, A., and M. L. Bekken. "Temperament Characteristics of Individuals Who Participate in Strenuous Sports." *Research Quarterly for Exercise and Sports* 57(1986):160.

Research and Forecasts, Inc. *The Miller Lite Report on American Attitudes toward Sports.* Milwaukee: Miller Brewing Co., 1983.

Riddle, P. K. "Attitudes, Beliefs, Behavioral Intentions and Behaviors of Women and Men toward Regular Jogging." *Research Quarterly for Exercise and Sports* 51(1980):663.

Rossman, J. R. "Participant Satisfaction with Employees Recreation." *Journal of Physical Education, Recreation and Dance* 54(1983):60.

Slava, S., D. R. Laurie, and C. B. Corbin. "The Long-Term Effects of a Conceptual Physical Education Program." *Research Quarterly for Exercise and Sports* 55(1984):161.

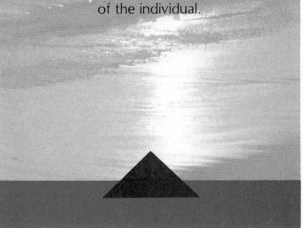

24

PLANNING YOUR EXERCISE PROGRAM

CONCEPT 24

In order to get maximal benefits from exercise, it is essential that a regular progressive program be planned to meet the specific needs of the individual.

INTRODUCTION

There is no single exercise program best suited to all people. In planning an exercise program it is important to consider your own unique needs and interests. Five steps to fitness program development are presented within this concept to aid you in your planning.

THE FACTS

There are five steps that should be considered in planning your personal exercise program.

Step 1—Identify your personal physical fitness needs.
If you have no medical problems, the first step in program planning is to test your physical fitness on each of the health-related components. Information concerning self-testing and physical fitness rating standards are presented in Lab 6D (cardiovascular fitness); Labs 8A and 8B (strength); Lab 9 (muscular endurance); Lab 11 (flexibility); Labs 13A and 13B (body composition); Labs 18A and 18B (posture and care of the back); and Lab 15 (skill-related physical fitness).

Fill out the physical fitness profile charts in Lab 24 (charts 24.1 and 24.2, pp. 282–283). These charts will help you identify your fitness strengths and weaknesses. This information can be used to help you select activities for your personal exercise program.

Step 2—Select the activities for your personal fitness program, including those that build all components of physical fitness.
Exercise is an excellent way to achieve physical fitness and one means of attaining good health. However, not all physical activities and exercises are good for developing physical fitness. Once you know what your fitness needs are, make sure you are aware of the facts concerning the kinds of exercise best suited to your personal needs.

To be sure that the exercises you select are safe, consult Concepts 4, 18, and 25. To be sure that the activities you select are done often enough (frequency), hard enough (intensity), and long enough (time) to build all parts of fitness, consult Concepts 6, 8, 9, 10, 11, and 13. Information concerning different exercise programs is included in Concepts 7, 10, 12, 16, and 18. The tables that summarize the specific fitness values of different activities will be especially valuable as you try to decide which exercise programs are best for your personal needs (see table 7.2 on p. 59; table 16.1 on p. 143; and table 16.3).

After reviewing these tables, write down all the activities you currently do on a regular basis. Next, write down a list of activities (new ones) that would be especially good for developing those components of fitness in which you need improvement. Use chart 24.3 on page 283 to write down the activities you plan to do.

Include activities from each of the following three areas: (1) activities you currently do; (2) new activities for specific aspects of fitness; and (3) activities you especially enjoy doing. It is important to include activities that build all parts of fitness, and also some that you simply enjoy doing. The best program in the world is not good unless you do it. If you don't enjoy it, you won't do it. You may want to check Concept 23 to get some ideas for making exercise more enjoyable.

Remember, no single activity can meet all your needs. Make sure you select exercise to build each of the physical fitness components.

Step 3—Write it down. Make up a personal weekly exercise program.

You are more likely to do your exercise program if you write it down. A sample weekly exercise program for a young adult is shown here. The Weekly Exercise Program on page 284 provides you with a chart just like the sample. Using the chart, write out a weekly personal exercise schedule. Be sure you give a specific day and time for each of the activities you listed in step 2.

Step 4—Do it.

Regularity is one of the keys to the success of an exercise program. A "hit or miss" program may turn into no program at all. From the beginning, set aside a specific time and place for your activity. Place a high priority on your exercise time. Don't allow anything to interrupt your exercise schedule. Build your exercise into your daily routine; make it as much a habit as taking a bath or eating regular meals. It is recommended that some form of exercise be done five to six days a week; three days should be the minimum.

Step 5—Periodically evaluate and modify your program.

The weekly program you wrote down in step 3 may be an excellent one. However, as time goes by, your needs, interests, and other factors change. For this reason, you should periodically evaluate and revise your personal program. If you become bored with certain activities, you may wish to drop them and add other new and interesting activities. Changes in the weather, the availability of facilities, and personal schedules may all require program changes. Each time you change your program, follow steps 1 through 4. It is not necessary to do the same program forever; the key is to have a program that meets your current needs and interests.

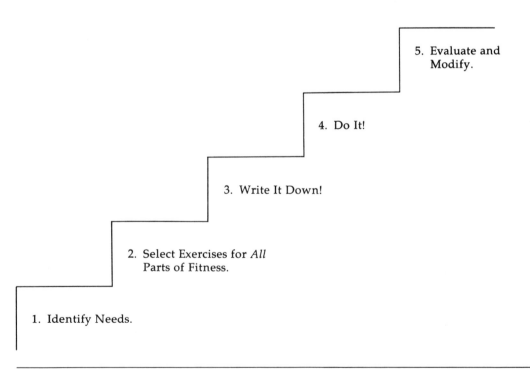

FIGURE 24.1 Five Steps of Program Planning

WEEKLY EXERCISE PROGRAM

Daily Schedules
(List the activities and times of day for each activity.)

Monday	Tuesday	Wednesday
7:00 a.m. "Special exercises" 5:30 p.m. Warm-up racquetball	7:00 a.m. "Special exercises" 12:30 p.m. Walk after lunch 5:30 p.m. Weight training (30 minutes)	7:00 a.m. "Special exercises" 5:30 p.m. Warm-up racquetball

Thursday	Friday	Saturday
7:00 a.m. "Special exercises" 12:30 p.m. Walk after lunch 5:30 p.m. Weight training (30 minutes)	7:00 a.m. "Special exercises" 12:30 p.m. Walk after lunch	afternoon – walk or swim Weight training (30 minutes)

Sunday	Warm-Up and Cool-Down Activities	Program Evaluation (Fill in after trying out your program.)
"Special exercises" when I get up. Other exercise if I have no other plans. If I can find a partner I may take lessons.	Calf stretcher toe touch leg hug side stretch two-minute walk **Special Exercises** sit-ups (bent knee) pectoral stretch Billig's exercise contract-relax routine before bed when I am tense	This seems to be working pretty well. I find I actually walk rather than swim because it is inconvenient to go to the pool. I am taking tennis lessons.

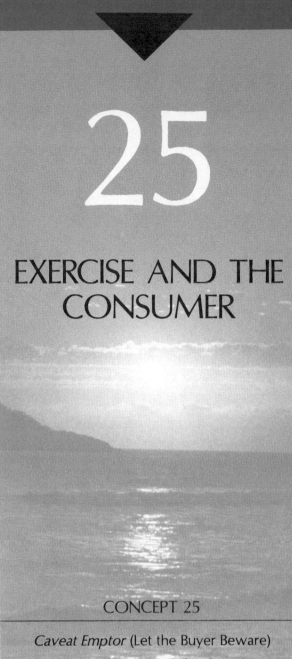

25

EXERCISE AND THE CONSUMER

CONCEPT 25

Caveat Emptor (Let the Buyer Beware)

is a good motto for the

consumer seeking advice

or a program for

developing or maintaining fitness.

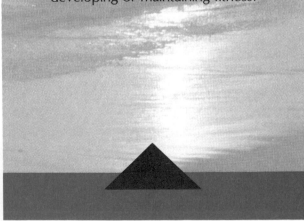

INTRODUCTION

People have always searched for the fountain of youth and the "easy," the "quick," and the "miraculous" route to health and happiness. This search has included the area of physical fitness, especially exercise and weight loss. Because of the popularity of these two subjects, the mass media have made it possible to convey as much *misinformation* as information. All people should seek the truth to protect their health as well as their pocketbooks. This concept discusses some myths and separates fact from fancy (also review Concepts 14 and 19 regarding drugs and supplements).

TERMS

AMA—Abbreviation for the American Medical Association.

Expert (in exercise and physical fitness)—person who has a degree(s) in physical education, exercise physiology, physical therapy, or corrective therapy from an accredited university and has specialized in exercise prescription and physical fitness.

FDA—Abbreviation for the Food and Drug Administration: A federal agency that recommends and enforces government regulations regarding certain foods and drugs.

Panacea—A cure-all; a remedy for all ills.

Passive—A type of exercise in which no voluntary muscle contraction occurs; some outside force moves the body part with no effort by the person.

Tonus—The most frequently misused and abused term in fitness vocabularies. It is "the resistance (tension) developed in a muscle as a result of passive stretch of a muscle. Tonus can not be determined by palpation or inspection of a muscle and has little or nothing to do with the voluntary strength of a muscle" (DeLateur, 1982).

FACTS ABOUT EXERCISE

*Exercise has many benefits, but is not a **panacea**.*

There are numerous benefits of exercise, many of which have been described throughout this book. However, some media accounts would have you believe the impossible. Those who contemplate beginning a fitness or weight reducing program are reminded of the following items:

1. The most satisfactory way to lose weight is to combine caloric reduction and exercise.
2. Exercise will *not* change the size of boney structures (e.g., ankles).

3. Exercise will *not* change the size of glands (e.g., breasts), however, chest/bust girth may be increased by strengthening chest muscles.
4. Exercise does *not* break up fatty deposits, though it does burn calories, thus fat will eventually be burned.
5. Exercise does *not ensure* good posture or good health, but it does help attain or maintain these attributes.
6. There is *no* such thing as "effortless exercise."

Exercise, even of an active nature, is not effective in promoting physical fitness unless it meets the appropriate threshold of training.

Some popular literature suggests that only a few minutes of exercise a day are necessary to develop total physical fitness. Research, however, indicates that total fitness (cardiovascular fitness, strength, muscular endurance, flexibility, and desirable body composition) can be attained only through considerable effort. As mentioned previously, exercise must be of sufficient frequency (daily or every other day), intensity, and time (at least fifteen to thirty minutes *each* day you exercise) for it to be effective. Programs that "promise" complete fitness but do not meet the necessary levels for frequency, intensity, and time of exercise should be strongly questioned.

Contrary to some claims, Hatha Yoga is not a good program for developing physical fitness.

Some advocates of Hatha Yoga claim that regular practice of the asanas (positions) will bring about improved flexibility, grace, serenity, relaxation, sleep, vitality, endurance, circulation; strength and firmness of muscles; strength of vital organs and glands; taut, smooth skin; ideal body weight; recovery, alertness, and clarity of mind; cure arthritis, the common cold, diabetes, gallstones, menstrual disorders, piles; and maintain good vision and hearing.

There is no scientific evidence to support most of these claims. Hatha Yoga will not help you lose weight, trim inches, remove flab, improve endurance, maintain proper circulation, strengthen glands and organs, or improve complexion. Neither will it cure diseases.

Hatha Yoga is considered useful for improving flexibility, although some positions are contraindicated (see Concept 19). Hatha Yoga is also useful in reducing stress reactions and in promoting neuromuscular relaxation. In some cases, it may be effective in lowering blood pressure in hypertensives. If a person has very weak muscles to begin with, mild strengthening and muscular endurance may develop from assuming and holding the positions.

Getting rid of cellulite does not require a special exercise, diet, or device, as some books and advertisements insist.

Cellulite is ordinary fat with a fancy name. You do not need a special treatment, a special device, or a special anything to get rid of it. Fat is fat. To decrease fat, eat fewer calories and exercise more.

"Jarming" isn't the road to fitness for every one.

Exercising with the arms only (jarming) has increased in popularity. It may be useful for the frail elderly or for the convalescing or disabled person, but the best aerobic exercise uses both the arms and the legs. Cross-country skiing, rowing, and swimming are highly recommended.

The value of using hand weights while walking and running is still open to question.

The practice of carrying small weights in the hands while walking, jogging, or aerobic dancing has been commercialized recently with a subsequent increase in popularity. There is very little research on the benefits or hazards of this practice. Theoretically, the additional weight increases the energy cost of the exercise and therefore the cardiovascular benefits. It is possible, however, that the additional weight may make the person walk, run, or climb stairs more slowly, so the energy used may be the same or less than without the weights. There is also the possibility of injury created by the change in rhythm, timing, and mechanics of the movement. Some experts believe this will result in increased stress on the muscles and joints.

FACTS ABOUT PASSIVE EXERCISE AND PASSIVE DEVICES

Passive exercise is not effective in weight reduction, spot reduction, increasing strength, or increasing endurance.

Passive exercise or devices come in a variety of forms.

1. *Rolling machines*—These ineffective wooden or metal rollers, operated by an electric motor, roll up and down the body part to which they are applied. They do *not* remove, break up, or redistribute fat.
2. *Vibrating belts*—These wide canvas or leather belts may be designed for the chin, hips, thighs, or abdomen. Driven by an electric motor, they jerk back and forth causing loose tissue of the body part to shake. They do *not* have any beneficial effect on fitness, fat, or figure, and they are potentially harmful if used on the abdomen (especially if used by women during pregnancy, menstruation, or while an IUD is in place). They might also aggravate a back problem.
3. *Vibrating tables and pillows*—Contrary to advertisements, these passive devices will not improve posture, trim the body, reduce weight, or develop

muscle **tonus.** For some people, vibration can help induce relaxation.

4. *Motor-driven cycles and rowing machines*—Like all mechanical devices that "do the work" for the individual, these motor-driven machines are *not* effective in a fitness program. They may help increase circulation, and some may even help maintain flexibility, but they are not as effective as active exercise. *Nonmotorized* cycles and rowing machines are very good equipment for use in a fitness program.

5. *Massage*—Whether done by a masseur or by a mechanical device, massage is passive, requiring no effort on the part of the individual. It can help increase circulation, induce relaxation, prevent or loosen adhesions, and serve other therapeutic uses when administered in the clinical setting for medical reasons, but massage has *no* useful role in a physical fitness program and will not alter your shape.

6. *Electrical muscle stimulators*—These devices, when applied to a muscle, cause the muscle to contract involuntarily. In the hands of qualified medical personnel, muscle stimulators are valuable therapeutic devices. They should never be used by the layperson and have *no* place in a reducing or fitness program. They can help prevent atrophy in a patient who is unable to move, and they may decrease spasticity and contracture, but they will *not* change your figure/physique. These devices can be harmful and may induce heart attacks; complicate gastrointestinal, orthopedic, kidney, and other disorders; and aggravate epilepsy, hernias, and varicose veins.

7. *Weighted belts*—Claims have been made that these belts reduce waists, thighs, and hips when worn for several hours under the clothing. In reality, they do none of these things and have been reported to cause actual physical harm. When used in a progressive resistance program, wristlet, anklet, or laced-on weights can help produce an overload and, therefore, develop strength or endurance.

8. *Inflated, constricting, or nonporous garments*— These garments include rubberized inflated devices ("sauna belts" and "sauna shorts") and paraphernalia that are airtight plastic or rubberized. Evidence indicates that their girth-reducing claims are *unwarranted*. If exercise is performed while wearing such garments, the exercise, *not* the garment, may be beneficial. You can *not* squeeze fat out of the pores *nor* can you melt it!

9. *Figure wrapping*—Some reducing salons, gyms, or clubs advertise that wrapping the body in bandages soaked in a "magic solution" will cause a permanent reduction in body girth. This so-called "treatment" is pure quackery. Tight, constricting bands can temporarily indent the skin and squeeze body fluids into other parts of the body, but the skin or body will regain its original size within minutes or hours. This practice may be dangerous to your health; at least one fatality has resulted.

FACTS ABOUT BATHS

Sauna, steam, and whirlpool baths are not effective in weight reduction nor in the prevention and cure of colds, arthritis, bursitis, backaches, sprains, and bruises.

The effect of such baths is largely psychological, although some temporary relief from aches and pains may result from the heat. The same relief, though, can be had by sitting in a tub of hot water at home. Sauna and steam baths are potentially dangerous for the elderly and persons suffering from diabetes, heart disease, or high blood pressure. They should not be used within an hour after eating or while under the influence of alcohol or such drugs as anticoagulants, stimulants, hypnotics, narcotics, or tranquilizers. Baths do not melt off fat!

FACTS ABOUT QUACKS

You can usually tell the difference between an expert and a quack because a quack does not use scientific methods.

Some of the ways to identify quacks, frauds, and rip-offs is to look for these clues:

1. They do not use the scientific method of controlled experimentation that can be verified by other scientists.
2. To a large extent, they use testimonials and anecdotes to support their claims rather than scientific methods.
3. They advise you to buy something you would not otherwise have bought.
4. They have something to sell.
5. They claim *everyone* can benefit from the product or service they are selling.
6. They promise "quick," "miraculous" results.
7. They may claim there is a conspiracy against them by "bureaucrats," "organized medicine," the **FDA,** the **AMA,** and other experts and governmental bodies.
8. Their credentials may be irrelevant to the area in which they claim expertise.
9. They use scare tactics, such as "if you don't do this, you will die of a heart attack"; or they may switch to being a sympathetic friend who wants to share with you a "new discovery."

10. They may quote from a scientific journal or other legitimate source, but they misquote or quote out of context to mislead you; or they may mix a little bit of truth with a lot of fiction.
11. They may cite research or quote from individuals or institutions that have questionable reputations for scientific truth.
12. They may claim it is a "new discovery" (usually it is said to have originated in Europe).
13. The product or organization name is often similar to that of a famous person or creditable institution (e.g., the Mayo Diet had no connection with the Mayo Clinic).
14. They often sell products through the mail, which does not allow you to examine the product personally.

"Spot reducing," or losing fat from a specific location on the body, is not possible. It is a fallacy.

When you exercise, calories are burned and fat is recruited from all over the body in a genetically determined pattern. You can not selectively exercise, bump, vibrate, or squeeze the fat from a particular spot. If you were flabby to begin with, local exercise could strengthen the local muscles, causing a change in the contour and the girth of that body part. But exercise affects the muscles, not the fat on that body part. General aerobic exercises are the most effective for burning fat, but you cannot control where the fat comes off.

FACTS ABOUT EQUIPMENT

The consumer who plans to purchase equipment should keep in mind certain guidelines to get the most for the money.

The following suggestions will help you select equipment:

1. Unless you are wealthy or just like to collect gadgets, there is no need to buy a lot of exercise equipment. A complete fitness program can be carried out with *no* equipment. If you learn to depend upon equipment, you may eventually feel like you cannot exercise unless you are at home or at a gym.
2. If you do not like jogging or swimming, and you hate calisthenics, then the minimal equipment you may want to consider is a bicycle (regular or stationary), treadmill, or rowing machine for cardiovascular fitness; and a set of weights, pulleys, or isokinetic device for strength and endurance.
3. Consult an expert if you want to know the effectiveness of a product. Individuals with college or university degrees in physical education, physical therapy, corrective therapy, and exercise physiology should be able to give you good advice.

4. Buy from a well-established, reputable company that will not disappear overnight and will back up warranties. Avoid mail order products. If the product is not available in a retail store where it can be examined, you probably should not buy it.

FACTS ABOUT "HEALTH CLUBS"

It is not necessary to join a club, spa, or salon to develop fitness, but if you are considering joining such an establishment, make your choice with care.

The consumer should observe these precautions before becoming a member of a club, spa, or salon.

1. Do not expect "miraculous" results as advertised.
2. Be prepared to haggle over prices and to resist a very hard sell for a long-term contract.
3. Choose a no-contract, pay-as-you-go establishment if possible. Otherwise, choose the shortest term contract available.
4. If there is a contract, read the fine print carefully and look for:
   a. the interest rate;
   b. "confession of judgment" clauses waiving your right to defend yourself in court;
   c. noncancelable clauses;
   d. "holder-in-due-course" doctrines allowing the establishment to sell your note to a collection agency;
   e. a waiver of the establishment's liability for injury to you on the premises.
5. Consult with an independent expert if you have questions about the programs offered by the establishment.
6. Do not accept diets, drugs, or food supplements from the club. Your physician will prescribe these if they are needed.
7. You do not have to conform to the program the club suggests for you. Do not perform dangerous exercises, passive exercises, or participate in fraudulent "treatments." Choose only those activities that meet the criteria explained in this book.
8. Refuse to be pestered by solicitations for new members.
9. Make a trial visit to the establishment during the hours when you would normally expect to use the facility to determine if it is open, if it is overcrowded, if the equipment is available, if the attendants are selling rather than assisting, and if you would enjoy the company of the other patrons.
10. Determine the qualifications of the personnel, especially of the individual responsible for programming you. Are they an expert as defined previously?

11. Make certain the club is a well-established facility that will not disappear overnight.
12. Check its reputation with the Better Business Bureau in your area.
13. Investigate the programs offered by the Y, local colleges and universities, and municipal park and recreation departments. These agencies often have excellent fitness classes at lower prices than commercial establishments and usually employ qualified personnel. For weight loss, investigate franchised clubs, such as Weight Watchers or TOPS, or affiliate with a hospital-based program.

FACTS ABOUT FITNESS BOOKS, MAGAZINES, AND ARTICLES

All fitness books do not provide scientifically sound, accurate, and reliable information.

Because publishers are motivated by profit and publishing is a highly competitive field, the choice of material to be printed is often selected on the basis of how popular or famous or attractive the author is or how sensational or unusual his or her ideas are. Movie stars, models, TV personalities, and even Olympic athletes are rarely experts in biomechanics, anatomy and physiology, exercise, and other foundations of physical fitness. Having a good figure/physique, being fit, or having gone through a training program does not, in itself, qualify a person to advise others.

If you have read the facts presented in the previous concepts, you should be able to distinguish between fact and fiction. To assist you further, however, there are ten guidelines listed in question form, which might help you evaluate whether or not a book, magazine, or article on exercise and fitness is valid, reliable, and scientifically sound. If the answer to each of the questions is not "yes," then you should be suspicious of the material. If in doubt, ask one or more experts or write to the American Alliance of Health, Physical Education, Recreation and Dance (AAHPERD) or the American College of Sports Medicine (ACSM) (see addresses in list of references). These organizations will refer your question to an appropriate expert.

▶ LAB RESOURCE MATERIALS (FOR USE WITH LAB 25, PAGE 285)

CHART 25.1 Exercise Evaluation*

	Yes	No		Yes	No
1. Is the article or book written by an expert as defined in Concept 25?	☐	☐	7. Is it an "active" exercise in which your own muscles contract?	☐	☐
2. Does the exercise employ the overload principle?	☐	☐	8. Are the benefits claimed for the exercise reasonable?	☐	☐
3. Does it employ the progression principle?	☐	☐	9. Are the authors trying to help you (rather than selling a product)?	☐	☐
4. Does it employ the F.I.T. principle?	☐	☐	10. Do they refrain from using terms such as "quick," "miraculous," "tone," "remove fat," "new discovery," or other gimmick words?	☐	☐
5. Does it employ the principle of specificity?	☐	☐			
6. Is it a safe exercise? (See Concept 19.)	☐	☐			

*If in doubt, you may seek an expert's opinion on some of these questions.

REFERENCES

American Alliance of Health, Physical Education, Recreation and Dance, 1900 Association Drive, Reston, Va. 22091.

American College of Sports Medicine, P.O. Box 1440, Indianapolis, In. 46206-1440.

Barrett, S. *The Health Robbers.* Philadelphia: George F. Stickley Co., 1980.

Bennet, W., and J. Gurin. *The Dieter's Dilemma.* New York: Basic Books, 1982.

Berland, T., and Editors of *Consumer Guide. Rating the Diets.* Skokie, Ill.: *Consumer Guide,* 1974.

Cohen, J. C., et al. "Altered Serum Lipoprotein Profiles in Male and Female Power Lifters Ingesting Anabolic Steroids." *Physician and Sportsmedicine* 14:6(June 1986):131.

"Congressional Panel to F.D.A.: Get Tough with Medical-Device Makers." *Medical World News* (16 August 1982):15.

Consumer Union, *Health Quackery.* Orangeburg, N.Y.: Consumer Reports Books, 1980.

Corbin, C., and R. Lindsey. *The Ultimate Fitness Book.* Champaign, Ill.: Leisure Press, 1984.

Delateur, B. J. "Therapeutic Exercise to Develop Strength and Endurance." In *Krusen's Handbook of Physical Medicine and Rehabilitation,* edited by Kotlke, Stillman, and Lehman. 3d ed. Philadelphia: W. B. Saunders Co., 1982.

Fahey, T. D., et al. "Influence of Sex Differences and Knee Joint Position on Electrical Stimulation-Modulated Strength Increases." *Medicine and Science In Sports and Exercise* 17:1(February 1985):144.

Fenner, L. "Cellulite: Hard to Budge Pudge." *F.D.A. Consumer* (May 1980):reprint.

"Foods, Drugs or Frauds?" *F.D.A. Consumer* (May 1985):reprint.

*Herbert, V., and S. Barrett. *Vitamins and Health Foods: The Great American Hustle.* Philadelphia: George F. Stickley Co., 1981.

Kuntzleman, C. T., and Editors of *Consumer Guide. Rating the Exercises.* New York: William Morrow and Co., 1978.

Lindsey, R. "Figure Wrapping: Would You Believe It?" *Fitness for Living* (1972).

Lindsey, R. *The Reducing Racket.* Unpublished book manuscript.

Maryland Center for Public Broadcasting. *Consumer Survival Kit: No Sweat.* Owings Mills, Md.: Maryland Center for Public Broadcasting.

"Medical Fraud/Quackery Rampant in U.S.A." *Food For Thought* (Orange County Nutrition Council) 12:2(January 1986):7.

Miller, R. W. "Critiquing Quack Ads." *F.D.A. Consumer* (November 1982):reprint.

Murphy, P. "Steroids Not Just For Athletes Anymore." *Physician and Sportsmedicine* 14:6(June 1986):48.

"New Shades of Risk at Tanning Salons." *Consumer Reports* (February 1986):73.

Romero, J. A., T. L. Sanford, R. V. Schroeder, and T. D. Fahey. "The Effect of Electrical Stimulation of Normal Quadriceps on Strength and Girth." *Medicine and Science in Sports and Exercise* 14(1982):194.

"Shearing the Suckers." *Consumer Reports* (February 1986):87.

Weltman, A., and B. Stamford. "Is Excessive Sweating Healthy?" *Physician and Sportsmedicine* 11:3(March 1983):195.

Willis, J. "About Body Wraps, Pills, and Other Magic Wands for Losing Weight." *F.D.A. Consumer* (November 1982): reprint.

Willis, J. "Diet Books Sell Well But . . ." *F.D.A. Consumer* (March 1985):reprint.

Willmore, J. H., et al. "Alterations in Body Size and Composition Consequent to Astro Trimmer and Slim Skins Training Programs." *Research Quarterly For Exercise and Sport* 56:1(1985):90.

THE LABS

LAB 1

A PHYSICAL ACTIVITY QUESTIONNAIRE

NAME _____ SECTION _____ DATE _____

PURPOSE

The purposes of this laboratory are:

1. To evaluate your feelings concerning physical activity.
2. To determine the specific reasons why you do or do not participate in regular physical activity.

PROCEDURE

1. Read each of the fourteen items in the physical activity questionnaire, chart 1.1 shown here or in the Lab Resource Materials for Concept 1 on page 6.
2. After each statement, check one box indicating whether you strongly agree, agree, disagree, or strongly disagree with it. If you are unsure of your answer, check "undecided."
3. When all fourteen items have been answered, use the scoring procedure on page 7 to score the physical activity questionnaire.

RESULTS

1. After you have determined seven different physical activity questionnaire scores and a total score, use chart 1.2, also in the Lab Resource Materials for Concept 1, to determine your rating for each score.
2. Check your rating for each of the seven reasons for exercising and your total score here.

	Ex	Good	Fair	Poor	VP
Health and fitness	☐	☐	☐	☐	☐
Fun and enjoyment	☐	☐	☐	☐	☐
Relaxation and tension release	☐	☐	☐	☐	☐
Challenge and achievement	☐	☐	☐	☐	☐
Social	☐	☐	☐	☐	☐
Appearance	☐	☐	☐	☐	☐
Competition	☐	☐	☐	☐	☐
Total Score	☐	☐	☐	☐	☐

CONCLUSIONS AND IMPLICATIONS

▶Read Concept 1 before completing this section. The seven scores on the physical activity questionnaire should reflect your reasons for participating in physical activity.

1. Do you think that the scores on which you were rated "excellent" or "good" accurately reflect the reasons why you might do regular exercise? Explain.

2. Do you think that the scores on which you were rated "poor" or "very poor" might be reasons why you would avoid physical activity? Explain.

3. Those who are physically active should score high on the total score. Is your total score a good reflection of your overall attitude about physical activity? Explain.

CHART 1.1 The Physical Activity Questionnaire

The term "physical activity" in the following statements refers to all kinds of activities, including sports, formal exercises, and informal activities, such as jogging and cycling. Check your answers first, then read the directions for scoring, found in the Lab Resource Materials for Concept 1 on page 6.

	Strongly Agree	Agree	Undecided	Disagree	Strongly Disagree	Score
1. Doing regular physical activity can be as harmful to health as it is helpful.	☐	☐	☐	☐	☐	_____
2. One of the main reasons I do regular physical activity is because it is fun.	☐	☐	☐	☐	☐	_____
3. Participating in physical activities makes me tense and nervous.	☐	☐	☐	☐	☐	_____
4. The challenge of physical training is one reason why I participate in physical activity.	☐	☐	☐	☐	☐	_____
5. One of the things I like about physical activity is the participation with other people.	☐	☐	☐	☐	☐	_____
6. Doing regular physical activity does little to make me more physically attractive.	☐	☐	☐	☐	☐	_____
7. Competition is a good way to keep a game from being fun.	☐	☐	☐	☐	☐	_____
8. I should exercise regularly for my own good health and physical fitness.	☐	☐	☐	☐	☐	_____
9. Doing exercise and playing sports is boring.	☐	☐	☐	☐	☐	_____
10. I enjoy taking part in physical activity because it helps me to relax and get away from the pressures of daily living.	☐	☐	☐	☐	☐	_____
11. Most sports and physical activities are too difficult for me to enjoy.	☐	☐	☐	☐	☐	_____
12. I do not enjoy physical activities that require the participation of other people.	☐	☐	☐	☐	☐	_____
13. Regular exercise helps me look my best.	☐	☐	☐	☐	☐	_____
14. Competing against others in physical activities makes them enjoyable.	☐	☐	☐	☐	☐	_____

LAB 2

PHYSICAL FITNESS

NAME _____ SECTION _____ DATE _____

▶Read Concept 2 before completing this lab.

PURPOSE

The purposes of this laboratory session are:

1. To help you identify different components of physical fitness. It is hoped that, through participation, you can begin to see the differences between the various aspects of physical fitness, especially the differences between health-related and skill-related physical fitness.
2. To help you to gain insight into the importance of various components of physical fitness and to help you evaluate them.

PROCEDURE

Perform all the physical fitness stunts described in chart 2.1 in the Lab Resource Materials for Concept 2 on pages 15–17. Record your results in the appropriate blank opposite each item.

RESULTS

The stunts you tried are *not* good tests of fitness, but attempting the stunts may help you see that fitness is not just one thing; it is many different things. Circle the numbers of the skill-related and health-related items you passed.

Skill-related   1   2   3   4   5   6

Health-related   7   8   9   10   11

CONCLUSIONS AND IMPLICATIONS

To really test your fitness, you will need to do many of the tests presented later in this text. Therefore, you may be especially interested in testing yourself in those areas in which you did not do well on various stunts. For your own well-being, you should want to do well in health-related fitness.

How did you do on the health-related fitness stunts?

Were you surprised or disappointed in your performance? Explain.

How did you do on the skill-related fitness stunts?

Were you surprised or disappointed in your performance? Explain.

LAB 3

HYPOKINETIC DISEASES
AND CONDITIONS

NAME _____   SECTION _____   DATE _____

▶Read Concept 3 before completing this lab.

PURPOSE

The purpose of this lab is to help you determine the extent to which hypokinetic diseases and conditions have a direct effect on your life at the present time.

PROCEDURE

1. Answer each of the questions in chart 3.1 shown here and in the Lab Resource Materials for Concept 3.
2. Determine the extent to which hypokinetic diseases or conditions directly affect your life by scoring each question on chart 3.1.

CHART 3.1 Incidence of Hypokinetic Diseases and Conditions

Listed here are various hypokinetic diseases and conditions. In the column beside each condition or disease, place a check (✔) if you possess it, if one of your close relatives possesses it, or if one of your close friends possesses it. Close relatives are the four or five people you consider to be closest to you, whether parents, brothers, sisters, grandparents, spouse, or children. Close friends are the four or five nonrelatives you care about most. You need not live close to the individual to classify him or her as a close friend or relative.

The Hypokinetic Disease or Condition	Self	Close Relative	Close Friend
1. Heart disease	☐	☐	☐
2. High blood pressure	☐	☐	☐
3. Back pain or problems	☐	☐	☐
4. Overfat or obese	☐	☐	☐
5. Ulcer	☐	☐	☐
6. Diabetes	☐	☐	☐
7. Insomnia	☐	☐	☐
8. Depression	☐	☐	☐
9. Type A personality	☐	☐	☐
Column Totals	_____	_____	_____

RESULTS

What is your own personal hypokinetic disease score? _____

What is the hypokinetic disease score of your relatives? _____

What is the hypokinetic disease score of your friends? _____

CONCLUSIONS AND IMPLICATIONS

How would you interpret the significance of these scores?

LAB 4A

PHYSICAL ACTIVITY READINESS

NAME   SECTION   DATE

▶ Read Concept 4 before completing this lab.

PURPOSE

The purpose of this lab is to help you determine your physical readiness for participation in a program of regular exercise.

PROCEDURE

1. Read the directions on "The PAR-Q and You" form shown here and in the Lab Resource Materials for Concept 4.
2. Answer each of the seven questions on the form.
3. If you answered "yes" to one or more of the questions, follow the directions in the lower left hand corner of the PAR-Q regarding medical consultation.
4. If you answered "no" to all seven questions, follow the directions at the lower right hand corner of the PAR-Q.
5. If you plan to participate in competitive sports or vigorous training, answer the five questions in chart 4.2.
6. Read chart 4.2—Physical Readiness for Sports or Vigorous Training. Check appropriate answers and then answer the questions in the Results section and the Conclusion section.

RESULTS

Physical Activity Readiness Questionnaire (PAR-Q)

Circle the number of yes answers that you had for the physical activity readiness questionnaire.

     0   1   2   3   4   5   6   7

Physical Readiness for Sports or Vigorous Training

Circle the number of yes answers that you had for the physical readiness for Sports or vigorous training questionnaire.

     0   1   2   3   4   5

Note: It is important that you answer all questions honestly. The PAR-Q is a scientifically and medically researched preexercise selection device. It complements exercise programs, exercise testing procedures, and the liability considerations attendant with such programs and testing procedures. PAR-Q, like any other preexercise screening device, will misclassify a small percentage of prospective participants, but no preexercise screening method can entirely avoid this problem.

CONCLUSIONS AND IMPLICATIONS

Based on the answers to the PAR-Q, should you seek medical consultation before beginning or modifying your exercise program? Why or why not?

Based on answers to the physical readiness for sports or vigorous training questionnaire, do you feel that you are physically ready for sports and vigorous training? Why or why not?

PHYSICAL ACTIVITY READINESS QUESTIONNAIRE (PAR-Q)*
A Self-administered Questionnaire for Adults

PAR Q & YOU

PAR–Q is designed to help you help yourself. Many health benefits are associated with regular exercise, and the completion of PAR-Q is a sensible first step to take if you are planning to increase the amount of physical activity in your life.

For most people physical activity should not pose any problem or hazard. PAR-Q has been designed to identify the small number of adults for whom physical activity might be inappropriate or those who should have medical advice concerning the type of activity most suitable for them.

Common sense is your best guide in answering these few questions. Please read them carefully and check the ☑ YES or NO opposite the question if it applies to you.

YES NO

☐ ☐ 1. Has your doctor ever said you have heart trouble?

☐ ☐ 2. Do you frequently have pains in your heart and chest?

☐ ☐ 3. Do you often feel faint or have spells of severe dizziness?

☐ ☐ 4. Has a doctor ever said your blood pressure was too high?

☐ ☐ 5. Has your doctor ever told you that you have a bone or joint problem such as arthritis that has been aggravated by exercise, or might be made worse with exercise?

☐ ☐ 6. Is there a good physical reason not mentioned here why you should not follow an activity program even if you wanted to?

☐ ☐ 7. Are you over age 65 and not accustomed to vigorous exercise?

If You Answered

YES to one or more questions

If you have not recently done so, consult with your personal physician by telephone or in person BEFORE increasing your physical activity and/or taking a fitness test. Tell him what questions you answered YES on PAR-Q, or show him your copy.

programs

After medical evaluation, seek advice from your physician as to your suitability for:
- unrestricted physical activity, probably on a gradually increasing basis.
- restricted or supervised activity to meet your specific needs, at least on an initial basis. Check in your community for special programs or services.

NO to all questions

If you answered PAR-Q accurately, you have reasonable assurance of your present suitability for:
- A GRADUATED EXERCISE PROGRAM - A gradual increase in proper exercise promotes good fitness development while minimizing or eliminating discomfort.
- AN EXERCISE TEST - Simple tests of fitness (such as the Canadian Home Fitness Test) or more complex types may be undertaken if you so desire.

postpone

If you have a temporary minor illness, such as a common cold.

* Developed by the British Columbia Ministry of Health. Conceptualized and critiqued by the Multidisciplinary Advisory Board on Exercise (MABE).

Reference: PAR-Q Validation Report, British Columbia Ministry of Health, May, 1978.

* Produced by the British Columbia Ministry of Health and the Department of National Health & Welfare.

CHART 4.2 Physical Readiness for Sports or Vigorous Training

Answer the PAR-Q before using this table. If you had one or more "yes" answers follow the directions for the PAR-Q concerning consultation with a physician. If you had all "no" answers on the PAR-Q, answer the additional questions below before beginning intensive training particularly for sports.

Yes   No

☐   ☐   1. Do you plan to participate on an organized team which will play intense competitive sports (i.e., varsity team, professional team).

☐   ☐   2. If you plan to participate in a collision sport (even on a less organized basis), such as football, boxing, rugby, or ice hockey, have you been knocked unconscious more than one time?

☐   ☐   3. Do you currently have pain from a previous muscle injury?

☐   ☐   4. Do you currently have symptoms of a previous back injury or do you experience back pain as a result of involvement in physical activity?

☐   ☐   5. Do you have any other symptoms during physical activity which give you reason to be concerned about your health?

If your answer to any of these questions is "yes," then you should consult with your physician by telephone or in person to determine if you have a potential problem with vigorous involvement in physical activity.

LAB 4B

THE WARM-UP AND COOL DOWN

NAME _____ SECTION _____ DATE _____

▶Read Concept 4 before completing this lab.

PURPOSE

The purpose of this lab is to familiarize you with a sample group of exercises that can be used as a warm-up or cool down for aerobic types of workout.

PROCEDURE

Perform the exercises described in Concept 4 on page 29.

RESULTS

1. In which of the stretches did you feel the most tightness?

	None	Moderate	Severe
Calf stretcher	☐	☐	☐
Toe touch	☐	☐	☐
Leg hug	☐	☐	☐
Side stretch	☐	☐	☐
Cardiovascular warm-up	☐	☐	☐

2. Did you notice an increase in heart rate during the cardiovascular warm-up? Yes ____ No ____

Do you think that the sample warm-up and cool-down program is adequate for the activities you plan to do as part of your exercise program? Yes ____ No ____ Explain.

Does the sport or activity you plan to do involve vigorous use of muscles not stretched by this program?
Yes ____ No ____   If so, what muscles or body parts will need special attention?

Read Concept 12 and consider those stretching exercises for your warm-up and cool down.

LAB 6A

COUNTING THE PULSE
(HEART RATE)

NAME _____ SECTION _____ DATE _____

▶Read Concept 6 before completing this lab.

PURPOSE

The purpose of this lab is to learn to count the pulse at two different locations: the carotid artery on the side of the neck and the radial artery near the wrist.

PROCEDURE

1. Practice counting the number of pulses felt for a given period of time at both the carotid and radial locations (see the Lab Resource Materials for Concept 6 on page 45 for directions on counting the pulse). Use a clock or watch to count for 15, 30, and 60 seconds. To establish your heart rate in beats per minute, multiply your 15-second count by four, and your 30-second count by two.
2. Practice locating your carotid and radial pulses quickly. This is important when trying to count your pulse after exercise. Counting pulse after exercise will be necessary in Labs 6B and 6C.
3. Practice counting the pulse of another person using both the wrist and carotid locations (do not use your thumb).

RESULTS

Record the various pulse counts you have taken in the spaces provided here.

Carotid Pulse Count (Self)   **Heart Rate Per Minute**

_____ 15 seconds × 4 _____

_____ 30 seconds × 2 _____

_____ 60 seconds × 1 _____

Carotid Pulse Count (Partner)   **Heart Rate Per Minute**

_____ 15 seconds × 4 _____

_____ 30 seconds × 2 _____

_____ 60 seconds × 1 _____

Radial Pulse Count (Self)   **Heart Rate Per Minute**

_____ 15 seconds × 4 _____

_____ 30 seconds × 2 _____

_____ 60 seconds × 1 _____

Radial Pulse Count (Partner)   **Heart Rate Per Minute**

_____ 15 seconds × 4 _____

_____ 30 seconds × 2 _____

_____ 60 seconds × 1 _____

CONCLUSIONS AND IMPLICATIONS

1. Which pulse did you find easiest to locate on yourself?
   (circle one)   Carotid   Radial

2. Which pulse did you find easiest to locate on your partner?
   (circle one)   Carotid   Radial

3. Which of the two methods of counting pulse do you think you would prefer to use when counting heart rate? Why?

LAB 6B

THE CARDIOVASCULAR
THRESHOLD OF TRAINING

NAME _____ SECTION _____ DATE _____

▶Read Concept 6 before completing this lab.

PURPOSE

The purposes of this laboratory session are:

1. To understand the threshold of training and target zone concepts.
2. To establish a personal minimal cardiovascular threshold of training.
3. To establish a personal target zone for cardiovascular fitness.
4. To determine the specific jogging speed necessary to elevate your heart rate to threshold of training and target zones.

PROCEDURE

To determine your cardiovascular fitness threshold and target heart rates, you will use your age and your resting heart rate.

1. Find your threshold of training and target zone on chart 6B.1 in the Lab Resource Materials for Concept 6 on page 45 and record it in the results section.
2. Select a partner.
3. One partner should run a quarter-mile, then the other partner should count her or his heart rate at the end of the run (use carotid pulse). Try to run at a rate that you think will keep the rate of the heart above the threshold of training and in the target zone. Use 15-second pulse counts and multiply by four to get heart rate in beats per minute (bpm). Record the bpm in the results section.
4. Repeat, alternating roles, the second person running and the first person counting heart rate. Record the results.
5. Repeat the test so each person runs a second time. Record the results.

RESULTS

What is your threshold of training (from chart 6B.1)? _____ bpm

What is your target zone (from chart 6B.1)? _____ bpm

What was your heart rate for the first run? (15 sec.) × 4 = _____ bpm

What was your heart rate for the second run? (15 sec.) × 4 = _____ bpm

How fast do you have to run to get your heart rate above threshold and into the target zone? Check the following.

First run speed just right ☐   Faster than the second run ☐

Faster than the first run ☐   Slower than the second run ☐

Slower than the first run ☐   Second run speed just right ☐

CONCLUSIONS AND IMPLICATIONS

Do you achieve the cardiovascular threshold in the course of a normal day? Yes ____ No ____

What would you suggest for yourself as a regular (3–5 times per week) cardiovascular exercise program? Explain.

LAB 6B SUPPLEMENT*

You may want to keep track of your heart rate over a week's time or longer to see if you are reaching the target zone in your workouts. Shade your target zone with a highlight pen and plot your exercise heart rate for each day of the week (see sample).

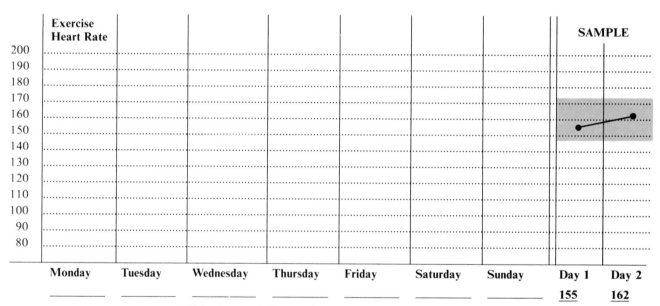

Write in your daily exercise heart rate on the lines above.

*Thanks to Ginnie Atkins for suggesting this lab supplement.

LAB 6C

CALORIES EXPENDED IN EXERCISE
(WEEKLY)

NAME   SECTION   DATE
_____

▶Read Concept 6 before completing this lab.

PURPOSE

The purpose of this lab is to determine how many calories you expend in exercise in a typical week. Because people who expend 2,000 to 3,500 calories per week have a reduced risk of heart disease, you may want to see if you meet this standard.

PROCEDURE

1. Write down each activity you do for each day of the week.
2. Use table 13.3 and Appendix C to determine how many calories you used in each activity. Use the calories for the body weight nearest your own. If the activity you performed is not listed, use the calories from an activity in the chart that you think is quite similar to the activity you performed.
3. Add up the calories expended per week.

RESULTS

Record amounts of times, names of activities, and calories on following list.

		Activities	Time (Mins.)	× Calories	= Total
Monday	1.	_____	_____	_____	_____
	2.	_____	_____	_____	_____
	3.	_____	_____	_____	_____
Tuesday	1.	_____	_____	_____	_____
	2.	_____	_____	_____	_____
	3.	_____	_____	_____	_____
Wednesday	1.	_____	_____	_____	_____
	2.	_____	_____	_____	_____
	3.	_____	_____	_____	_____
Thursday	1.	_____	_____	_____	_____
	2.	_____	_____	_____	_____
	3.	_____	_____	_____	_____
Friday	1.	_____	_____	_____	_____
	2.	_____	_____	_____	_____
	3.	_____	_____	_____	_____
Saturday	1.	_____	_____	_____	_____
	2.	_____	_____	_____	_____
	3.	_____	_____	_____	_____
Sunday	1.	_____	_____	_____	_____
	2.	_____	_____	_____	_____
	3.	_____	_____	_____	_____
	Totals		_____	_____	_____

CONCLUSIONS AND IMPLICATIONS

If you DID NOT expend 2,000 to 3,500 calories in recreational activities for the week, answer these questions.

1. Do you have an active job?   Yes ☐ No ☐
2. Do you think your job and your recreational activities together would require you to expend 2,000 to 3,500 calories in a week?   Yes ☐ No ☐
3. Do you think (realistically) that it is possible to increase your activity levels to equal 2,000 to 3,500 on a regular basis?   Yes ☐ No ☐

If you DID expend 2,000 to 3,500 calories in recreational activities for the week, answer these questions.

1. Do you think the week for which you kept records is typical of your activity patterns?   Yes ☐ No ☐
2. Do you have an active job?   Yes ☐ No ☐
3. Do you think that you expend 2,000 to 3,500 in recreational exercise and your job activities in a typical week?   Yes ☐ No ☐

To what extent do you think that you are active enough to reduce the risk of heart disease through your regular exercise? Explain.

LAB 6D

EVALUATING CARDIOVASCULAR FITNESS

NAME _____ SECTION _____ DATE _____

▶Read Concept 6 before completing this lab.

PURPOSE

The purposes of this laboratory are:

1. To acquaint you with several methods for evaluating cardiovascular fitness.
2. To help you evaluate and rate your own cardiovascular fitness.

PROCEDURE

Perform one or more of the three cardiovascular fitness tests described in the Lab Resource Materials for Concept 6 on pages 45–47. Determine your ratings on the test(s) using the rating charts provided.

RESULTS

Record the information obtained from taking the cardiovascular fitness test(s) (one or more) in the space provided.

Twelve-Minute Run

Distance _____ miles

Rating _____

The Step Test

Heart Rate _____ bpm

Rating _____

The Bicycle Test

Workload _____ kpm

Heart Rate _____ bpm

Weight _____ lbs.

Weight in kg _____

(Weight in lbs. ÷ 2.2)

ml/O_2/kg _____

Rating _____

CONCLUSIONS AND IMPLICATIONS

If you took more than one test, were the ratings for each similar? Yes ____ No ____ If so, were the ratings what you expected them to be?

If not, which rating do you think is really the best indicator of your cardiovascular fitness? Explain.

If you took only one test, do you think your rating is really representative of your cardiovascular fitness?
Yes ____ No ____ Explain.

Is your cardiovascular fitness what you think it ought to be? Yes ____ No ____ Explain.

LAB 7A

JOGGING/RUNNING

NAME _____ SECTION _____ DATE _____

▶Read Concept 7 before completing this lab.

PURPOSE

The purposes of this laboratory session are:

1. To give you an opportunity to experience one type of jogging program that can be used to develop and maintain cardiovascular fitness.
2. To acquaint you with basic jogging techniques.

PROCEDURE

1. Work with a partner and evaluate each other on jogging techniques. Make notes on chart 7A.1, describing any problems in your technique.
   a. Stand twenty yards in front of your partner while he/she jogs toward you; watch his/her arm and leg swing and foot placement.
   b. Jog along ten yards behind your partner while he/she is jogging and watch for arm and leg swing and foot placement.
   c. Stand ten yards to one side as your partner jogs past you; watch for body position and foot placement.
2. Using proper jogging technique, jog for fifteen minutes at your own individual cardiovascular threshold of training. (Determine your threshold of training using chart 6B.1, page 45.)

RESULTS

What is your cardiovascular target zone heart rate? _____ bpm

What was your heart rate after your fifteen-minute jog? _____ bpm

During your fifteen-minute jog, did you reach your threshold of training? Yes _____ No _____

With the help of a partner, note on chart 7A.1 any problems in technique. (Read the information on jogging in Concept 7, page 57, before evaluating your partner's jogging technique.

CHART 7A.1 Jogging Technique

Source of Problem	Problem		Nature of the Problem
	Yes	No	Describe the Problem
Foot placement			
Length of stride			
Arm movement			
Body position			

CONCLUSIONS AND IMPLICATIONS

Do you have any jogging problems? Yes ____ No ____

Do you feel that you can solve any jogging problems you have? Yes ____ No ____ Explain.

Do you think that jogging is a good type of exercise for you? Yes ____ No ____ Explain.

Do you think that you will include jogging in your exercise program for use in later life? Yes ____ No ____ Explain (if different from answer above).

LAB 7B

AEROBIC AND ANAEROBIC EXERCISES

NAME _____   SECTION _____   DATE _____

▶ Read Concept 7 before completing this lab.

PURPOSE

The purposes of this laboratory session are:

1. To give you an opportunity to experience an aerobic or anaerobic exercise program that is particularly good for developing cardiovascular fitness and aiding in fat reduction.
2. To familiarize you with an exercise program that can be continued as part of your normal life's pattern.

PROCEDURE

1. Select a sample program for some form of aerobic or anaerobic exercise and try it out. It can be earning points according to Cooper's Aerobics Chart (p. 51), trying the sample calisthenics program (pp. 52 and 53), or performing a sample of any of the other forms of aerobic or anaerobic exercise discussed in Concept 7. For example, you may want to try a sample speed play program, an interval training program, a rope jumping routine, or a circuit weight program.

    If you would like to repeat this lab more than once doing a different activity each time, space is provided in the results section for four descriptions.

RESULTS

Name the activity in which you participated and briefly describe and evaluate your experience.

Activity name _____

Time spent _____ minutes

Description and evaluation

Activity name _____

Time spent _____ minutes

Description and evaluation

Activity name _____

Time spent _____ minutes

Description and evaluation

Activity name _____

Time spent _____ minutes

Description and evaluation

CONCLUSIONS AND IMPLICATIONS

Did you like the activity or activities you performed? Yes ____ No ____
Do you think you would choose to make one or more of these activities part of your regular exercise program?
Yes ____ No ____ Explain.

If you did more than one activity, which one did you most enjoy? _____
Why?

Of all the activities discussed in Concept 7, which ones do you think you would be most likely to include in your regular exercise program?

LAB 7C

DANCE AEROBICS

NAME _____ SECTION _____ DATE _____

▶Read Concept 7 before completing this lab.

PROCEDURE

1. Perform the sample dance aerobics program shown below. See pages 54–56 for specific details as to how to perform the routine.
2. Review the suggestions in the table below before you begin.

DANCE AEROBIC ROUTINE

16 counts	Jog in place. Clap your hands.
32 counts	8 Schottische steps, alternate right and left.
32 counts	8 Jesse polka steps, alternate right and left.
32 counts	8 Schottische steps, alternate right and left.
32 counts	8 Jesse polka steps, alternate right and left.
32 counts	16 Side lunges, alternate left and right.
32 counts	16 Ponies.
32 counts	16 Backward lunges.
32 counts	8 Schottische steps, alternate right and left.
32 counts	8 Jesse polka steps, alternate right and left.
32 counts	16 Twists, alternate right and left.
32 counts	Jog and double-time clap.
32 counts	8 Schottische steps, alternate right and left.
32 counts	8 Jesse polka steps, alternate right and left.

GENERAL SUGGESTIONS FOR USING THIS ROUTINE

1. Warm-up before and cool down after the routine.

2. If the routine is too vigorous for you, jog in place or eliminate arm movements for several counts.

3. Learn the skills first, then try the routine.

4. Learn the foot steps first, then add arm movements.

5. Perform the routine to Lionel Richie's "Dancing on the Ceiling" or another 4-count song.

RESULTS

Did you have difficulty with any of the dance aerobics steps. Yes ____ ?   No ____ ? Explain.

In general, was the dance aerobics routine too easy ____ just right ____ too hard ____ ? Explain.

Did you like the dance aerobics routine? Yes? or No? Do you think you would make dance aerobics part of your exercise program. Yes? No? Explain.

LAB 8A

EVALUATING ISOTONIC STRENGTH

NAME _____ SECTION _____ DATE _____

▶Read Concept 8 before completing this lab.

PURPOSE

The purpose of this lab is to evaluate the strength of four muscle groups using self-testing stunts.

PROCEDURE

1. Attempt the stunt groups found in the Lab Resource Materials for Concept 8 (pp. 68–71) in any order, starting with the stunt in each grouping that you believe is the most difficult one that you are likely to pass. If you can pass it, try the next most difficult one in that same group, and so forth. If you cannot pass it, try the next lower stunt, the next, and so on.
2. Give yourself the score of the most difficult stunt that you can pass in each group.
3. Record your scores and your rating in the results section of this report.
4. When you have attempted all of the tests, perform the isotonic exercises in Concept 10.

RESULTS

Record your score for each part of the test and then total all scores.

Best score, test I   _____

Best score, test II   _____

Best score, test III   _____

Best score, test IV   _____

Total score   _____

Find your total score on the rating chart (chart 8A.1 in the Lab Resource Materials for Concept 8).
Rating _____

What muscle groups are involved in each of the tests?

Test I _____

Test II _____

Test III _____

Test IV _____

CONCLUSIONS AND IMPLICATIONS

Explain what the tests told you about the strength of those muscles, and suggest some exercises you might do to correct any strength deficiencies.

LAB 8B

EVALUATING ISOMETRIC STRENGTH

NAME _____ SECTION _____ DATE _____

▶Read Concept 8 before completing this lab.

PURPOSE

The purpose of this lab is to evaluate the isometric strength of several muscle groups.

PROCEDURE

All individuals will be tested on four isometric strength tests: right-hand grip strength, left-hand grip strength, back strength, and leg strength. Testing procedures are found on page 70 of the Lab Resource Materials for Concept 8. Measurements are made with dynamometers. If time permits, three measures on each test should be taken and the best score recorded in the results section of this report.

RESULTS

Isometric strength scores:

Grip strength (right)   Grip strength (left)   Back strength   Leg strength

_____   _____   _____   _____

Total score = _____ (Sum of four figures)

To determine strength per pound of body weight, divide the *total score* by the body weight.

Strength per lb. of wt. _____

Check your rating on isometric strength using chart 8B.1 in the Lab Resource Materials for Concept 8. Note that there are different charts for men and women.

	High Performance	**Good Fitness**	**Marginal**	**Poor**
Right grip	☐	☐	☐	☐
Left grip	☐	☐	☐	☐
Back strength	☐	☐	☐	☐
Leg strength	☐	☐	☐	☐
Total score	☐	☐	☐	☐
Per lb./wt.	☐	☐	☐	☐

CONCLUSIONS AND IMPLICATIONS

Which hand is the strongest? Right ＿＿ Left ＿＿ What is your explanation for this?

Do you need to perform strength exercises (regularly)? Yes ＿＿ No ＿＿ Explain.

What isometric exercises would you choose to correct any deficiencies found today?

What other muscle groups might also need isometric strength exercises?

LAB 9

EVALUATING MUSCULAR ENDURANCE AND POWER

NAME _____ SECTION _____ DATE _____

▶Read Concept 9 before proceeding with this lab.

PURPOSE

The purpose of this laboratory session is to evaluate the muscular endurance of two muscle groups and the power of the legs.

PROCEDURE

1. Perform the sitting tucks, chins or bent-arm hang, and jump tests described in the Lab Resource Materials for Concept 9 on page 77.
2. When not being tested, perform muscular endurance exercises in Concept 9 using a light weight and many repetitions. If you wish to work on power, use more weight and greater speed.
3. Record your tests scores in the results section. Determine and record your rating from charts 9.1, 9.2, and 9.3 in the Lab Resource Materials for Concept 9.

RESULTS

Record your scores below.

Sitting tucks _____ Chins _____ Hang _____ (seconds) Jump _____
Check your ratings below.

	High Performance	**Good Fitness**	**Marginal**	**Poor**
Sitting tucks	☐	☐	☐	☐
Chins	☐	☐	☐	☐
Power (jump)	☐	☐	☐	☐
For Those Who Cannot Do a Chin				
Making progress toward a chin	☐			

CONCLUSIONS AND IMPLICATIONS

Do you need to perform muscular endurance exercises regularly for the muscle groups tested in this lab? Yes ___ No ___ Explain.

What muscular endurance exercises do you think you need to perform regularly?

Do you need to perform power exercises for the leg muscles? Yes ___ No ___ Explain.

What power exercises do you think you need to perform regularly?

LAB 10

WEIGHT TRAINING
FOR STRENGTH

NAME _____ SECTION _____ DATE _____

▶ Read Concepts 8 and 10 before proceeding with this lab.

PURPOSE

1. To give you an opportunity to experience a sample weight training program.
2. To acquaint you with a strength program that can be continued throughout your life.
3. To give you an opportunity to experiment with free weights and weight machines.

PROCEDURE

1. Read Concepts 8 and 10 to learn about strength and weight training.
2. Perform the exercises in chart 10.1 following. Choose either the exercises listed in the free weight column, or if you have machines, perform those listed in the weight machine column. If you have both free weights and machines available, choose one or the other, but not both on the same day. You might want to try one program one day and the other on another day so that you may compare them. Use the weight amount listed in the final columns. (The names and numbers of the exercises shown in chart 10.1 correspond with the detailed exercises shown in Concept 10 on pp. 84–89.)
3. Use three sets of six repetitions with the load suggested. *Note:* This is only a "get acquainted" program and is not suitable for adoption as your regular program. (Follow the guidelines in Concept 8 to develop your own program to fit your individual needs.)

CHART 10.1 Sample Weight Training Program

Free Weight Exercise		Weight Machine Exercise		Suggested Weight	
Name	Number	Name	Number	Men	Women
Shoulder shrug	1	Hamstring curl	9	40	30
Military press	2	Bench press	6	50	40
Half squat	3	Leg press	3	60	40
Biceps curl	4	Biceps curl	1	40	30
Triceps curl	5	Triceps curl	5	25	15
Toe raises	6	Ankle press	7	60	40
Pull to chin	7	Seated rowing	2	30	30

RESULTS

Which program did you choose? _____

List the muscles you exercised by choosing this program.

How long did it take you to complete the program? _____ minutes.

CONCLUSIONS AND IMPLICATIONS

Were the weights suggested too heavy for you? Yes ____ No ____

Were the weights suggested too light for you? Yes ____ No ____

Briefly give your reaction to weight training as a potential program for you to use to develop your own fitness (strength or endurance).

LAB 11

EVALUATING FLEXIBILITY

NAME _____ SECTION _____ DATE _____

▶ Read Concept 11 before completing this lab.

PURPOSE

The purpose of this laboratory session is to evaluate your flexibility in several joints.

PROCEDURE

1. Take the flexibility tests as outlined on pages 105 and 106 of the Lab Resource Materials for Concept 11.
2. Record your scores in the results section.
3. Use Chart 11.1 in the Lab Resource Materials for Concept 11 to determine your rating on both of the flexibility tests, then record your rating in the results section.

RESULTS

	Test 1	Test 2 Right up	Left up	Test 3
What were your flexibility scores?	_____	_____	_____	_____

Check your rating below.

	High Performance	Good Fitness	Marginal	Poor
Test 1	☐	☐	☐	☐
Test 2 Right Up	☐	☐	☐	☐
Left Up	☐	☐	☐	☐
Test 3	☐	☐	☐	☐

Do any of these muscle groups need stretching?

	Yes	No
Back of the thighs and knees (hamstrings)	☐	☐
Calf muscles	☐	☐
Lower back (lumbar region)	☐	☐
Front of right shoulder	☐	☐
Back of right shoulder	☐	☐
Front of left shoulder	☐	☐
Back of left shoulder	☐	☐
Most of the body	☐	☐

Note: Read Concept 12 and Lab 12 for exercises to improve your flexibility.

CONCLUSIONS AND IMPLICATIONS

Discuss your current flexibility and your flexibility needs for the future.

LAB 12

STRETCHING EXERCISES

NAME _____ SECTION _____ DATE _____

▶Read Concept 12 before performing this lab. Also review Concept 11.

PURPOSE

The purposes of this laboratory session are:

1. To give you an opportunity to experience different flexibility exercises.
2. To acquaint you with a flexibility program that can be continued throughout your life.
3. To help you distinguish between the types of flexibility exercises.

PROCEDURE

1. Review the stretching exercises in Concept 12 on pages 109–113.
2. Perform each of the exercises to your threshold (or slightly below if you have not been exercising regularly). See Concept 11 for your threshold level.

RESULTS

List the exercises that you found difficult to perform.

Which exercises would you include in your stretching program?

Explain.

LAB 13A

EVALUATING BODY FATNESS

NAME _____   SECTION _____   DATE _____

▶Read Concept 13 before completing this lab.

PURPOSE

The purposes of this laboratory session are:

1. To determine your percent body fat using skinfold and/or body circumference measurements.
2. To learn to use skinfold calipers to make skinfold measurements.
3. To learn to use body circumference measurements.

PROCEDURE

1. If calipers, a tape measure, and a scale are available determine your body fatness using the procedures described here.
2. Read the directions for making skinfold and/or body circumference measures described on pages 116 and 124.
3. If possible, observe a demonstration of the proper procedures for measuring skinfolds and body circumferences at each of the different body locations. In the future, you may wish to help a person of the same or opposite sex take measurements, so you may wish to learn how to make all the measurements.
4. Work with a partner if possible. Take several measurements on your partner at each of the different skinfold and body circumference locations. Allow your partner to make the appropriate measurements on you.
5. If possible, have an expert make measurements on you and your partner so that you can compare your measurements.
6. Record each of the measurements in the results section.
7. Calculate your body fatness from skinfolds by summing the appropriate skinfold values (chest, abdominal, and thigh for men; triceps, iliac crest, and thigh for women). Using your age and the sum of the appropriate skinfolds, determine your body fatness using chart 13A.1 (men) and 13A.2 (women).
8. Calculate your body fatness from body circumferences using chart 13A.3 (women) and 13A.4 (men). For women, locate hip girth and height values on the chart. For men, locate the waist and weight values on the chart. Connect the two points with a straight edge and determine the percent fat on the scale in the middle of the chart.
9. Rate your fatness using chart 13A.5 on page 125. If you do both skinfold and circumference measures, you will have two different estimates of body fatness. You may wish to compare the two.
10. If different types of calipers are available to you, practice making measurements with each type so that comparisons of results can be made.
11. Remember that body composition measurements are confidential information. Care should be taken not to discuss another person's results. Results are intended to be useful information to the people being tested. Take the skinfold testing seriously.

RESULTS

Write your skinfold measurements in the blanks provided. In some cases, all measurements may not be possible. Provide results for the tests you were able to complete. List the name of the caliper used.

| **Males** | **Females** |
| (Skinfolds) | (Skinfolds) |

Measurement by Partner	**Measurement by Partner**
Chest _____ mm	Tricep _____ mm
Abdominal _____ mm	Iliac Crest _____ mm
Thigh _____ mm	Thigh _____ mm
Sum _____	Sum _____
Percent Body Fat _____	Percent Body Fat _____
Rating _____	Rating _____
Caliper Used _____	Caliper Used _____

Measurement by the Instructor (if possible)	**Measurement by the Instructor (if possible)**
Chest _____ mm	Tricep _____ mm
Abdominal _____ mm	Iliac Crest _____ mm
Thigh _____ mm	Thigh _____ mm
Sum _____	Sum _____
Percent Body Fat _____	Percent Body Fat _____
Rating _____	Rating _____
Caliper Used _____	Caliper Used _____

| **(Circumferences)** | **(Circumferences)** |

Measurement by Partner (or Self)	**Measurement by Partner (or Self)**
Waist Circumference _____ in.	Hip Circumference _____ in.
Weight _____ lbs.	Height _____ in.
Percent Body Fat _____	Percent Body Fat _____
Rating _____	Rating _____

Measurement by Instructor (if possible)	**Measurement by Instructor (if possible)**
Waist Circumference _____ in.	Hip Circumference _____ in.
Weight _____ lbs.	Height _____ in.
Percent Body Fat _____	Percent Body Fat _____
Rating _____	Rating _____

CONCLUSIONS AND IMPLICATIONS

If you did more than one assessment of fatness, were the results consistent? Yes ____ No ____ Explain.

Is your fatness (percent body fat) what you would like it to be? Yes ____ No ____ Explain.

What do you think you will need to do in the future to obtain or maintain a desirable level of body fatness?

LAB 13B

DETERMINING "DESIRABLE" BODY WEIGHT

NAME _____ SECTION _____ DATE _____

▶Read Concept 13 and complete Lab 13A before doing this lab.

PURPOSE

The purposes of this laboratory session are:

1. To determine desirable weight.
2. To compare two different methods for determining desirable body weight.

PROCEDURE

1. Measure percent of body fat (see Lab 13A), height (without shoes), and weight (with indoor clothing and shoes).
2. Determine your frame size (small, medium, or large) using the following procedure. With a tape, measure the smallest girth of your wrist just above the styloid process (boney bump on wrist). Pull the tape snugly (but not tight enough to indent the skin) around the wrist as you measure. Look up your frame size on Chart 13B.1 in the Lab Resource Materials for Concept 13 on page 125.
3. Determine your desirable weight. Locate your height in inches on the left and your frame size across the top. Find the desirable weight for your height and your frame size. Men are to use chart 13B.2 and women are to use chart 13B.3, both of which are in the Lab Resource Materials for Concept 13 on page 125.
4. Determine your desirable weight using a different procedure. Locate your actual body weight on the left and your percent body fat (from Lab 13A) across the top. Find the desirable weight for your weight and body fat percent. Men are to use chart 13B.4; women are to use chart 13B.5. Both charts are in the Lab Resource Materials for Concept 13.
5. Step 4 may have to be repeated twice if you arrive at different body fat percent values for skinfolds and circumferences.

RESULTS

Record your scores below:

Percent body fat _____ (skinfold) Percent body fat _____ (circumference)

Weight (indoor clothes) _____ lbs.

Height (without shoes) _____ in.

Frame size   small _____ medium _____ large _____

Desirable weight (Chart 13B.2 or 13B.3) _____ lbs.

Desirable weight (Chart 13B.4 or 13B.5) _____ lbs. (skinfolds)

Desirable weight (Chart 13B.4 or 13B.5) _____ lbs. (circumferences)

Is your desirable weight as determined from the height-weight chart what it should be?   Yes ____ No ____

Is your desirable weight as determined from percent body fat (skinfolds) what it should be?   Yes ____ No ____

Is your desirable weight as determined from percent body fat (circumferences) what it should be?   Yes ____ No ____

Is there a discrepancy between your answers?   Yes ____ No ____

LAB 14A

NUTRITION ANALYSIS

NAME _____ SECTION _____ DATE _____

▶Read Concept 14 before proceeding with this lab.

PURPOSE

1. To determine the nutritional quality of your diet.
2. To determine your average daily caloric intake.
3. To determine necessary changes in eating habits.

PROCEDURE

1. a. Record your dietary intake for three days using the dietary record sheet (chart 14A.3) on page 134 (make three copies). Record intake for two weekdays and one weekend day.
   b. Include the actual foods eaten, the amount (size of portion in teaspoons, tablespoons, cups, oz. or other standard units of measurement). Be sure to include all drinks (coffee, tea, soft drinks, etc).
   c. Include *all* foods eaten including sauces, gravies, dressings, toppings, spreads, etc.
   d. Determine your calorie consumption for each of the three days. Use Appendix B to assist you.
   e. Check the number of servings from each food group.
   f. Estimate the proportion of complex carbohydrate, simple carbohydrate, protein, and fat in each meal and snacks.
2. a. Answer the questions in chart 14A.1 (on page 252) using information from each of the three dietary record sheets.
   b. Score one point for each yes answer on chart 14A.1.
   c. Use the chart 14A.2 to rate your dietary habits. Circle the appropriate rating.

RESULTS

Record the number of calories consumed for each of the three days.

Day 1 _____ Day 2 _____ Day 3 _____

Circle your Dietary Habits score on the Rating Chart below.

CHART 14A.2 Dietary Habits *Rating Scale*

Score	Rating
14–15	Very Good
12–13	Good
10–11	Marginal
9 or less	Poor

CHART 14A.1 Dietary Habits Questionnaire

Yes	No	
☐	☐	1. Do you eat regular meals?
☐	☐	2. Do you eat a good breakfast daily?
☐	☐	3. Do you eat lunch regularly?
☐	☐	4. Does your diet contain about 55 percent–60 percent carbohydrates with a high concentration of fiber?
☐	☐	5. Are less than ¼ of the carbohydrates you eat simple carbohydrates?
☐	☐	6. Does your diet contain 10–15% protein?
☐	☐	7. Does your diet contain less than 30% fat?
☐	☐	8. Do you limit the amount of saturated fat in your diet?
☐	☐	9. Do you limit salt intake to acceptable amounts?
☐	☐	10. Do you get adequate amounts of vitamins in your diet without a supplement?
☐	☐	11. Do you eat regularly from all food groups?
☐	☐	12. Do you drink adequate amounts of water?
☐	☐	13. Do you get adequate minerals in your diet without a supplement?
☐	☐	14. Do you limit your caffeine consumption to acceptable levels?
☐	☐	15. Is your average calorie consumption for the three day period reasonable for your body size and for the amount of calories you normally expend?

CONCLUSIONS

Are changes in your eating habits necessary? If so, what changes? If not, explain.

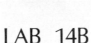

LAB 14B

EXERCISE FOR CALORIC EXPENDITURE

NAME _____ SECTION _____ DATE _____

▶ Read Concept 14 and perform Lab 14A before performing this lab.

PURPOSE

1. To experience an exercise period that will expend as many calories as are consumed at lunch.
2. To relate caloric consumption (eating) with caloric expenditure (exercise).

PROCEDURE

1. From chart 14A.1, record the foods you consumed at lunch on the first day recorded on your diet record. (If you did not eat lunch on that day, use the record for day 2.) Also record the number of calories for each food item. Copy this data on the following chart.

Lunch Food—Day 1	Calories	Check Off

2. From Appendix C select one or more activities and perform them until you have expended enough calories to equal the lunch item with the fewest calories. When you have done that, check off that item on the list, then continue to exercise until another food item has been equaled in caloric output and check that item off, until all have been checked off or until the period is ended.
3. To determine the number of calories expended (in number 2), multiply the hours, or fractions of hours, times the number of calories, times the body weight. If you wish to convert the caloric cost of an exercise into minutes rather than hours, divide the calories-per-hour-per-pound by sixty to obtain calories-per-minute-per-pound.

RESULTS

1. How many calories were you able to expend ("burn") in this exercise period? _____
2. Were you able to expend enough calories to burn off your lunch? Yes ____ No ____

CONCLUSIONS AND IMPLICATIONS

Do you feel that you exercise enough each day to expend the calories you consume each day?
Yes ____ No ____
Do you believe that exercise alone is the method you could use to balance your caloric input and output?
Yes ____ No ____

Explain your answer.

CHART 14A.3 Diet Record

Day _____				
Breakfast Food	**Amount**	**Calories**	**Basic Food Servings**	**Food Content**
			Dairy group ☐ ☐ Meat/Fish/Eggs ☐ ☐ Vegetables/Fruits ☐ ☐ ☐ ☐ Breads/Cereals ☐ ☐ ☐ ☐	% Protein ————— % Fat ————— % Complex Carbohydrate ————— % Simple Carbohydrate —————
Lunch Food	**Amount**	**Calories**	**Basic Food Servings**	**Food Content**
			Dairy group ☐ ☐ Meat/Fish/Eggs ☐ ☐ Vegetables/Fruits ☐ ☐ ☐ ☐ Breads/Cereals ☐ ☐ ☐ ☐	% Protein ————— % Fat ————— % Complex Carbohydrate ————— % Simple Carbohydrate —————
Dinner Food	**Amount**	**Calories**	**Basic Food Servings**	**Food Content**
			Dairy group ☐ ☐ Meat/Fish/Eggs ☐ ☐ Vegetables/Fruits ☐ ☐ ☐ ☐ Breads/Cereals ☐ ☐ ☐ ☐	% Protein ————— % Fat ————— % Complex Carbohydrate ————— % Simple Carbohydrate —————
Snack Food	**Amount**	**Calories**	**Basic Food Servings**	**Food Content**
			Dairy group ☐ ☐ Meat/Fish/Eggs ☐ ☐ Vegetables/Fruits ☐ ☐ ☐ ☐ Breads/Cereals ☐ ☐ ☐ ☐	% Protein ————— % Fat ————— % Complex Carbohydrate ————— % Simple Carbohydrate —————
Total Calories for Day				

LAB 15

EVALUATING SKILL-RELATED
PHYSICAL FITNESS

NAME _____ SECTION _____ DATE _____

▶Read Concept 15 before completing this lab.

PURPOSE

The purpose of this lab is to help you evaluate your own skill-related fitness, including agility, balance, coordination, power, speed, and reaction time. This information may be of value in planning your personal fitness program and in deciding which sports may be best, based on your own skill-related fitness.

PROCEDURE

1. Read the directions for each of the skill-related fitness tests presented on pages 138–140 of the Lab Resource Materials for Concept 15.
2. Take as many of the tests as possible, given the time and equipment available.
3. Be sure to warm up before and to cool down after the tests.
4. It is alright to practice the test before trying them. However, you should decide ahead of time which trial you will use to test your skill-related fitness.
5. After completing the tests, write your scores in the appropriate places in the results section.
6. Determine your rating for each of the tests from the rating charts on pages 138–140 of the Lab Resource Materials for Concept 15.

RESULTS

Place a check in the box for each of the tests you completed.

Agility (Illinois run)   ☐

Balance (Bass test)   ☐

Coordination (stick test)   ☐

Power (vertical jump)   ☐

Reaction time (stick drop test)   ☐

Speed (three-second run)   ☐

Record your score and rating (from charts 15.1–15.6 in the Lab Resource Materials for Concept 15) in the following spaces.

	Score	Rating	
Agility	_____	_____	(Chart 15.1, p. 138)
Balance	_____	_____	(Chart 15.2, p. 139)
Coordination	_____	_____	(Chart 15.3, p. 139)
Power	_____	_____	(Chart 15.4, p. 139)
Reaction Time	_____	_____	(Chart 15.5, p. 140)
Speed	_____	_____	(Chart 15.6, p. 140)

CONCLUSIONS AND IMPLICATIONS

Discuss your strengths and weaknesses in these skill-related fitness tests. How do you account for your strengths and what can you do to eliminate your weaknesses?

Sports require different components of skill-related fitness. Which sports seem best suited for you, given your skill-related fitness scores? Why?

LAB 16A

SPORTS FOR PHYSICAL FITNESS

NAME _____   SECTION _____   DATE _____

▶Read Concept 16 before completing this lab.

PURPOSE

The purpose of this lab is to explore the use of different sports as a part of your personal physical fitness program.

PROCEDURE

1. On chart 16A.1 check any of the ten most popular sports in America in which you especially like to participate.
2. Also on chart 16A.1 check the sports in which you feel you are skilled (ones in which you have enough skill to enjoy playing a game without more lessons).
3. Perform, in or out of class, two or three different sports, each for thirty to sixty minutes.
4. On chart 16A.2 in the results section list the sports you played.
5. Check the fitness parts in which you think you might improve by playing the sport. Refer to table 16.1, page 143.

RESULTS

CHART 16A.1 Sports Interests and Proficiencies

Sports	Check If Interested	Check If Proficient
Bowling	☐	☐
Tennis	☐	☐
Basketball	☐	☐
Softball	☐	☐
Baseball	☐	☐
Golf	☐	☐
Volleyball	☐	☐
Football	☐	☐
Frisbee	☐	☐
Table Tennis	☐	☐
Others (write in)		
_____	☐	☐
_____	☐	☐

CHART 16A.2 Fitness Benefits

Benefit	Sport _____	Sport _____	Sport _____
Cardiovascular fitness	☐	☐	☐
Flexibility	☐	☐	☐
Body leanness	☐	☐	☐
Strength	☐	☐	☐
Muscular endurance	☐	☐	☐

CONCLUSIONS AND IMPLICATIONS

Which sports do you feel you might actually include in your exercise program for a lifetime?

Why did you choose them?

LAB 16B

PREPLANNED
EXERCISE PROGRAMS

NAME _____ SECTION _____ DATE _____

▶Read Concept 16 before completing this lab.

PURPOSE

The purposes of this laboratory session are:

1. To give you an opportunity to experience an exercise program that is preplanned.
2. To familiarize you with an exercise program that can be continued as part of your normal life's pattern.

PROCEDURE

Try the Sample **XBX** and 5BX Exercise Program on pages 145–148 in Concept 16 or you may want to try the aqua dynamics or another preplanned program with which you are familiar.

RESULTS

List the activity you tried in the space provided and briefly discuss what you did during that exercise period.

Activity name _____

Time spent _____ minutes

Description

Activity name _____

Time spent _____ minutes

Description

Activity name _____

Time spent _____ minutes

Description

Activity name _____

Time spent _____ minutes

Description

CONCLUSIONS AND IMPLICATIONS

Did you enjoy the activity you performed? Yes ____ No ____

Do you think you would choose to make this activity part of your regular exercise program?

Yes ____ No ____ Why or why not?

If you did more than one preplanned program, which one did you like best? _____

Why?

Of all the preplanned exercise programs, which ones do you think you would be most likely to include as a part of your own personal exercise program?

LAB 18A

CARE OF THE BACK

NAME _____ SECTION _____ DATE _____

▶Read Concepts 17 and 18 before completing this lab.

PURPOSE

The purposes of this laboratory session are:

1. To determine if you have some muscle imbalance.
2. To learn exercises suitable for preventing or correcting lordosis and preventing or alleviating low back pain.

PROCEDURE

1. Secure a partner and administer the muscle tests to each other. (Details appear on page 165 of the Lab Resource Materials for Concept 18.) Record results of tests in the results section of this laboratory.
2. Determine your rating by circling your score on chart 18A.1.
3. Under the direction and supervision of the instructor, perform the following exercises described in Concept 18, numbers 9–16 and 19. For the purposes of this lab, two or three repetitions of each exercise will be adequate.

RESULTS

1. On test 1, was there evidence that you have shortened lumbar and/or hip flexor muscles? Yes _____ No _____
2. a. On test 2, was there evidence that you have short hamstrings? Yes _____ No _____ Right _____ Left _____
   b. Was there evidence of short lumbar and/or hip flexor muscles? Yes _____ No _____
3. On test 3, was there evidence that you have short hip flexors? Yes _____ No _____ Right _____ Left _____
4. Did you have difficulty performing any of the exercises? Yes _____ No _____

   If so, which ones?

Circle your overall rating on chart 18A.1.

CHART 18A.1 Back "Health" *Rating Scale*

Rating	Number of Tests Passed
Good Fitness Zone	3
Marginal Zone	2
Poor Zone	0–1

CONCLUSIONS AND IMPLICATIONS

If you had difficulty with any of the exercises, explain why. If you had no difficulty, how do you account for it?

What specific exercises might help correct your muscle imbalance?

LAB 18B

POSTURE

NAME   SECTION   DATE

▶Read Concepts 17 and 18 before completing this lab.

PURPOSE

The purposes of this laboratory session are as follows:

1. To learn to recognize postural deviations and thus become more posture conscious.
2. To determine your posture limitations in order to institute a preventive and corrective program.

PROCEDURE

1. Wear as little clothing as possible (bathing suits are recommended) and remove shoes and socks.
2. Work in groups of two or three, with one person acting as the "subject" while partners serve as "examiners"; alternate roles.
   a. Stand by a vertically hung plumb line.
   b. Use chart 18B.1 found in the Lab Resource Materials for Concept 18 on page 166. Check any deviations and indicate their severity as follows: 0—none; 1—slight; 2—moderate; 3—severe.
   c. Total the score and determine your posture rating from chart 18B.2 in the Lab Resource Materials.
3. If time permits, perform the following ten exercises from Concept 18: 1–8; 18, 19.

RESULTS

Record your posture score. ────────────────

Circle your posture rating of chart 18B.2.

CHART 18B.2 Posture *Rating Scale*

Classification	Total Score
Excellent	0–2
Very good	3–4
Fair	5–7
Poor	8–11
Very poor	12 or more

CONCLUSIONS AND IMPLICATIONS

Were you aware of the deviations that were found? Yes _____ No _____

List the deviations that were moderate or severe.

What program will you follow to build or maintain good posture? List specific exercises from Concept 18 that you need to practice to correct each deviation you have identified.

If you were checked as having some of the symptoms of scoliosis, see your instructor for a more thorough examination and possible referral to a physician.

LAB 19

QUESTIONABLE EXERCISES

▶ Read Concept 19 before performing this lab.

PURPOSE

To experience some "good" exercises that can accomplish the purpose of some "questionable" exercises.

PROCEDURE

1. Look at the illustrations of questionable exercises in Concept 19, then review the exercises suggested as good alternatives.
2. For each questionable exercise listed, there is one (or more) good alternative to accomplish the same purpose without harm to the individual. Perform the good exercises listed.

RESULTS

1. List the questionable exercises that you have used in the past.

_____   _____   _____
_____   _____   _____
_____   _____   _____
_____   _____   _____

2. List the good exercises that you have used in the past.

_____   _____   _____
_____   _____   _____
_____   _____   _____
_____   _____   _____

CONCLUSIONS AND IMPLICATIONS

List the names of the exercises that you will use as alternatives in the future.

LAB 20A

EVALUATING YOUR STRESS LEVEL

NAME   ·   SECTION   DATE

▶Read Concept 20 before proceeding with this lab.

PURPOSE

The purpose of this laboratory is to help you evaluate your current stress level. Research shows that when people are stressed, they are more susceptible to certain diseases. Some stress-related diseases include heart disease, ulcers, allergies, hypertension, and insomnia. People with high stress levels need to recognize the causes and effects of stress and to consider ways of avoiding, coping with, or reducing stress. Exercise and relaxation are important therapeutic techniques.

PROCEDURE

1. Look at the list of stressful life events in table 20A.1 or table 20A.2 shown in the Lab Resource Materials for Concept 20. If you are a full-time college student under twenty-five years of age, use table 20A.1. If you are older than twenty-five, use table 20A.2. Circle the score opposite each event that seems to be true for you in the last twelve months.
2. Add up all the circled numbers. Record your score.
3. Look up your rating on chart 20A.1. (Use the same rating scale for either table.)
4. Interpret your score by answering the following questions.

CHART 20A.1 *Rating Scale* for Stressful Life Events

Rating	Score	Implication for Illness
Low stress	150 or less	35% chance of getting a stress-related disease in the next two years
Moderate stress	151–300	51% chance of getting a stress illness in the next two years
High stress	301 or higher	80% chance of getting a stress illness in the next two years

RESULTS

Record your score on the test _____

What is your rating? _____

CONCLUSIONS AND IMPLICATIONS

What does your stress score suggest in terms of possible future illnesses?

Do you feel that you need to do anything to reduce your stress level? Yes _____ No _____ Explain.

TABLE 20A.1 Stressful Life Events for College Students*

	Event	Score		Event	Score
_____	Death of a close family member	100	_____	Problems with your boss or professor	25
_____	Jail term	80	_____	Outstanding personal achievement	25
_____	Final year or first year in college	63	_____	Failure in some course	25
_____	Pregnancy (to you or caused by you)	60	_____	Final exams	20
_____	Severe personal illness or injury	53	_____	Increased or decreased dating	20
_____	Marriage	50	_____	Change in working conditions	20
_____	Any interpersonal problems	45	_____	Change in your major	20
_____	Financial difficulties	40	_____	Change in your sleeping habits	18
_____	Death of a close friend	40	_____	Several-day vacation	15
_____	Arguments with your roommate (more than every other day)	40	_____	Change in eating habits	15
_____	Major disagreements with your family	40	_____	Family reunion	15
_____	Major change in personal habits	30	_____	Change in recreational activities	15
_____	Change in living environment	30	_____	Minor illness or injury	15
_____	Beginning or ending a job	30	_____	Minor violations of the law	11

Adapted from the Social Readjustment Scale devised by Thomas Holmes and Richard Rahe. Used by permission.

TABLE 20A.2 Stressful Life Events*

Event	Score	Event	Score
Death of spouse	100	Son/daughter leaves home	29
Divorce	73	Trouble with in-laws	29
Marital separation	65	Outstanding achievement	28
Jail term	63	Spouse begins work	26
Death of close family member	63	Start or finish school	26
Personal injury/illness	53	Change in living conditions	25
Marriage	50	Revision of personal habits	24
Fired from work	47	Trouble with boss	23
Marital reconciliation	45	Change in work hours, conditions	20
Retirement	45	Change in residence	20
Change in family member's health	44	Change in schools	20
Pregnancy	40	Change in recreational habits	19
Sex difficulties	39	Change in church activities	19
Addition to family	39	Change in social activities	18
Business readjustment	39	Mortgage/loan under $10,000	18
Change in financial status	38	Change in sleeping habits	16
Death of close friend	37	Change in number of family gatherings	15
Change in number of marital arguments	35	Change in eating habits	15
Mortgage/loan over $10,000	31	Vacation	13
Foreclosure of mortgage/loan	30	Christmas season	12
Change in work responsibilities	29	Minor violation of law	11

This test is adapted from the Social Readjustment Scale devised by Thomas Holmes and Richard Rahe. Used by permission.

LAB 20B

RESPONSE TO STRESS

NAME _____ SECTION _____ DATE _____

▶Read Concept 20 before proceeding with this lab.

PURPOSE

The purposes of this laboratory session are as follows:

1. To observe and compare the effects of a variety of physical and emotional stressors.
2. To determine the amount of time required to recover from the stressors.

PROCEDURE

(You may work with or without a partner)

1. Determine your resting heart rate by counting your pulse for thirty seconds, and record it on the chart provided.
2. Next, you will be exposed to a stressor by your instructor.*
3. Immediately after the stressor is applied, count your heart rate for thirty seconds and record.
4. Three minutes or more will be allowed for recovery, then another stressor will be applied.
5. Continue to record your thirty-second pulse after each stressor.

*Note: Instructor should refer to the Instructor's Manual.

RESULTS

Resting heart rate: Self ____bpm   Partner ____ bpm
Record stressors and thirty-second heart rates on the chart that follows.

Stressor	Heart Rate	
	Self	Partner
1. _____	_____	_____
2. _____	_____	_____
3. _____	_____	_____
4. _____	_____	_____
5. _____	_____	_____

Graph your own heart rate on the following graph by drawing a line across each bar at the level of your heart rate. Then darken the bar with a pen or felt marker.

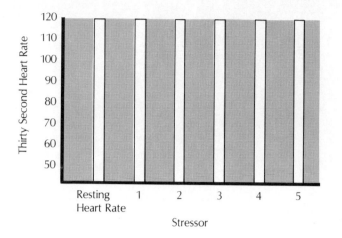

CONCLUSIONS AND IMPLICATIONS

Indicate which type of stressor affected your heart rate most by checking the appropriate blank.

Emotional _____ Physical _____

Did you react more to the stressor than did your partner? Yes _____ No _____

Could your present (last twenty-four hours) physical or emotional state affect the way you responded today?

Yes _____ No _____

Explain.

Could your previous experiences affect the way you responded to these stressors? Yes _____ No _____

Explain.

LAB 20C

EVALUATING NEUROMUSCULAR TENSION

NAME _____ SECTION _____ DATE _____

▶Read Concept 20 before proceeding with this lab.

PURPOSE

The purpose of this laboratory session is to learn to recognize signs of excess tension in yourself and in others by symptomatic mannerisms and by manually testing your ability to relax. If time permits, perform the relaxation exercises in Concept 20 before executing the lab.

PROCEDURE

1. Choose a partner. Designate one partner as the subject and the other as the tester. Alternate roles.
2. The subject should lie supine in a comfortable position and consciously try to relax as described in Concept 20. This may be done alone, or the instructor may wish to direct the entire group in this procedure.
3. The tester should kneel beside the subject's right hand and remain very still and quiet while the subject is concentrating.
4. After five minutes have elapsed, the tester should observe the subject for signs of tension according to the procedures outlined on page 182 of the Lab Resource Materials for Concept 20. Record signs of tension in chart 20C.1 on page 272.
5. Record your relaxation rating in the results section of this report. (Use chart 20C.2 on page 272.)

RESULTS

What is your tension score? _____

What is your relaxation rating? _____

CONCLUSIONS AND IMPLICATIONS

	Yes	No
Were you aware of your own tensions?	Yes ___	No ___
Was it more difficult to relax than you expected?	Yes ___	No ___
Did your awareness of your partner make it more difficult to concentrate?	Yes ___	No ___
Can you concentrate on your breathing without altering its rhythm?	Yes ___	No ___

Could you learn to release muscular tension consciously with additional practice? Yes ___ No ___

Could you learn to release tension while sitting or standing with your eyes open? Yes ___ No ___

Do you think your score today is typical of your normal tension level? Yes ___ No ___

What implications does this concept have for you in terms of your daily life (e.g., sleeping, studying, taking exams, performing on stage, and so on).

CHART 20C.1 Signs of Tension Observed by Tester

	No	Yes
A. Visual Symptoms		
Frowning	☐	☐
Twitching	☐	☐
Eyelids fluttering	☐	☐
Breathing	☐	☐
shallow	☐	☐
rapid	☐	☐
irregular	☐	☐
Mouth tight	☐	☐
Swallowing	☐	☐
B. Manual Symptoms		
Assistance (subject helps lift arm)	☐	☐
Resistance (subject resists movement)	☐	☐
Posturing (subject holds arm in raised position)	☐	☐
Perseveration (subject continues upward movement)	☐	☐

Total number of yes checks _____

CHART 20C.2 Tension-Relaxation Rating Scale

Classification	Total Score
Excellent (relaxed)	0
Very good (mild tension)	1–3
Fair (moderate tension)	4–6
Poor (tense)	7–9
Very poor (marked tension)	10–12

LAB 20D

RELAXING TENSE MUSCLES

NAME _____   SECTION _____   DATE _____

▶Read Concept 20 before completing this lab.

PURPOSE

To learn how to relax tense muscles.

PROCEDURE

Part I

Perform each of the exercises in the box in Concept 20, page 180.

Part II

1. Sit in a chair or lie on your back in a quiet, nondistracting atmosphere while you are learning this relaxation technique. (Later you will want to be able to use the technique in public, everyday situations, while you are at work, or any time you are under stress.) Get as comfortable as possible.
2. Do the contract-relax routine for relaxation in Concept 20, page 181. Contract the muscles to a moderate level of tension (do not use maximum contractions) as you inhale for five to seven seconds. Study where you are feeling the tension. Try to keep the tension isolated to the designated muscle group without allowing it to spill over to other muscles. Use the dominant side of body first; repeat on the nondominant side.
3. Next, release the tension completely, instantly relaxing the muscles, and exhale. Extend the feeling of relaxation throughout your muscles for twenty to thirty seconds before contracting again. Think of relaxing expressions like "warm," "calm," "peaceful," and "serene."
4. If time permits, you should practice each muscle group two to five times (until tension is gone) before going on to the next group. In a class situation, you may have time for only one trial. For home practice, do the routine twice a day for fifteen minutes.

Note: You will need your textbook to do this lab.

Did you find the relaxation exercises effective? Yes _____ No _____

Do you think you would find them useful as part of your normal daily routine? Yes _____ No _____ Explain.

Did you find the contract-relax exercise routine relaxing? Yes _____ No _____

Do you think you would find them useful as part of your normal daily routine? Yes _____ No _____ Explain.

LAB 21

ASSESSING HEART DISEASE
RISK FACTORS

NAME _____   SECTION _____   DATE _____

▶Read Concept 21 before completing this lab.

PURPOSE

The purpose of this lab is to assess your risk of developing coronary heart disease.

PROCEDURE

1. Complete the ten questions on the heart disease risk factor questionnaire (shown here or on page 186 in the Lab Resource Materials for Concept 21) by circling the answer that is most appropriate for *you*.
2. Look at the top of the column for each of your answers. In the space provided at the right of each question, write down the number of risk points for that answer.
3. Determine your unalterable risk score by adding the risk points for questions 1, 2, and 3.
4. Determine your alterable risk score by adding the risk points for questions 4 through 10.
5. Determine your total heart disease risk score by adding the scores obtained in steps 3 and 4.
6. Look up your risk ratings on chart 21.1 (shown here or on page 187 in the Lab Resource Materials for Concept 21).

RESULTS

Write your risk scores and risk ratings in the appropriate blanks below.

	Score	Rating
Unalterable risk	_____	_____
Alterable risk	_____	_____
Total heart disease risk	_____	_____

CHART 21.1 Heart Disease Risk *Rating Scale*

Rating	Unalterable Score	Alterable Score	Total Score
Very High	9 or More	21 or More	31 or More
High	7–8	15–20	26–30
Average	5–6	11–14	16–25
Low	4 or Less	10 or Less	15 or Less

CONCLUSIONS AND IMPLICATIONS

The higher your score on the heart disease risk questionnaire, the greater your heart disease risk. Which of the risk factors do you need to try to control to reduce your risk of heart disease? Why?

Heart Disease Risk Factor Questionnaire*

Circle the appropriate answer to each question.

	Risk Points				
	1	**2**	**3**	**4**	**Score**
Unalterable Factors					
1. How old are you?	30 or less	31–40	41–54	55+	_____
2. Do you have a history of heart disease in your family?	none	grandparent with heart disease	parent with heart disease	more than one with heart disease	_____
3. What is your gender?	female		male		_____
				Total Unalterable Risk Score	_____
Alterable Factors					
4. What is your percent of body fat?	F = 20%↓ M = 15%↓	25%↓ 20%↓	30%↓ 25%↓	35%↑ 30%↑	_____
5. Do you have a high-fat diet?	no	slightly high in fat	above normal in fat	eat a lot of meat, fried and fatty foods	_____
6. What is your blood pressure? (systolic or upper score)	120↓	121–135	136–155	155↑	_____
7. Do you have other hypokinetic diseases?	no	ulcer	diabetes	both	_____
8. Do you exercise regularly?	4–5 days a week	3 days a week	less than 3 days a week	no	_____
9. Do you smoke?	no	cigar or pipe	less than 1/2 pack a day	more than 1/2 pack a day	_____
10. Are you under much stress?	less than normal	normal	slightly above normal	quite high	_____
				Total Alterable Risk Score	_____
				Grand Total Risk Score	_____

Adapted from W. J. Stone, CAD Risk Factor Scoring Scale Tempe: Arizona State University, 1984.

LAB 22

PHYSICAL ACTIVITY
FOR A LIFETIME

NAME _____ SECTION _____ DATE _____

▶ Read Concept 22 before performing this lab.

PURPOSE

The purposes of this laboratory session are:

1. To estimate your fitness needs twenty years from now.
2. To plan a program for your use twenty years from now.
3. To determine the difference in exertion for your current program and your program for later life.

PROCEDURE

1. Assume that your age is twenty years more than it is today. Look up your cardiovascular threshold of training for that specific age. Estimate your resting heart rate (it tends to go up as you get older and less fit). Record it in the results section.
2. Estimate what exercise would make you reach the cardiovascular threshold of training for a person of your assumed age. Think of a person you know (perhaps a parent) as you plan the program. Write this exercise down in the results section and note the rate (e.g., one mile in seven minutes).
3. List three flexibility exercises and three strength or muscular endurance exercises that you think you should be performing (list only those you really think you could do at that age). Record this in the results section.
4. Perform the cardiovascular exercise for fifteen minutes and do the flexibility and strength-muscular endurance exercises.

RESULTS

What age have you assumed? _____ years

What will be your cardiovascular target zone at the age you have assumed? _____ bpm

What exercise(s) would you do to get your heart rate above the level noted for the age you have assumed?

List three flexibility exercises you would do at the age you have assumed.

Exercise	Repetitions
1. _____	_____
2. _____	_____
3. _____	_____

List three strength or muscular endurance exercises you would do at the age you have assumed.

Exercise	**Repetitions**
1. _____	_____
2. _____	_____
3. _____	_____

CONCLUSIONS AND IMPLICATIONS

How much easier for you were these exercises than the exercises in your own program?

Do you really think you will be fit enough to do the listed exercises at the age you have assumed? Yes ____ No ____ Could your parent of the same sex or a relative of an age similar to the one you have assumed do the exercises you have selected? Yes ____ No ____ Why or why not?

At the age you have assumed, do you expect to be more or less fit than the typical person at that age? More Fit ____ Average ____ Less Fit ____ Explain.

Could you help a person of the age you have assumed plan an exercise program? Yes ____ No ____ Explain.

LAB 23

A PHYSICAL ACTIVITY QUESTIONNAIRE: A REEVALUATION

NAME _____ SECTION _____ DATE _____

▶Read Concept 23 before performing this lab.

PURPOSE

The purpose of this laboratory session is to help you to detect any change in feelings about physical activity that may have developed from the time you completed questionnaire 1 (Concept 1) to the completion of questionnaire 2 (Concept 23).

PROCEDURE

1. Read each of the fourteen items in the physical activity questionnaire shown here and on page 197 of the Lab Resource Materials for Concept 23.
2. After each statement, check one box indicating whether you strongly agree, agree, disagree, or strongly disagree with it. If you are unsure of your answer, check undecided.
3. When all fourteen items have been answered, use the procedures on page 198 to score the physical activity questionnaire.

RESULTS

After scoring your test, write your rating in the chart provided for each scale of the questionnaire under rating 2. Then look up your rating from the first time you took the test (chart 1.1) and record that under rating 1. Check whether your score increased ($+$), decreased ($-$), or stayed the same.

	Rating 1	Rating 2	+	Same	−
Health and fitness	_____	_____	____	____	____
Fun and enjoyment	_____	_____	____	____	____
Relaxation and tension release	_____	_____	____	____	____
Challenge and achievement	_____	_____	____	____	____
Social	_____	_____	____	____	____
Appearance	_____	_____	____	____	____
Competition	_____	_____	____	____	____
Total Score	_____	_____	____	____	____

CONCLUSIONS AND IMPLICATIONS

Discuss any changes in your feelings about physical activity between questionnaire 1 and questionnaire 2. If changes occurred, how do you account for them?

If changes did not occur, why?

CHART 23.1 The Physical Activity Questionnaire

The term "physical activity" in the following statements refers to all kinds of activities, including sports, formal exercises, and informal activities, such as jogging and cycling. Check your answers first, then read the directions for scoring, found in the Lab Resource Materials for Concept 23 on page 198.

	Strongly Agree	Agree	Undecided	Disagree	Strongly Disagree	Score
1. Doing regular physical activity can be as harmful to health as it is helpful.	☐	☐	☐	☐	☐	_____
2. One of the main reasons I do regular physical activity is because it is fun.	☐	☐	☐	☐	☐	_____
3. Participating in physical activities makes me tense and nervous.	☐	☐	☐	☐	☐	_____
4. The challenge of physical training is one reason why I participate in physical activity.	☐	☐	☐	☐	☐	_____
5. One of the things I like about physical activity is the participation with other people.	☐	☐	☐	☐	☐	_____
6. Doing regular physical activity does little to make me more physically attractive.	☐	☐	☐	☐	☐	_____
7. Competition is a good way to keep a game from being fun.	☐	☐	☐	☐	☐	_____
8. I should exercise regularly for my own good health and physical fitness.	☐	☐	☐	☐	☐	_____
9. Doing exercise and playing sports is boring.	☐	☐	☐	☐	☐	_____
10. I enjoy taking part in physical activity because it helps me to relax and get away from the pressures of daily living.	☐	☐	☐	☐	☐	_____
11. Most sports and physical activities are too difficult for me to enjoy.	☐	☐	☐	☐	☐	_____
12. I do not enjoy physical activities that require the participation of other people.	☐	☐	☐	☐	☐	_____
13. Regular exercise helps me to look my best.	☐	☐	☐	☐	☐	_____
14. Competing against others in physical activities makes them enjoyable.	☐	☐	☐	☐	☐	_____

LAB 24

PLANNING YOUR PERSONAL
EXERCISE PROGRAM

NAME _____   SECTION _____   DATE _____

▶Read Concept 24 before completing this lab.

PURPOSE

The purpose of this lab is to plan a personal fitness program using the five steps outlined in Concept 24.

PROCEDURE

Answer the questions and fill in the charts following the five steps outlined below.

1. Identify Your Personal Fitness Needs

In chart 24.1, darken the boxes of your self-test rating for each of the tests you have taken. (Refer to the appropriate rating charts to determine your ratings.) If you did not take a test, darken the "no result" box.

In chart 24.2, darken one box for each component of fitness. Make only *one* rating for each by combining ratings from chart 24.1. If you took more than one test for a particular fitness component, use your own judgment in determining your single ratings. Use ratings 1–3 for cardiovascular fitness, 4–5 for strength, 6 for muscular endurance, 7 for flexibility, and 8 for fatness. Make only one rating for skill-related fitness using ratings 9–14 from chart 24.1. Make only one rating for fitness of the back and posture using ratings 15–16 from chart 24.1. Connect the darkened boxes to create your own personal fitness profile. The completed profile will give you important information for planning your program.

2. Select Activities

Fill in chart 24.3. In the top part of the chart, list the activities you currently do on a regular basis that you would like to continue. In the middle section, write down some new activities that would be especially good for developing fitness in the areas in which you have a weakness or special need (see chart 24.2). Finally, in the bottom section of the chart, list some new activities you would especially like to try because you enjoy them (even if they do not meet your special fitness needs). After each, note the component of fitness developed by the activity. You should have at least one activity for each of the health-related fitness components. You should be especially careful to include exercise for the components of fitness for which you have low ratings.

3. Write Down a Personal Schedule

Fill in chart 24.4. For each day of the week, write down the activities you plan to do on that particular day. Select the activities from chart 24.3. A special place is provided for your warm-up and cool-down activities. In this section, write down the activities you will do to warm up and cool down each day. (You do not need to list these each day on the daily schedules. Another section is provided for "special exercises" that you may do on a regular basis.) These may include exercises for the back, or just a set of calisthenics or exercises you plan to do. Once you list these activities in the "special exercise section," you need only refer to them in your daily schedule as "special exercises," rather than write them on each day's schedule.

4. Try It Out

Actually perform your program for at least one week and for several weeks if possible. You may perform the exercises for one or more days of the program during class time.

5. Evaluate and Modify Your Program

After you have tried your program, either in class or on your own, evaluate it. Note your comments in the appropriate section of Chart 24.4. *Remember, even the best program needs periodic evaluation and modification.*

CHART 24.1 *Ratings* for Fitness Self-Tests

Rating Chart	Rating				
	High Performance Zone	Good Fitness Zone	Marginal Zone	Low Zone	No Results
1. Twelve-Minute Run Chart 6D.1, page 46	☐	☐	☐	☐	☐
2. Step Test Chart 6D.2, page 47	☐	☐	☐	☐	☐
3. Bicycle Test Chart 6D.3, page 47	☐	☐	☐	☐	☐
4. Isotonic Strength Chart 8A.1, page 70	☐	☐	☐	☐	☐
5. Isometric Strength (average) Chart 8B.1, page 71	☐	☐	☐	☐	☐
6. Muscular Endurance Chart 9.1, page 77	☐	☐	☐	☐	☐
7. Flexibility Chart 11.1, page 106 Test 1 Test 2 Test 3	☐ ☐ ☐	☐ ☐ ☐	☐ ☐ ☐	☐ ☐ ☐	☐ ☐ ☐
8. Fatness Rating (skinfold) Chart 13A.3, page 124 (circumference)	☐ ☐	☐ ☐	☐ ☐	☐ ☐	☐ ☐
9. Agility Chart 15.1, page 138	☐	☐	☐	☐	☐
10. Balance Chart 15.2, page 139	☐	☐	☐	☐	☐
11. Coordination Chart 15.3, page 139	☐	☐	☐	☐	☐
12. Power Chart 15.4, page 139	☐	☐	☐	☐	☐
13. Reaction Time Chart 15.5, page 140	☐	☐	☐	☐	☐
14. Speed Chart 15.6, page 140	☐	☐	☐	☐	☐
15. Fitness of the Back Chart 18A.1, page 166	☐	☐	☐	☐	☐
16. Posture Chart 18B.1, page 166	☐	☐	☐	☐	☐

CHART 24.2 A Profile of Personal Fitness

Rating Chart	Rating				
	High Performance Zone	**Good Fitness Zone**	**Marginal Zone**	**Low Zone**	**No Rating**
Cardiovascular	☐	☐	☐	☐	☐
Endurance	☐	☐	☐	☐	☐
Strength	☐	☐	☐	☐	☐
Flexibility	☐	☐	☐	☐	☐
Fat Control	☐	☐	☐	☐	☐
Skill-Related Fitness	☐	☐	☐	☐	☐
Posture and Fitness of the Back	☐	☐	☐	☐	☐

CHART 24.3 Personal Physical Activities

Current Activities
(List activities in which you currently participate.)

Activity	Fitness Components Developed by Activity
1. _____	_____ _____
2. _____	_____ _____
3. _____	_____ _____
4. _____	_____ _____
5. _____	_____ _____

Proposed New Activities for Fitness
(List new activities for meeting fitness needs.)

Activity	Fitness Components Developed by Activity
1. _____	_____ _____
2. _____	_____ _____
3. _____	_____ _____
4. _____	_____ _____
5. _____	_____ _____

New Activities Just for Fun
(List new activities that you think you might especially enjoy, but that may not be good for developing fitness.)

Activity

1. _____
2. _____
3. _____

WEEKLY EXERCISE PROGRAM

Daily Schedules
(List the activities and times of day for each activity.)

Monday	Tuesday	Wednesday

Thursday	Friday	Saturday

Sunday	Warm-Up and Cool-Down Activities	Program Evaluation (Fill in after trying out your program.)
	Special Exercises	

LAB 25

EXERCISE AND THE CONSUMER

NAME _____ SECTION _____ DATE _____

▶ Read Concept 25 before completing this lab.

PURPOSE

To practice evaluating exercises found in popular literature.

PROCEDURE

1. Read a popular book or magazine and find an exercise that claims to improve your health, fitness, figure, or posture. If possible, attach a copy of the programs to this lab sheet.
2. Use chart 25.1 to evaluate the exercises in the program. Check "yes" or "no" for each item. Then record your scores in the result section.
3. Describe the exercises you evaluated in the space provided in chart 25.2.

CHART 25.1 Exercise Evaluation*

	Yes	No
1. Is the article or book written by an expert as defined in Concept 25?	☐	☐
2. Does the exercise employ the overload principle?	☐	☐
3. Does it employ the progression principle?	☐	☐
4. Does it employ the F.I.T. principle?	☐	☐
5. Does it employ the principle of specificity?	☐	☐
6. Is it a safe exercise? (See Concept 19.)	☐	☐
7. Is it an "active" exercise in which your own muscles contract?	☐	☐
8. Are the benefits claimed for the exercise reasonable?	☐	☐
9. Are the authors trying to help you (rather than selling a product)?	☐	☐
10. Do they refrain from using terms such as "quick," "miraculous," "tone," "remove fat," "new discovery," or other gimmick words?	☐	☐

CHART 25.2 Exercise Description

_____

_____

_____

_____

_____

_____

_____

_____

_____

*If in doubt, you may seek an expert's opinion on some of these questions.

RESULTS

1. Give the program you are evaluating one point for a "yes" answer on questions 1, 8, 9, and 10.
   _____ (Score 1)
2. Give the program one point for a "yes" answer on questions 2, 3, 4, 5, 6, and 7. _____ (Score 2)
3. Total of score 1 and score 2. _____ (Total score)

CONCLUSIONS AND IMPLICATIONS

1. A high score 1 total (3 or 4) in the results section indicates that the authors of the program know what they are talking about.
2. A high score 2 total (5 or 6) indicates that the program is consistent with good exercise theory.
3. A high total score (8 to 10) suggests that the program is sound for at least some aspects of fitness.

Using this information, write an assessment here of the program from the book or magazine you read.

APPENDIX A

PAR$_x$

PHYSICAL ACTIVITY PRESCRIPTIONS*

PAR$_x$ is a checklist of medical conditions requiring that a degree of precaution and/or special advice be considered for adults undertaking physical activities. Three categories are provided, and conditions are grouped by system or otherwise as appropriate. Comments under Special Prescriptive Conditions/Advice are general, since details and alternatives require clinical judgment in each individual instance.

ABSOLUTE CONTRAINDICATIONS	RELATIVE CONTRAINDICATIONS	SPECIAL PRESCRIPTIVE CONDITIONS/ ADVICE		System
• Permanent restriction, or temporary restriction until condition is treated, stable, and/or past acute phase.	• Highly variable. Value of exercise testing and/or program may exceed risk. Activity may be restricted. • Desirable to maximize control of condition. • Direct or indirect medical supervision of exercise program may be desirable.	• Individualized prescriptive advice generally appropriate: • limitations imposed and/or • special exercises prescribed • May require medical following and/or initial medical supervision in exercise program.		Comments
☐ aortic aneurysm (dissecting) ☐ aortic stenosis (severe) ☐ congestive heart failure ☐ crescendo angina ☐ myocardial infarction (acute) ☐ myocarditis (active or recent) ☐ pulmonary or systemic embolism – acute ☐ thrombophlebitis ☐ ventricular tachycardia and other dangerous dysrhythmias (e.g. multi-focal ventricular activity)	☐ aortic stenosis (moderate) ☐ subaortic stenosis (severe) ☐ marked cardiac enlargement ☐ supraventricular dysrhythmias (uncontrolled or high rate) ☐ ventricular ectopic activity (repetitive or frequent) ☐ ventricular aneurysm ☐ hypertension – untreated or uncontrolled severe (systemic or pulmonary)	☐ aortic (or pulmonic) stenosis – mild angina pectoris and other manifestations of coronary insufficiency (e.g. post-acute infarct) ☐ cyanotic heart disease ☐ shunts (intermittent or fixed) ☐ conduction disturbances • complete AV block • left BBB • Wolff-Parkinson-White syndrome ☐ dysrhythmias – controlled ☐ fixed rate pacemakers	• clinical exercise test may be warranted in selected cases, for specific determination of functional capacity and limitations and precautions (if any). • slow progression of exercise to levels based on test performance and individual tolerance. • consider individual need for initial conditioning program under medical supervision (indirect or direct)	Cardiovascular
		☐ intermittent claudication	progressive exercise to tolerance	
		☐ hypertension: systolic 160-180; diastolic 105+	progressive exercise; care with medications (serum electrolytes; post-exercise syncope; etc.)	
☐ acute infectious disease (regardless of etiology)	☐ subacute/chronic/recurrent infectious diseases (e.g. malaria, others)	☐ chronic infections	variable as to condition	Infections
PHYSICAL ACTIVITY RECOMMENDATIONS	☐ uncontrolled metabolic disorders (diabetes, thyrotoxicosis, myxedema)	☐ renal, hepatic & other metabolic insufficiency	variable as to status	Metabolic
		☐ obesity (25-50+ pounds overweight)	dietary moderation, and initial light exercises with slow progression (walking, swimming, cycling)	
Provided as a physician checklist or patient handout	☐ complicated pregnancy (e.g. toxemia, hemorrhage, incompetent cervix, etc.)	☐ advanced pregnancy (late 3rd trimester)	taper off intensity near term	Pregnancy
		☐ chronic pulmonary disorders ☐ obstructive lung disease ☐ asthma ☐ "exercise-induced asthma"	special relaxation and breathing exercises; breath control during endurance exercises to tolerance; avoid polluted air; avoid hyperventilation during exercise	Lung
		☐ anemia – severe (< 10 Gm/dl) ☐ electrolyte disturbances	control preferred; exercise as tolerated	Blood
		☐ hernia	minimize straining and isometrics; strengthen abdominal muscles	Hernia
		☐ convulsive disorder not completely controlled by medication	minimize exercise in hazardous environments and/or exercising alone (e.g. swimming, mountain climbing, etc.)	CNS
		☐ low back conditions (pathological, functional) ☐ arthritis–acute (infective, rheumatoid; gout) ☐ arthritis – subacute ☐ arthritis – chronic (osteoarthritis and above conditions ☐ orthopedic	avoid forced extreme flexion, extinsion, and violent twisting, correct posture, proper back exercises treatment, plus judicious blend of rest, splinting and gentle movement progressive increase of active exercise therapy maintenance of mobility and strength; endurance exercises to minimize joint trauma (e.g. cycling, swimming, etc.) highly variable and individualized	Musculoskeletal
		☐ antianginal ☐ antiarrhythmic ☐ antihypertensive ☐ anticonvulsant ☐ beta-blockers ☐ digitalis preparations ☐ diuretics ☐ ganglionic blockers ☐ others	NOTE: consider underlying condition. Potential for: exertional syncope, electrolyte imbalance, bradycardia, dysrhythmias, impaired coordination and reaction time, heat intolerance. May alter resting and exercise ECG's and exercise test performance.	Medications
		☐ post-exercise syncope ☐ heat intolerance ☐ temporary minor illness	moderate program; prolong cool-down with light activities postpone until recovered	Other

---

PHYSICAL ACTIVITY RECOMMENDATIONS

If you have been cleared by your physician for unrestricted activity and/or a progressive exercise program, these key points may be of assistance to you.

☐ Components of a balanced exercise program (the 3S's)
  • Strength – arms, shoulders, back, abdomen and legs
  • Suppleness – stretch and relaxation of body and limbs
  • Stamina – endurance fitness through aerobic activities (large muscle action that increases the heart rate)

☐ Progression – slow and easy; gradually increase the volume and vigor of your activities over several weeks.

☐ Warm-up and cool-down – quiet entry and exit of a few minutes each, such as with calisthenics and light activities.

☐ FITT is a guide to your Stamina (endurance) activities.

FREQUENCY	INTENSITY	TIME	TYPE
3 to 5 times per week	Work up to and sustain a target heart rate (for your age) during exercise	Once your body is accustomed to exercise, attempt to keep moving for at least 15 minutes (even if it means slowing down a little)	Any endurance exercise – walking, jogging, swimming, cycling, skipping, vigorous ball games, ski touring, etc.

☐ Pulse count is a good method to assess your response to aerobic exercises. Count for 10 seconds *immediately* after stopping your activity. Have your physician or exercise professional show you how to count your pulse. The chart below is age-adjusted. Be content to work at the lower FIT START heart rate initially until your condition improves, then slowly increase the intensity of your activity until your heart rate is reaching the KEEP FIT level. Remember, enter and exit your activity gently.

FIT START			KEEP FIT	
AGE	HEART RATE		AGE	HEART RATE
20 - 29	118		20 - 29	146 - 164
30 - 39	112	Progress Slowly	30 - 39	138 - 156
40 - 49	106		40 - 49	130 - 148
50 - 59	100		50 - 59	122 - 140
60 - 69	94		60 - 69	116 - 132

Derived from the "Half-As-Much" approach, B.C. Department of Health

* REFER TO SPECIAL PUBLICATIONS FOR ELABORATION AS REQUIRED.

MAJOR REFERENCES FOR PAR$_x$ CHART:

1. Fox, S.M. III, Naughton, J.P., and Haskell, W.C. Physical Activity and the Prevention of Coronary Heart Disease. Ann. Clin. Res. 3: 404-432, 1971.
2. American College of Sports Medicine. Guidelines for Graded Exercise Testing and Exercise Prescription. Lea and Febiger. 1975.
3. Committee on Exercise and Physical Fitness. Evaluation for Exercise Participation – The Apparently Healthy Individual. JAMA 219: 900-01, 1972.
4. Cooper, K.H. Guidelines in the Management of the Exercising Patient. JAMA 211: 1663-67, 1970.
5. Licht, S. Therapeutic Exercise Volume III. Waverly Press, 1965.
6. Recommendations and Guidelines of the Canadian Heart Foundation for Exercise Testing and Exercise Programmes for Improving Cardiopulmonary and General Physical Fitness. 1975.

PAR-X

Physical Activity Readiness Examination

Par-X is the medical complement to Par-Q, the Physical Activity Readiness Questionnaire. Please refer to "Guide To Use" below.

NAME
ADDRESS

BIRTHDATE	SEX	TELEPHONE

S.I. No.	MEDICAL No.

PAR-Q

	No	Yes	Comments / Additional History
Q1 Heart Trouble	☐	☐	
Q2 Chest Pain	☐	☐	
Q3 Dizziness	☐	☐	
Q4 Blood Pressure	☐	☐	
Q5 Musculoskeletal	☐	☐	
Q6 Other reason	☐	☐	
Q7 Over 65 Years	☐	☐	
Medications (relevant)	☐	☐	

ACTIVITY LEVEL

	L	M	H
Job	☐	☐	☐
Leisure	☐	☐	☐

Fitness Program
☐ Regular
☐ Sporadic
☐ None

ACTIVITY INTERESTS

☐ Recreation ☐ Sports
☐ Fitness Program
☐ Other

PHYSICAL EXAM

Ht. _____ Wt. _____ BP ___ / (___ / ___)

☐ Cardiovascular

☐ Respiratory

☐ Musculoskeletal

☐ Other

TESTS AS INDICATED

☐ ECG

☐ Exercise Test

☐ X-Ray   ☐ Hemoglobin   ☐ Urinalysis

☐ Other

STATUS

PLAN

Recommend ☐ Unrestricted Activity
☐ Progressive Exercise Program

Prescribe ☐ Avoid _____
☐ Add _____
☐ Medically Supervised Program
☐ Physiotherapy _____
☐ Further Investigation
☐ Exercise Contraindicated
☐ Indefinite   ☐ Temporary

GUIDE TO USE

Most adults are able to readily participate in physical activity and fitness programs. PAR-Q by itself is adequate for the majority of adults. However, some may require a medical evaluation and specific advice (exercise prescription).

PAR-X is an exercise-specific checklist for clinical use for persons with positive responses to PAR-Q or when further evaluation is otherwise warranted. In addition, PAR-X can serve as a permanent record. Its use is self explanatory.

Following evaluation, generally a PLAN is devised for the patient by the examining physician. To assist in this, three additional sections are provided:

- PHYSICAL ACTIVITY RECOMMENDATIONS (overleaf) with selected advice and pointers for most adults who are suited to participate in any activity and/or a progressive exercise conditioning program.

- PHYSICAL ACTIVITY PRESCRIPTIONS (PAR$_x$ overleaf) is a chart-type checklist of conditions requiring special medical consideration and management.

- PHYSICAL ACTIVITY READINESS form (to right) is an optional tear-off tab for verifying clearance, restrictions, etc., or for making a referral.

PAR-Q, PAR-X and PAR$_x$ were developed by the British Columbia Department of Health. They were conceptualized and critiqued by the Multidisciplinary Advisory Board on Exercise (MABE). Translation, reproduction and use of each in its entirety is encouraged.

The tear-off tab below is made available for use at the discretion of the Physician.

PHYSICAL ACTIVITY READINESS

Based upon a current review of health status, _____

_____ is considered suitable for:

☐ Unrestricted Activity

☐ Progressive Exercise Program

  ☐ with no restrictions/special exercises

  ☐ with avoidance of _____
  _____

  ☐ with addition of _____
  _____

☐ Only a medically supervised exercise program until further medical clearance

☐ Physiotherapy

Special Concerns (if any):

_____ M.D.

_____ 19 _____
              (Date)

Further Information:

☐ Attached

☐ To Be Forwarded

☐ Available Upon Request

REPRINTED FROM B.C. MEDICAL JOURNAL – Vol. 17, No. 11, November, 1975 Courtesy B.C. Ministry of Health & Dept. of National Health & Welfare

APPENDIX B

CALORIE GUIDE TO COMMON FOODS*

Beverages
Coffee (black)	3
Coke (12 oz.)	137
Hot chocolate, milk (1 cup)	247
Lemonade (1 cup)	100
Limeade, diluted to serve (1 cup)	110
Soda, fruit flavored (12 oz.)	161
Tea (clear)	3

Breads and Cereals
Bagel (1 half)	76
Biscuit (2″ × 2″)	135
Bread, Pita (1 oz.)	80
Bread, raisin (½″ thick)	65
Bread, rye	55
Bread, white enriched (½″ thick)	64
Bread, whole wheat (½″ thick)	55
Bun (hamburger)	120
Cereals, cooked (½ cup)	80
Corn flakes (1 cup)	96
Corn Grits (1 cup)	125
Corn muffin (2½″ diam.)	103
Crackers, graham (1 med.)	28
Crackers, soda (1 plain)	24
English muffin (1 half)	74
Macaroni, with cheese (1 cup)	464
Muffin, plain	135
Noodles (1 cup)	200
Oatmeal (1 cup)	150
Pancakes (1–4″ diam.)	59
Pizza (1 section)	180
Popped corn (1 cup)	54
Potato chips (10 med.)	108
Pretzels (5 small sticks)	18
Rice (1 cup)	225
Roll, plain (1 med.)	118
Roll, sweet (1 med.)	178
Shredded wheat (1 med. biscuit)	79
Spaghetti, plain cooked (1 cup)	218
Tortilla (1 corn)	70
Waffle (4½″ × 5″)	216

Dairy Products
Butter, 1 pat (1½ tsp.)	50
Cheese, cheddar (1 oz.)	113
Cheese, cottage (1 cup)	270
Cheese, cream (1 oz.)	106
Cheese, Parmesan (1 tbsp.)	29
Cheese, Swiss natural (1 oz.)	105
Cream, sour (1 tbsp.)	31
Dairy Queen Cone (med.)	335
Frozen custard (1 cup)	375
Frozen yogurt, vanilla (1 cup)	180
Ice cream, plain (prem.) (1 cup)	350
Ice cream soda, choc. (large glass)	455
Ice milk (1 cup)	184
Ices (1 cup)	177
Milk, chocolate (1 cup)	185
Milk, half-and-half (1 tbsp.)	20
Milk, malted (1 cup)	281
Milk, skim (1 cup)	88
Milk, skim dry (1 tbsp.)	28
Milk, whole (1 cup)	166
Sherbet (1 cup)	270
Whipped topping (1 tbsp.)	14
Yogurt (1 cup)	150

Desserts and Sweets
Cake, angel (2″ wedge)	108
Cake, chocolate (2″ × 3″ × 1″)	150
Cake, plain (3″ × 2½″)	180
Chocolate, bar	200–300
Chocolate, bitter (1 oz.)	142
Chocolate, sweet (1 oz.)	133
Chocolate, syrup (1 tbsp.)	42
Cocoa (1 tbsp.)	21
Cookies, plain (1 med.)	75
Custard, baked (1 cup)	283
Doughnut (1 large)	250
Gelatin, dessert (1 cup)	155
Gelatin, with fruit (1 cup)	170
Gingerbread (2″ × 2″ × 2″)	180
Jams, jellies (1 tbsp.)	55
Pie, apple (1/7 of 9″ pie)	345
Pie, cherry (1/7 of 9″ pie)	355
Pie, chocolate (1/7 of 9″ pie)	360
Pie, coconut (1/7 of 9″ pie)	266
Pie, lemon meringue (1/7 of 9″ pie)	302
Sugar, granulated (1 tsp.)	27
Syrup, table (1 tbsp.)	57

Fruit

Apple, fresh (med.)	76
Applesauce, unsweetened (1 cup)	184
Avocado, raw (½ peeled)	279
Banana, fresh (med.)	88
Cantaloupe, raw (½, 5″ diam.)	60
Cherries (10 sweet)	50
Cranberry sauce, unsweetened (1 tbsp.)	25
Fruit cocktail, canned (1 cup)	170
Grapefruit, fresh (½)	60
Grapefruit, juice, raw (1 cup)	95
Grape juice, bottled (½ cup)	80
Grapes (20–25)	75
Nectarine (1 med.)	88
Olives, green (10)	72
Olives, ripe (10)	105
Orange, fresh (med.)	60
Orange juice, frozen diluted (1 cup)	110
Peach, fresh (med.)	46
Peach, canned in syrup (2 halves)	79
Pear, fresh (med.)	95
Pears, canned in syrup (2 halves)	79
Pineapple, crushed in syrup (1 cup)	204
Pineapple (½ cup fresh)	50
Prune juice (1 cup)	170
Raisins, dry (1 tbsp.)	26
Strawberries, fresh (1 cup)	54
Strawberries, frozen (3 oz.)	90
Tangerine (2½″ diam.)	40
Watermelon, wedge (4″ × 8″)	120

Meat, Fish, Eggs

Bacon, drained (2 slices)	97
Bacon, Canadian (1 oz.)	62
Beef, hamburger chuck (3 oz.)	316
Beef, pot pie	560
Beef steak, sirloin or T-bone (3 oz.)	257
Beef and vegetable stew (1 cup)	185
Chicken, fried breast (8 oz.)	210
Chicken, fried (1 leg and thigh)	305
Chicken, roasted breast (2 slices)	100
Chili, without beans (1 cup)	510
Chili, with beans (1 cup)	335
Egg, boiled	77
Egg, fried	125
Egg, scrambled	100
Fish and Chips (2 pcs. fish; 4 oz. chips)	275
Fish, broiled (3″ × 3″ × ½″)	112
Fish stick	40
Frankfurter, boiled	124
Ham (4″ × 4″)	338
Lamb (3 oz. roast, lean)	158
Liver (3″ × 3″)	150
Luncheon meat (2 oz.)	135
Pork chop, loin (3″ × 5″)	284
Salmon, canned (1 cup)	145
Sausage, pork (4 oz.)	510
Shrimp, canned (3 oz.)	108
Tuna, canned (½ cup)	185
Veal, cutlet (3″ × 4″)	175

Nuts and Seeds

Cashews (1 cup)	770
Coconut (1 cup)	450
Peanut butter (1 tbsp.)	92
Peanuts, roasted, no skin (1 cup)	805
Pecans (1 cup)	752
Sunflower seeds, (1 tbsp.)	50

Sandwiches
(2 slices of bread—plain)

Bologna	214
Cheeseburger (small McDonald's)	300
Chicken salad	185
Egg salad	240
Fish Filet (McDonald's)	400
Ham	360
Ham and cheese	360
Hamburger (small McDonald's)	260
Hamburger, Burger King Whopper	600
Hamburger, Big Mac	550
Hamburger (McDonald's Quarter Pounder)	420
Peanut butter	250
Roast Beef (Arby's Regular)	425

Sauces, Fats, Oils

Catsup, tomato (1 tbsp.)	17
Chili sauce (1 tbsp.)	17
French dressing (1 tbsp.)	59
Margarine (1 pat)	50
Mayonnaise (1 tbsp.)	92
Mayonnaise-type (1 tbsp.)	65
Vegetable, sunflower, safflower oils (1 tbsp.)	120

Soup, Ready to Serve

Bean (1 cup)	190
Beef noodle	100
Cream	200
Tomato	90
Vegetable	80

Vegetables

Alfalfa sprouts (½ cup)	19
Asparagus (6 spears)	22
Bean sprouts (1 cup)	37
Beans, green (1 cup)	27
Beans, lima (1 cup)	152
Beans, navy (1 cup)	642
Beans, pork and molasses (1 cup)	325
Broccoli, fresh cooked (1 cup)	60
Cabbage, cooked (1 cup)	40
Cauliflower (1 cup)	25
Carrot, raw (med.)	21
Carrots, canned (1 cup)	44
Celery, diced raw (1 cup)	20
Coleslaw (1 cup)	102
Corn, sweet, canned (1 cup)	140
Corn, sweet (med. ear)	84
Cucumber, raw (6 slices)	6
Lettuce (2 large leaves)	7
Mushrooms, canned (1 cup)	28
Onions, french fried (10 rings)	75
Onions, raw (med.)	25
Peas, field (½ cup)	90
Peas, green (1 cup)	145
Pickles, dill (med.)	15
Pickles, sweet (med.)	22
Potato, baked (med.)	97
Potato, french fried (8 stick)	155
Potato, mashed (1 cup)	185
Radish, raw (small)	1
Sauerkraut, drained (1 cup)	32
Spinach, fresh, cooked (1 cup)	46
Squash, summer (1 cup)	30
Sweet pepper (med.)	15
Sweet potato, candied (small)	314
Tomato, cooked (1 cup)	50
Tomato, raw (med.)	30

Note: For a complete listing of foods, the reader is referred to: *Nutritive Value of Foods,* U.S. Department of Agriculture, Washington, D.C., Home and Gardens Bulletin, No. 72. (Available in most libraries, university bookstores, and Home Economics departments.)

APPENDIX C
CALORIES PER MINUTE
IN ACTIVITY

(Approximate Number of Calories Used Per Pound of Body Weight)

Activity	Calories Per Minute Per Pound
Daily Activities	
Lying	
Sleeping	.0066
Resting	.0079
Sitting	
Quietly; reading	.0080
Viewing T.V.; conversing; hand sewing; eating	.0116
Writing	.0120
Typing (manual)	.0166
Driving a car	.0150
Playing piano	.0150
Standing	
Dressing; undressing; grooming	.0133
Cooking; dishwashing; ironing	.0150
Household tasks (cleaning, dusting, sweeping, etc.)	.0200
Singing	.0190
Washing clothes	.0190
Showering	.0230
Making bed	.0270
Exercise and Sports	
Archery	.0340
Basketball	.0470
Bicycling (level) 5.5 mph	.0330
(uphill)	.0410
(downhill)	.0180
Bowling	.0440
Calisthenics	.0330
Dancing (moderately)	.0270
(vigorously)	.0460
Football	.0670
Golf	.0360
Squash; racquetball	.0690
Table tennis	.0260
Tennis	.0460
Walking slowly (level)	.0183
(uphill)	.0560

INDEX